Healthy Cities

To Tapas, Ratna, Sarika, Rini and Angelina;
Maggie, Chloe and Sam;
Anne, David, Owen and Daniel.
We are each indebted to, supported by and made wise by our families.

Healthy Cities

Public Health through Urban Planning

Chinmoy Sarkar

School of Medicine and School of Planning and Geography, Cardiff University, UK

Chris Webster

Faculty of Architecture, University of Hong Kong

John Gallacher

School of Medicine, Cardiff University, UK

Edward Elgar

Cheltenham, UK • Northampton, MA, USA

Published by
Edward Elgar Publishing Limited
The Lypiatts
15 Lansdown Road
Cheltenham
Glos GL50 2JA
UK

Edward Elgar Publishing, Inc.
William Pratt House
9 Dewey Court
Northampton
Massachusetts 01060
USA

A catalogue record for this book
is available from the British Library

Library of Congress Control Number: 2013954347

This book is available electronically in the ElgarOnline.com
Social and Political Science Subject Collection, E-ISBN 978 1 78195 572 7

MIX
Paper from responsible sources
FSC® C013056

ISBN 978 1 78195 571 0 (cased)

Typeset by Servis Filmsetting Ltd, Stockport, Cheshire
Printed and bound in Great Britain by T.J. International Ltd, Padstow

Contents

Foreword

> And now let doctors leave the centre stage
> And usher in the prophylactic phase.
>
> (From 'Superfluous Doctors', a poem written in prisoner-of-war camp by Archie Cochrane)

In the privileged West we have come a long way since Edwin Chadwick and Southwood Smith challenged the authorities in the 1840s about the living conditions and the lack of sanitary provision for 'the labouring population'. Their work led to the formation of the Health of Towns Association in 1844, and to the passing of the Public Health Act 1848 under which the collection of sewage, the supply of water and the cleansing of streets became a statutory duty of the local authorities. We have come a long way from these, and from the surveys of Charles Booth in the 1890s in which streets were classified on a scale from 'lowest class, vicious and semi-criminal', through 'very poor, casual, chronic want' to 'fairly comfortable, good ordinary earnings' and 'upper classes, wealthy'.

While one could argue that these major battles have been largely won in the West in relation to infectious disease, there are still substantial differences in chronic disease incidence and death rates attributable to social class and to area of residence. Furthermore, as McKeown argued, after the early successes public policy on health in Britain and in many other countries became dominated by a treatment rather than a prevention orientation. Indeed it could be argued that, in the UK at any rate, the major objective in many departments of public health has become the monitoring and evaluation of therapeutic services, rather than a focus on the preservation of health and prevention of disease.

Nevertheless, the Healthy Cities Initiative in 1986 by the World Health Organization has provided a framework for what some have termed 'the New Public Health', in that it brings together environmental changes and personal preventive measures, with a focus on public policy and individual lifestyle. This recognition of the built environment as a 'first cause' (alongside genetics and the socio-economic environment) of chronic disease has profound implications, as it brings into context the foundational importance of the built environment and urban planning. To be able to design environments, including redesigning and retrofitting parts of cities in the West that are past their due date and creating brand new cities in developing countries, which promote health across chronic as well as infectious disease will affect global health for generations to come, just as the reshaping of cities since the first Public Health Acts did over a century ago.

Against this background this work of Sarkar, Webster and Gallacher is highly opportune. Their application of objective built environment assessment to cohort data represents a step-change in rigour. It is an essential step towards quantifying the effect of the built environment on chronic disease in individuals over the life course. It is also a modern milestone in the construction of an evidence base for healthy town planning. The empirical part of the book draws on results from a small town, but one that has become one of the best international epidemiologic laboratories. It is rather remarkable that significant urban design effects have been found in such a small town and population. The Caerphilly study results are encouraging, therefore, but more data await the analysis of this team. The automation of their methods has allowed their application to large-scale data sets, and work is under way to apply their built environment metrics to the UK Biobank (a flagship UK epidemiology study of half a million people) and other cohorts. This work holds enormous promise.

The records of the Health of Towns Association of late-nineteenth-century England show that the Association members argued and debated and the early medical officers of health were branded as troublemakers. A new round of debate is upon us with very different types of urban public health concerns, notably obesity, mental health and an ageing population. Therefore – let the work continue and the evidence-based arguments begin.

Peter Elwood
Cardiff University
July 2013

Preface

Mounting scientific evidence generated over the past decade points to the significant role played by the myriad attributes of our cities' built environments in shaping our health and well-being. Nonetheless, the attainment of healthy cities still remains a massive unmet challenge to urban societies at all levels of development. The production and socio-spatial distribution of health originate as a result of a complex interplay between contextual socio-economic, built and natural environmental as well as individual- and population-level factors; and this complexity is tricky to unravel. We undertook to write this book with this challenge in mind. In particular, we wanted to bring together the disciplines of urban planning, public health and epidemiology and show how once again in the modern history of urban planning they have need of each other. The modern era of urban planning in the UK, and the West as a whole, started under the influence of public health studies and policy concerns. We believe that it is time to reunite the two fields in more than a rhetorical manner.

To decipher the impact of healthy (or unhealthy) places upon health outcomes, the book hypothesizes that the constituent components of the built environment, especially the configuration and design of land uses and street networks, govern the distribution of resources and services and configure neighbourhood activity space. They thereby influence individual physical activity behaviour, social interactions, general well-being and specific health such as weight outcomes and mental health. The underlying causal hypothesis in the book, and in the field of studies that it reviews and extends, is that the configuration of urban space and the distribution of opportunities within its subspaces influence physical activity and influence exposure to health-enhancing and -subtracting factors.

The transport networks of a city, particularly its road grid, can be thought of as distributing the benefits and costs of living together in a city. For this reason, property prices are highly correlated with the accessibility conferred by the grid. The urban grid also distributes health risks. If this is so, then it should be possible to use urban accessibility measured from the road network to both explain and predict individual health variations within cities.

Chapters 1–4 conceptualize the *urban health niche* as a novel holistic and spatially explicit paradigm in health-related urban planning and public health planning, and propose a method for empirically modelling the healthy city. Chapters 5–8 demonstrate how this paradigm, informed by accumulated research evidence, can be used to structure empirical studies and provide scientific evidence much needed to support healthy-city policy and planning. These empirical chapters show how we have created and integrated multi-level data sets pertaining to health, socio-economic, built and natural environments to constitute a high-resolution health niche database. We call this a *spatial Design Network Analysis for Urban Health* model (*sDNA-UH*) after the sDNA spatial network analysis tool that conceptually and empirically underlies the implemented health niche model (http://www.cardiff.ac.uk/sdna/). The sDNA-UH model reported in this book has been developed for the assembly constituency of Caerphilly, an assembly constituency of South Wales in the UK.

State-of-the-art spatial and network analysis performed on UK Ordnance Survey MasterMap data layers creates objective measurements of urban built environment accessibility (morphological metrics – *morphometrics*). These are used to investigate fine-scale associations between urban configuration and individual health. We employ health data from the Caerphilly Prospective Study, a long-standing and internationally prominent cohort study of adult men. Using the morphometrics and the health data, we construct a series of multi-level cross-sectional and longitudinal models in Chapters 5–8 to examine the association between built environment configuration and individual health outcomes.

The conceptual and empirical chapters (Chapters 1–4 and 5–8 respectively) are intended to point to a more focused and evidence-based approach to investigating and designing for healthy cities. We hope that the book will encourage a new generation of scholars to pursue the new opportunities now available through innovations in data and spatial and network data analysis methods and technology.

The book is intended to be of interest to an interdisciplinary body of scholars, practitioners and policy makers within the domains of urban planning, spatial epidemiology, health geography, sociology, public health and psychology. The empirical studies in Chapters 5–8 are especially intended for advanced undergraduate and postgraduate scholars and urban health researchers who may want to integrate readily accessible spatial data with health data in constructing robust spatial epidemiological and public health models.

We wish to thank several individuals who helped us in the writing of this book. Our ideas for the book have been refined over time under the influence of contributions from many scholars, including some of the works cited in the References. In particular we would like to thank Professor Peter Elwood, Professor Stephen Palmer and Professor Lawrence Frank for their encouragement during the course of the project. Professor Elwood's influence goes back to the start of the careers of two members of the authoring team (Chris Webster and John Gallacher), and this is a good opportunity to thank him for shaping our respective intellectual journeys. We also thank our students and colleagues at Cardiff University for being a constant source of challenge and renewal in our academic pursuits. Special thanks are due to the anonymous respondents of the Caerphilly Prospective Study, whose health we study in this book. We further wish to thank the UK Ordnance Survey for the MasterMap data layers that formed the base for the construction of built environment metrics in this project. Thanks are also due to the UK Economic and Social Research Council and UK Biobank for their support of the authors' WHealth modelling project (ESRC grant reference: ES/L003201/1 under its Transformative Research Programme) and UK Biobank Built Environment project (entitled Morphometric Analysis of the Built Environment in UK Biobank). The work presented in this book provided a pilot run for the scaled-up version in these research projects. At the same time, the ESRC project provided resources towards the completion of the book, which contains the fullest statement in print of the methodology underlying the WHealth modelling paradigm. We express our thanks to Jo Betteridge, Caroline Cornish, Emily Neukomm and Alex Pettifer at Edward Elgar for their patient help with the editing of the original manuscript. Last but not the least, we owe special gratitude to our families for their constant encouragement and support, as well as for patiently enduring this project with us.

Chinmoy Sarkar
Chris Webster
John Gallacher

Abbreviations

ACEs	active community environments
AIC	Akaike information criterion
APGAR	adaptation, partnership, growth, affection, resolve
ARI	acute respiratory infections
ARIC	Atherosclerosis Risk in Communities
ASA	angular segment analysis
BALTS	Baltimore Active Living Teens Study
BATS	Bay Area Travel Survey
BE	built environment
BEAT	Built Environment Assessment Tool
BEPAS	Belgian Environmental Physical Activity Study
BESSC	Built Environment Site Survey Checklist
BG	block group
BIC	Bayesian information criterion
BMI	body mass index
BRFSS	Behavioural Risk Factor Surveillance System
CAAL	Child/Adolescent Activity Log
CaPS	Caerphilly Prospective Study
CAS	complex adaptive systems
CATI	computer-assisted telephone interview
CBD	central business district
CCD	census collection district
CCHS	Canadian Community Health Survey
CDC	Centers for Disease Control and Prevention
CES-D	Center for Epidemiologic Studies Depression Scale
CHD	coronary heart disease
CHS	Community Health Survey (New York City)
CI	confidence interval
CIS-R	Revised Clinical Interview Schedule
CMSA	consolidated metropolitan statistical area
CO	carbon monoxide
CO_2	carbon dioxide
COPD	chronic obstructive pulmonary disease
Cred.I	credible interval

CVD	cardiovascular disease
DALYs	disability-adjusted life-years
DHAs	district health authorities
DSSI	Duke Social Support Index
DTM	digital terrain model
DZ	data zone
ETS	environmental tobacco smoke
FAR	floor area ratio
GDP	gross domestic product
G–E	gene–environment
GGHB	Greater Glasgow Health Board
GHQ	General Health Questionnaire
GIS	geographic information system
GLLAMM	generalized linear latent and mixed models
GP	general practitioner
GWAS	genome-wide association studies
HADS	Hospital Anxiety and Depression Scale
HANAH	Housing and Neighbourhood and Health
HCl	hydrogen chloride
HHI	Herfindahl–Hirschman Index
HIMS	Health in Men Study
HIV	human immunodeficiency virus
HNC	household–neighbourhood–city
HNO_2	nitrous acid
HNO_3	nitric acid
HRQoL	health-related quality of life
HSE	Health Survey for England
ICSU	International Council for Science
IHD	ischaemic heart disease
IPAQ	International Physical Activity Questionnaire
IPS	International Physical Activity Prevalence Study
ITN	Integrated Transport Network
LA	local authority
L.A.FANS	Los Angeles Family and Neighborhood Study
LARES	Review of European Housing and Health Status
LGA	local governing area
LSOA	lower super output area
LU	land use
LUM	land use mix
MCMC	Markov Chain Monte Carlo
MESA	Multi-Ethnic Study of Atherosclerosis
METS	metabolic syndrome

MI	myocardial infarction
MoNAT	Montreal Neighbourhood Assessment Tool
MSOA	middle super output area
MVPA	moderate to vigorous physical activity
NALP	Neighbourhood Active Living Potential
NBZ	network buffer zone
NDVI	Normalized Difference Vegetation Index
NEWS	Neighbourhood Environment Walkability Scale
NHANES	National Health and Nutrition Examination Survey
NHS	National Health Service
NHTS	National Household Travel Survey
NICE	National Institute for Health and Clinical Excellence
NIHL	noise-induced hearing loss
NO_2	nitrogen dioxide
NOx	oxides of nitrogen
NPAQ	Neighbourhood Physical Activity Questionnaire
NPTS	National Personal Transportation Survey
NQLS	Neighbourhood Quality of Life Study
O_3	ozone
OPCS	Office of Population Censuses and Surveys
OR	odds ratio
OS	Ordnance Survey
OSM	Ordnance Survey MasterMap
PA	physical activity
PACW	physically active commuting to work
PANES	Physical Activity Neighbourhood Environment Survey
PCS	postcode sector
PEDS	Pedestrian Environmental Data Scan
PERI	Psychiatric Epidemiological Research Instrument
PLACE	Physical Activity in Localities and Community Environments
PM	particulate matter
POR	prevalence odds ratio
ppm	parts per million
PR	prevalence ratio
QoL	quality of life
REAT	Residential Environment Assessment Tool
RESIDE	RESIDential Environment project
SAD	seasonal affective disorder
SAR	sample of anonymized records
SD	standard deviation
sDNA	spatial Design Network Analysis

sDNA-UH	spatial Design Network Analysis for Urban Health
SE	standard error
SEAs	state economic areas
SEID1	Study of Environmental and Individual Determinants
SES	socio-economic status
SHAPE	Senior Health and Physical Exercise
SMARTRAQ	Strategies for Metropolitan Atlanta's Regional Transportation and Air Quality
SofC	sense of community
SOV	single-occupant vehicle
SPACES	Systematic Pedestrian and Cycling Environmental Scan
spc	standardized path coefficient
SVOCs	semi-volatile organic compounds
SWAT	Scottish Walkability Assessment Tool
SWEAT	Senior Walking Environmental Assessment Tool
TAZ	traffic analysis zone
TIA	transient ischaemic attack
TREC-IDEA	Trans-disciplinary Research on Energetics and Cancer – Identifying Determinants of Eating and Activity
UMBECS	University of Miami Built Environment Coding System
USEPA	US Environmental Protection Agency
VHT	vehicle hours of travel
VIFs	variance inflation factors
VOCs	volatile organic compounds
WBC	Walkable and Bikeable Communities
WHO	World Health Organization
WIMD	Welsh Index of Multiple Deprivation
WOMAN	Women on the Move through Activity and Nutrition
WPS	Walkable Places Survey

1. Introduction

> For in general you will find assimilated to the nature of the land both the physique and the characteristics of the inhabitants.
>
> (Hippocrates, 1948: 137)

The first decade of the twenty-first century was for British urban planning something of a rerun of the first decade of the twentieth century: planning was heralded as a powerful new antidote to urban public health problems. A hundred years ago, the cause was the abysmal conditions in cities that had emerged by the middle of the nineteenth century and the consequent successive waves of public health-related legislation that eventually gave rise to the modern British planning system at the dawn of the new century. This time around, it was an epidemic in obesity allied with growing concerns over the health outcomes of unequal cities, marginalized groups and problem neighbourhoods and a shift in perspective amongst epidemiologists that favoured a holistic view of health, health problems and interventions and led them to view urban planning as the ultimate public health intervention:

> Understanding the urban factors that are risk or protective factors for health can capitalize on the positive aspects of urban living and lead to the development of appropriate interventions and preventive measures. Given the growing predominance of the urban living, interventions that take into account features of the urban environment have the potential to be widely applicable and to influence the health of vast number of people. (Vlahov and Galea, 2003)

In the United Kingdom, the relationship between urban planning and public health has come under renewed focus by medical and planning academics (H. Barton and Tsourou, 2000; Kidd, 2007; H. Barton, 2009; Herrick, 2009; Townshend and Lake, 2009; B. Evans et al., 2012) and public health and planning policy makers (National Heart Forum, 2007; Department of Health, 2008; NICE, 2008; RTPI, 2009). Britain is not alone in this: the same connections are being made across Europe, Australia, New Zealand (National Heart Foundation of Australia, 2004; Public Health Advisory Committee, 2008; Healthy Spaces and Places, 2009; WHO Europe, 2010) and the USA (Greenberg et al., 1994; Diez Roux, 2001, 2002; Dannenberg et al., 2003; Frank et al., 2003; Corburn,

2004; Sallis et al., 2012). The developed world has been rediscovering one of the forgotten fundamental purposes of city planning. The modern scholarship picks up from that of the early pioneering ecological health studies aimed at deciphering the disparities in health and mortality. The earliest studies were conducted in the seventeenth century; John Graunt ([1662] 1939) reported on the social distribution of death from plague in London, while William Petty enumerated the costs of mortality (Petty and Hull, 1899). Towards the late nineteenth century (1886–91), Charles Booth (1889), a social reformer, conducted a detailed survey to measure and map the incidence and causes of poverty in inner London, which formed the basis of the contemporary Registrar General's social class scheme.

The relationship between health and urban development pattern has not had to be rediscovered in countries at a less advanced stage of economic and urban development. Cities in developing countries, as with European cities 150 years ago, have always been intrinsically unhealthy. The proportion of urban population increased from slightly below 20 per cent to 36 per cent over the period 1960–2000 in both Asia and Africa (Bloom et al., 2008). Increasing competition for space in the cities results in socio-spatial stratifications wherein residents of the poorer neighbourhoods typically experience inadequate housing and sanitation, lack of access to potable water, overcrowding, pollution, substance use, crime and the associated health costs. Induced behavioural changes result in sedentary lifestyles manifested by physical inactivity, psychosocial stress, increased dependence on junk or otherwise poor-quality food, and tobacco use: potential precursors for chronic non-communicable diseases. For example, the estimated mortality from cardiovascular disease in 1990 was 70 per cent higher in the developing countries (at 8–9 million fatalities) relative to developed countries at 5.3 million deaths over the same period (A.D. Lopez, 1993). A study found comparatively higher incidence rates of hypertension in the urban areas of India and sub-Saharan Africa than in the rural areas (Srinath Reddy et al., 2005; Addo et al., 2007). Another study, conducted in China, indicates that the propensity to report poor health increases with increasing degree of urbanization. Incidence rates of obesity and hypertension were also comparatively higher in urban populations than their rural counterparts (Van de Poel et al., 2012). Another longitudinal study, conducted in eight provinces of China, reported a 14 per cent increase in car ownership between 1989 and 1997 and an associated 1.8 kilogram greater weight gain, while the likelihood of becoming obese during that time period doubled (A.C. Bell et al., 2002; F.B. Hu, 2011). The world's slum population is increasing despite the rapid progress in urban environmental quality made in some parts of the developing world. The population of slum dwellers has risen from 0.75 billion in 1990 to 1 billion today, and this has been projected to further rise to 1.4 billion by 2020 (Lopez Moreno and Warah, 2006). The ubiquitous slum and informal settlement problems that accompany rapid urban and economic development have usually helped keep sanitation and health improvement a fundamental objective of urban planning in such countries. Even in China, where there are no informal squatter settlements, the wholesale redevelopment of the so-called 'villages in the city' is driven in part by public health concerns and exactly mirrors the slum removal and city beautification and modernization movement of early- and mid-twentieth-century Europe (Wu et al., 2010).

The ongoing link between built environment and health in developing countries and the rediscovery of the same in developed countries are a challenge for urban planners, not least because they have spent very little time during the last hundred years of fashioning their craft developing a parallel science of healthy cities. This is especially so of planning in the West. Most urban planning scholarship in the universities has very little to do with empirically testing the relationship between built-form parameters (referred to as urban *morphometrics* in this book) and urban performance parameters such as health outcomes. That is something that is thankfully beginning to be redressed, and one of the aims of this book is to review progress to date and point the way forward in particular directions. First, however, we place the problem in a broader context of a simple model of urban costs and benefits in order to make the point that urban public health is something that should be optimized, not necessarily maximized.

Cities exist as a result of individuals co-locating in pursuit of wealth and welfare. They form and grow because of the economies of agglomeration. For firms, labour is cheaper in cities than in dispersed locations, as are the specialized inputs needed to make things and deliver services. For individuals, consuming is cheaper in cities because of economies in scale in consumption, producing better education and better health care, for example. Competition among consumers makes cities more innovative than dispersed locations, as producers of services and goods have to be creative in meeting people's needs and wants in order to stay in business. Competition among producers of goods and services keeps prices lower in cities than in small settlements. The advantages of living in cities over living in dispersed locations are also advantages of living in larger cities over smaller cities. Choice and price of inputs, products and services are all improved, in principle, as the number of individuals and firms clustering together in ever greater concentration rises. Economics and spatial optimization drives urban growth and, as an urban economy deepens, so does the division of labour, as people are able to develop more and more specialized skills (C. Webster and Lai, 2003). They invest in their own skills in pursuit of a labour premium but can only do this as far as they find ways

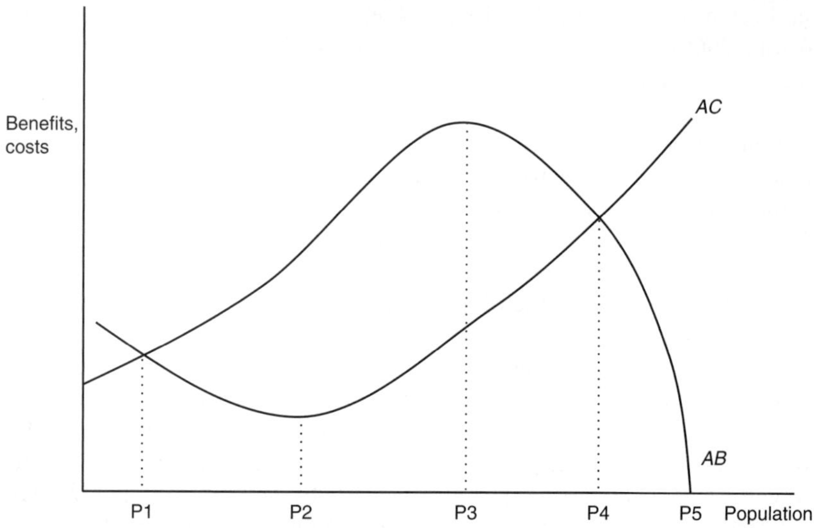

Notes: P1 = minimum city size, P2 = lowest-cost city size, P3 = city size giving maximum welfare to existing citizens, P4 = optimal city size, AB = average net benefits, AC = average costs.

Source: Derived from Alonso (1971); Richardson (1978); reproduced from Webster and Lai (2003).

Figure 1.1 Urban efficiency and city size

of meeting the demands of other individuals for ever more specialized goods and services. This virtuous deepening and diversification of human interaction is the blessing of the city. The city also has its curse, however. The curse of the city is the congestion (crowding) costs that set in at certain points as population density increases. Figure 1.1 is a classical model (after Alonso, Richardson and others) that hypothesizes the relationship of costs and benefits of agglomeration as a city grows in size. The average benefits (costs) of city living are the total benefits (costs) divided by the number of people and could be measured empirically in a number of ways.

Up to P3, the average benefits of living in the city continue to rise. After P3, each additional person has the effect of reducing the average benefits, because *crowding* effect has set in. Hospitals, clinics, general practitioner (GP) practices, and primary and secondary schools at some stage all get congested, like the roads that carry people to such services and enable people to live apart from their workplace. Investment in additional health care services and facilities, schools and roads moves P3 to the right, but, for any fixed stock of services and physical infrastructure, it is reasonable to suppose that an inflection point is reached after which average benefits decline. Once a city is built, the cost of renewing and expanding infrastructure is a function of land price, which is itself a function of demand and therefore population and population density, so it becomes problematic to reinvest to avert the inflection point. All cities have their own demise built into their DNA. Set against the benefits curve in the figure is a cost curve – the cost of supplying urban infrastructure and services divided by the number of people sharing the costs. Up to P2, cost per person falls, as the cost of a fixed stock of infrastructure is shared by more people. At some stage, however, the average costs rise, as it becomes increasingly more expensive to purchase land, build facilities, manage them, diversify them, and innovate to meet increasingly demanding expectations. P3 is the optimal city size from the point of view of those who live in the city: the point of maximum distance between benefits and costs. It is the NIMBY size so vigorously pursued by so many local authorities in the South-East of England, for example. P4 is the socially optimal city size from the point of view of society as a whole: compared to P3, it has accommodated P4 – P3 additional people, all of whom experience net benefits. Beyond P4, the costs exceed the benefits. Rational people would not move to this city, and a rational and all-powerful government would stop a city at this size and start another one. A more enlightened rational and powerful government might insist that all cities stop at P3. Many cities in the world have clearly exceeded P4. Migrants keep flocking to them, however, because of the future value they place on urban life – the jobs they expect to get and the education and jobs they expect for their children. In the most crowded and extensive cities of the world, the health costs feature as a very significant part of the diseconomy of urban life beyond P4. The costs and benefits of size are unevenly distributed to a city's population spatially and socially. The urban sprawl and associated real estate developments in the megacities of the developing world create two contrasting configurations: the peripheral regions typically characterized by informal settlements lacking basic infrastructure and public services, with the suburban sprawl also accommodating the creation of mixed residential zones for high- and middle-income groups coexisting with high-priced commercial and retail complexes. Such spatial disparity in wealth and quality of life aggravates socio-economic segregation and health inequity with significant health costs (Frumkin, 2002; Frumkin et al., 2004). According to the latest projected estimates for 2015, the urban agglomerations of Lagos (20 501.35), Metro Manila (20 086.98), Mumbai (19 337.99), Surat (17 119.91) and Seoul (15 967.40) will have the highest population densities in persons per square kilometre (United Nations, 2012). Each of them belongs to a developing country in Asia or Africa. They could well be out-of-control primate cities with no hope of servicing their populations adequately. They illustrate the power of the hope that governs mass rural–urban migration and the reality of hope deferred or lost as the net real benefits of urban living remain static or are squeezed beyond P4 in Figure 1.1 – squeezed towards parity with rural subsistence living (the ultimate alternative and opportunity cost facing the urban poor) or worse (since the transaction costs of relocating are high for most urban poor families and they are therefore, to a degree, trapped).

What, then, may be said about public health and urban planning on the basis of this simple but profound and resilient model?

First, at low levels of per capita investment in urban physical and social infrastructure, health risks soon surface as a limiting constraint to the benefits of urban agglomeration. This is where London was at the end of the nineteenth century and modern cities in less developed countries have been during the last 50 years or so of massive urbanization. Cities in developing countries typically find it difficult to raise sufficient tax revenues to provide for the health standards that the West has become accustomed to.

Second, the West also finds it difficult to sustain the standards it has become accustomed to. Owing to rising labour costs, rising costs of medical technology, changing demographics and the high costs of organizing health care supply, for example, the cost of sustaining a city at P4 are probably on the increase (AC moves upwards). This leads to the intriguing hypothesis that rising health care costs imply the need for smaller cities. This is because higher health care costs that do not raise the benefits of urban living commensurately raise the general costs of supporting an urban population, and the higher the general costs the lower the population that can be efficiently accommodated for a given set of agglomeration benefits. It should be noted in this respect that, despite the huge inflow of public funds into the British National Health Service over the last decade (NHS expenditure increased by 70 per cent from £60 billion to £102 billion in the first decade of the twenty-first century), total UK NHS productivity has gone down by an average of 0.2 per cent per year over the period 2000–01 to 2010–11. Over the same period, productivity in hospitals fell by 1.4 per cent per year (Comptroller and Auditor General, 2010). The scientific relationship between health, health care costs and settlement size is an under-researched issue.

Third, investments in health care technology (as opposed to labour-related and other unproductive cost inflation) raise the benefits of living in cities (moving AB upwards in Figure 1.1). Specialized health and hospital services and the latest medical technology are classical agglomeration benefits represented by the AB curve. They are found in cities because of economies of consumption and production: larger concentrations of people create demand for more costly and more diverse services and equipment, which can be provided in cities at a cheaper unit price.

Fourth, a long-standing and widespread urban planning doctrine (not a scientific principle) is to design cities at the neighbourhood scale around core services, especially primary schools, but also primary health care such as GP surgeries and clinics. Physical layouts of new urban development in many cities across the world are planned under certain assumptions about the numbers of homes and people efficiently clustered around a set of core neighbourhood services. One definition of a healthy city (in the sense of being well provided with health care facilities) is one in which health care services and facilities are organized in size and location in a way that optimizes their effectiveness. If the horizontal axis of Figure 1.1 is reinterpreted as being the population co-consuming a given health service or facility, then P4 is the optimal population catchment. If there are many such services in a city or region, then one of the tasks of urban planners working with health care planners is to coordinate with each other to ensure an optimal allocation of services across the population: something that inevitable leads to a hierarchy of services with local services nested within the catchment of services that require a larger threshold for efficient provision. This is never a perfectly efficient process, however, since health care facilities are lumpy and the services provided within them inevitably either over- or, more likely, under-supply the urban population, which is never exactly equal to the breakeven threshold of the bundle of services provided at a facility. It may be noted that market-like institutions introduced into public health organizations over recent decades can improve the efficiency of the spatial health economy. If health care buyers representing patients in one city can buy services supplied in another and patients assume some of the costs of being mobile customers, then there need not be such a closely matched or tightly designed configuration of health services and population and the intrinsic inefficiencies of inevitably lumpy health facility planning can be mitigated.

Fifth, and most important for the focus of this book, health problems are part of the cause of the benefits inflection in Figure 1.1. Some health problems are directly caused by crowding. Respiratory problems, stress and mental illness can be caused, or exacerbated, by living near or using overcrowded roads, for example (Babisch et al., 1990, 1999; Oftedal et al., 2003; Nordling et al., 2008; Pujades-Rodríguez et al., 2009). Mental health problems result from congestion in the labour and housing market. High-density living is associated with diseases related to dampness, airborne pollution, exposure to industrial waste-borne toxins and so on (Ginns and Gatrell, 1996; Elliott et al., 1999; Gómez-Jacinto and Hombrados-Mendieta, 2002).

This brings us to the main focus of the book: investigating the relationship between urban design (or, put another way, built environmental configuration or urban morphology) and health. Chapter 4 reviews this relationship at a fine level of detail. The aim is to offer a definitive review at this point of time which tries to capture all that is currently known of any significance about the relationship.

We preface the scientific review in Chapter 4 with the observation that there seems to be a widespread intuitive belief that the design of the built environment has an effect on health outcomes. It is not surprising that urban planners have readily accepted this, since it bolsters their professional justification. That the epidemiological and medical practitioner community has accepted the belief is more significant in the sense that these professions have nothing to gain and possibly something to lose by admitting the built environment into the lexicon of their associative and causal models and intervention mechanisms. The relationship is an intuitive one: it is plausible and makes sufficient common sense for journalists to rally to the cause. The scientific basis for this belief is controvertible, however. Urban planners tend to work by doctrine, not by science. One objective of the book is to lay the science before the planning community and propose theoretical and empirical models that will help establish an empirical evidence base for healthy city planning. At most, there is a weak relationship between urban morphology and health outcomes. Weak relationships are important nevertheless. They can still guide our urban designs, plans and policies, thereby acting as crucial public health interventions aimed at minimizing health risks and hence costs. What we should be doing is to try to measure them more accurately so that we can progressively build up a knowledge base about healthy city attributes and performance.

To this end, the book introduces an approach to measuring morphometrics that goes beyond any other study yet published in terms of level of spatial detail and matching of this to individual health records. The book revolves around an ongoing research project based at Cardiff University, the University of Hong Kong and Cambridge University, the first phase of which involved what we have called the *spatial **D**esign **N**etwork **A**nalysis for **U**rban **H**ealth* (*sDNA-UH*), a high-resolution GIS and network analysis model comprising a series of built environment (BE) morphological metrics (morphometrics) coupled with socio-demographic, lifestyle and health variables. The first phase of this study focused on one of the UK's most comprehensively studied epidemiology laboratories: the assembly constituency of Caerphilly, South Wales (83 600 inhabitants over 114.54 square kilometres, with a density of 727 inhabitants per square kilometre). UK Ordnance Survey MasterMap (OSM) data layers – the Topography

Layer, Integrated Transport Network (ITN) Layer and Address Layer 2 of Caerphilly – were employed as the base sources for built environment data, and a robust set of morphometrics were measured at the dwelling level as well as within specified street network buffers around an individual respondent's dwelling unit. GIS-based spatial analysis and network models have been employed to construct more than 100 objectively measured BE morphometrics for each member of the epidemiological study cohort, broadly categorized as: dwelling level, land use, street network accessibility, physical environment and area-level deprivation variables. These have been matched to individual socio-demographic and health data from a long-established panel study of elderly men to test the effects of the built environment on individual health within this sub-population at multiple spatial scales.

Chapter 2 traces the origins of public health and city planning and describes the evolving paradigms of epidemiology as definitions of health have changed in response to emerging social costs of urbanization and changing disease aetiology. It concludes by highlighting the contemporary shift towards a paradigm that is holistic and multidisciplinary, giving due credence to both biomedical and contextual (social, built and natural environmental) determinants of health.

Drawing together diverse strands of research evidence, we introduce the concept of the urban *health niche* as a fundamental public health planning paradigm in Chapter 3. The framework endeavours to integrate four key elements: (1) the multiple spatial scales at which various health-defining processes function; (2) levels of organization for studying health, from the individual to the population level; (3) the health-promoting and -inhibiting attributes of space; and (4) temporal dynamism. Given the complexity of the notion of a healthy city, we employ the concept of urban health niche to conceptualize a bottom-up model that incorporates and integrates the multiple, multi-level health determinants existing at the different spatial hierarchies in a city system.

Chapter 4 provides a systematic review of the epidemiologic, public health and health geography literature on built environment and health, following the urban health niche model. Determinants of health are discussed in detail at the housing, neighbourhood and city levels.

Chapter 5 discusses the methodology involved in the development of the spatial Design Network Analysis for Urban Health and its component morphometrics. State-of-the-art spatial and network analysis techniques are employed to quantify various facets of the urban environment that have the potential to influence an individual's health.

To illustrate the evidence-based approach to healthy city planning advocated in the early chapters of the book, Chapters 6–8 present a series of epidemiological models that attempt to measure the degree of association between various parameterized features of the built environment and various health outcomes, specifically obesity and mental health outcomes.

In conclusion, Chapter 9 reflects on what has been achieved by the conceptual and empirical innovations presented in the book, sets out elements for an ongoing research agenda, and poses challenges for researchers, students, professionals and policy makers working in the healthy cities field.

2. Tracing the ever-evolving relationship between urban planning and public health

2.1 INTRODUCTION

The advent of urbanization and associated problems endemic to it led to the evolution of the disciplines of public health and town planning. Although emerging from a common necessity to cope with the demands of urbanization and the resulting health issues, over the course of the past 200 years the relationship between the two disciplines has waxed and waned. Earlier, the good health of an individual had been simply synonymous with the non-existence of any identifiable serious disease, while a nation's health was reflected solely by measures such as infant mortality, mortality of middle-aged persons, prevalence of infectious diseases like tuberculosis, malnutrition in infants and expecting mothers, incidences of epidemic outbreaks, and so on. The multifold increases in population in Britain from the early or mid-nineteenth century and the West more generally over the next 100 years, and the ensuing accelerated urban expansion have been accompanied by increasing complexity of the urban health issues.

As the aetiology of the disease shifted from *infectious* to *chronic*, the notion of health no longer remained intrinsically synonymous with the existence or non-existence of disease(s). It shifted away from the original unidimensional disease-focused model to a more holistic model comprising multiple dimensions of analysis, diagnosis and prescription in the form of well-being, quality of life and the so-called positive health agenda. The counterproductiveness of following purely *unidirectional* (*biomedical*) thinking has been eloquently summarized by Tinetti and Fried in the *American Journal of Medicine*: 'The changed spectrum of health conditions, the complex interplay of biological and non-biological factors, the aging population, and the inter-individual variability in health priorities render medical care that is centred primarily on the diagnosis and treatment of individual diseases at best out of date and at worst harmful' (Tinetti and Fried, 2004). This was anticipated in the more comprehensive definition of health proposed by the World Health Organization (WHO) in

1948: 'Health is a state of complete physical, mental and social well-being and not merely the absence of disease or infirmity. The enjoyment of the highest attainable standard of health is one of the fundamental rights of every human being without distinction of race, religion, political belief, economic or social condition' (WHO, 2005a).

Nonetheless, the onslaughts of subsequent changes in demography as well as patterns of illness accompanying rapid urbanization have meant that the definition has often been unproductive and, in some cases, counterproductive (Huber et al., 2011). The French physician Georges Canguilhem in his book *Le normal et le pathologique* (1966) introduced the notion of health as an individual's ability to adapt and self-manage. This was a much more realistic formulation, as health depends on an individual's circumstances and includes both animate and inanimate environments in addition to physical, mental and social dimensions of human life (Editorial, 2009). More recently, health has been parameterized in terms of frailty in an ageing population (D.M. Jones et al., 2004; Rockwood et al., 2005). Others have associated health with the idea of human rights (Susser, 1993) and justice, demanding the ability to live a life of value (Sen, 2009). At the same time, the near impossibility of defining health on account of its multidimensional nature has been highlighted by several authors (Paine, 2005; Jadad and O'Grady, 2008).

In this chapter, we trace the pre-war and post-war origins of public health and urban planning movements, highlighting the evolution of epidemiological paradigms to cater to new challenges of urban health. The chapter concludes by highlighting a current resurgence of the uniting links between the disciplines of public health and urban planning and a thrust towards a more holistic approach in public health planning.

2.2 THE PRE-WAR ERA

A brief look back at the epidemiological records of the past indicates that the cities of medieval and early modern Europe were regarded as unhealthy places, consistently characterized by higher rates of mortality than the adjoining rural areas. The urban historian Bairoch (1988) concluded:

> By the beginning of the nineteenth century, the urban death rate was distinctly higher than that recorded in rural districts – as was also the case with infant mortality, which of course contributed to the overall pattern. The difference between urban and rural mortality, large at the start of the nineteenth century, gradually decreased until it vanished during the first years of the twentieth century. The average difference, which around 1810–1830 seems to have been on the order of 40–60%, fell to around 10–30% by about 1890. From the start

> of the twentieth century, the difference disappeared altogether or had even reversed its direction. (pp. 233–4)

The term *urban penalty* or *le handicap urbain* was employed to highlight the comparatively higher rates of mortality in cities than rural areas. The twin processes of industrialization and urbanization resulted in overcrowding, pollution, and lack of sanitation and the corresponding increased burden of communicable diseases, especially tuberculosis (Kearns, 1988; R. Woods, 2003; Harpham, 2009). As an example, between the period 1862 and 1880, the crude death rates in towns of Imperial Germany (erstwhile Prussia) were on average 10 per cent higher than in rural areas (Vögele, 2000). The pattern was similar in nineteenth-century British cities as the urban population increased steadily 25 to 66 per cent (Szreter and Mooney, 1998). Life expectancy at birth in England and Wales remained low at 40–41 years over the first half of the nineteenth century, while a slight increase of six years was observed in the second half (Wrigley et al., 1997). In 1861, the life expectancy at birth for a male was only 26 years in Liverpool, in contrast to the much higher 57 years for a baby born in rural Okehampton, Devon (W.I. Woods and Woodward, 1984).

The first quarter of the nineteenth century witnessed the emergence of the sanitary movement and the evolution of *miasma* as the predominant theory to cope with the urban health challenge. The rapid urbanization was identified as the root cause, as eloquently highlighted by Wrigley (1969):

> It is perhaps more accurate to say that high mortality was caused by urbanization rather than by industrialization. It was in the bigger cities that mortality was so very high. Most of these big cities were not heavily engaged in the new industries, but were administrative and commercial centres. Paris, Berlin, Marseilles, and Liverpool all had high death rates and low expectation of life, though none was a typical product of the industrial revolution in the narrow sense. In a broader sense, of course, all were able to develop only because of the improvements in transport and growth in productive capacity which characterize the industrial revolution. To a notable extent, but now in a different context, mortality was still density-dependent. Wherever there were large cities there were slum areas with very high densities of population and severe overcrowding which allowed diseases like tuberculosis to spread very widely and exposed children and young people to a great range of infectious illness. (Reproduced from Bairoch, 1988, p. 236)

Thus foul pollutants emanating from the physical environment (air, water and soil) as well as overcrowding were believed to be the main causes of mortality and morbidity. Overall data on sickness and death were collected from the unhygienic inner cities of Europe to study the emergent spatial patterns. Special importance was laid on ecological mapping of overall mortality and morbidity, rather than on the causality and attributes of specific ailments. Mortality was mapped in relation to specific diseases, housing conditions, industries and occupations. The English Births and Deaths Registration Act was passed in 1836, and the Registrar General's Office was subsequently set up. William Farr, as the head of the statistical department in the English Registrar General's Office, introduced in 1839 the diagnostic classifications for national mortality statistics. His pioneering contributions to vital statistics provided much required direction to the efforts of sanitary reformers. His studies on cholera in London identified significant district-level variations in mortality with respect to housing quality, air quality and residential elevation above the sea level (Farr, 1885). This period also witnessed significant metamorphosis of the social fabric of England as it made its transition from an agricultural to an industrial economy. The Reform Bill of 1832 and the Municipal Corporations Act 1835 were important developments that eventually led to social reforms aimed at improving health. Edwin Chadwick spearheaded the social medicine movement and led the commission of inquiry into the working of poor laws that resulted in the Poor Law Amendment Act 1834. He emphasized the significant social value of public housing and improved sanitation in the neighbourhoods, especially as a means to eradicate poverty. In one of the most extensive reports of the epoch he stressed that the contextual health inequalities originating from the physical environmental factors resulted in poverty and deprivation (Chadwick, 1842). Subsequently, Friedrich Engels studied the health of the factory workers of Manchester in 1844 and reported twice the mortality rate among the workers living in poor housing as among those in well-off housing conditions. He reversed Chadwick's causality, arguing that poverty resulted in disease (Engels, [1845] 1987). John Snow conducted extensive ecological analysis of the geographical distribution of cholera in London. He was able to map the spatial distribution of deaths from cholera in the Broad Street district of London, where more than 500 mortalities were recorded within just ten days of September 1854 (Snow, 1936). He termed his map the 'cholera field'; its centre was a pump in Broad Street near Golden Square, while the 'field' was bounded by four streets: Great Marlborough Street, Dean Street, Brewer Street and King Street. This remains to this date a classic study in the domain of geographical epidemiology.

During this era, the professions of city planning and public health functioned in unison in both Europe and America to produce initiatives that were mostly preventive in nature. These included closure of open drainage and sewer systems, systemized waste disposal, and public baths built to inhibit contamination, as well as public housing and designed parks and playgrounds to contain the miasma (Duffy, 1990). These were to some extent successful in bringing about major improvements in health and hygiene, especially in the control of leprosy and smallpox. Nonetheless, social epidemiology was more oriented to the understanding of causes and prevention of disease at the population levels rather than targeting the real biological agents responsible.

The second part of the nineteenth century witnessed the evolution of germ theory as a predominant paradigm in public health. Jacob Henle ([1840] 1938) was in all probability the first to articulate the pathogenic cause of contagious diseases, associating miasma with contagion. In the first chapter of his treatise entitled *Pathologische Untersuchingen* (Henle, 1840), he classified contagious diseases into two groups: epidemic and endemic. He further classified them into three subgroups: diseases caused by miasmas, miasmatic contagious diseases, and pure contagion. He argued that the propagation of the latter two was a result of *contagium animatum*, a substance excreted by the diseased organism, which on transmission to a healthy organism has the capacity to multiply and produce the same disease (Henle, [1840] 1938). Almost 13 years later, John Snow (1853) published *On Continuous Molecular Changes, More Particular in Their Relation to Epidemic Diseases*, which elaborated a similar hypothesis about the causes of contagious diseases. Based on his observations of the cholera epidemic, he concluded that infections commenced in the alimentary canal subsequent to the ingestion of contaminated water. He subtly emphasized the implicit role of microbial agents and metabolic processes (coined as *continuous molecular changes*) in the infection, multiplication and propagation of communicable diseases (Snow, 1936; Winkelstein, 1995).

This period constituted a transitional phase, heralding the new era of infectious disease epidemiology accompanying the novel advances in microbiology of the time. Almost a quarter-century after Henle's first proposition, Louis Pasteur in 1865 demonstrated the role of living organisms in the causation of epidemic in silkworms (Vallery-Radot and Devonshire, 1901). The ensuing rapid advances in microbiological research over the subsequent decades eventually usurped the position of the miasma theory as the dominant paradigm and ushered in the era of germ theory. The 1870s were associated with the isolation of pathogenic agents responsible for leprosy and anthrax; and over the 1880s the germs for typhoid, tuberculosis, cholera, diphtheria and meningococcal meningitis were identified, and those for plague and malaria during the 1890s. The period of medical discovery driven by the microbial paradigm was an equivalent one to the present one emanating from the genetic paradigm.

The principal tenets of the germ theory were based on Robert Koch's postulates which hypothesized that a single pathogenic germ was invariably associated with a specific disease (A.S. Evans, 1976). Diagnosis and treatment involved identification of the micro-organisms, their isolation and culture from the disease sites, experimental inoculation and reproduction of lesions. The overall strategy was *germ*-centric, aimed at minimizing the spread through vaccination and isolation of the affected and eventual clinical treatment through antibiotics and chemotherapy.

The enhanced cooperations between the disciplines of planning and public health and the population-based preventive interventions of the sanitary age were reoriented to laboratory-based bacteriology, often manifested through individual clinical interventions such as vaccinations and doses of antibiotics for epidemic control and cure (Duhl and Sanchez, 1999).

Despite its accurate causal explanations of several infectious diseases, germ theory held a mono-aetiological model of causation of infectious diseases, with focus exclusively on the attributes of pathogenic agents (G.T. Stewart, 1968). It failed to explain why some individuals were more susceptible to a particular illness while others were not (also termed as the doctrine of specific aetiology). Interpretation of diseases implicitly based on the aetiology of infection proved to be a logical fallacy, as it failed to take into consideration the other equally important co-determinants, especially age, sex, genetic predispositions, behavioural factors, nutritional factors, social and hygienic factors, and so on. Thus germ theory had no causal hypothesis for prevalent non-pathogenic disease, especially those arising from nutritional deficiencies and occupational exposures. Furthermore, it failed to provide suitable interpretation of complex causality, especially when infections caused by pathogens remained in a latent state until some physiological or environmental factors acted as triggers, thereby activating its pathogenicity.

Towards the beginning of the twentieth century, considerable transformations in economic and social landscapes accompanied the advancing industrialization and urban expansion. It was during this era that city planning and design eventually established itself as a more formal discipline striving to overcome the negative health impacts of the Victorian industrial city characterized by urban sprawl and pollution. The world's first university urban planning school (University of Liverpool's Department of Civic Design) was founded in 1909. Between the years 1870 and 1914, most British cities had acquired some form of public transport system. This was initially in the form of horse trams and buses, which were subsequently replaced by motor buses and electric trams. London even had electrified suburban lines as early 1905–09. This had significant consequences with respect to the dynamics of urbanization. The areal extent of the city was virtually fixed as the population doubled between 1800 and 1851; however, the city began to expand in all directions post-1850 as the railway networks grew, manifested by its initial and abiding dendritic form. However, with the evolution of a more accelerated public transport system in the form of electric trains, by 1939 London had begun to experience a more uniform growth, so that its form had by that time attained an almost circular shape, 12–15 miles in radius. Similar urban patterns of expansion were observed in other major cities of Europe. Such rapid urbanization came with severe public health consequences, especially negative effects originating from high density, overcrowding, unhygienic living conditions and poor quality of the environment. The term *smog* was coined by a Londoner in 1905 to describe the hazardous combination of fog and smoke from industries and traffic. Londoners were periodically prone to the detrimental health effects of smog events, also called *pea-soupers*, eventually culminating in the Great Smog of 1952, which was responsible for approximately 12 000 mortalities (M.L. Bell et al., 2004).

In the US, the phenomenon of urban expansion occurred via the twin processes of annexation and consolidation. During the annexation phase, the city expanded by adding unincorporated land, while consolidation was accompanied by the institutional merger of adjoining government municipalities (Frank et al., 2003). Major waves of annexation and consolidation had occurred in Philadelphia (1854), St Louis (1856), Chicago (1889), New York (1898) and Detroit (1880–1918). The boom in car usage and cheap electricity resulted in two simultaneous processes. On the one hand, there was increased mechanization and lesser dependence on human labour, resulting in a marked decline in the farm population from 32 per cent in 1900 to 23 per cent in 1940 and almost 3 per cent in 1980. On the other hand, many planners, including Frank Lloyd Wright, advocated reduced dependence on the urban centres and increased dispersion of both homes and jobs. Wright proposed a dispersed planning approach characterized by low-density urban spread, also called the *Broadacre City*, wherein he conceptualized each home to be surrounded by an acre of agricultural land and connected to the mass transit system (Wright, 1935). The peripheral regions of the urban centres became the areas of targeted growth, expanding at a rate almost twice that of the urban core in 96 of the largest US cities over the decade 1920 to 1930 (Jackson, 1985). The offshoot of such a policy saw the emergence of low-density suburban form characterized by less expensive properties built on larger plots with comparatively lower land use diversity, job density and street-level accessibility (Heimlich and Anderson, 2001; Frumkin et al., 2004). Thus, in contrast to the case in European cities, the process of urban expansion in the US occurred at a larger scale (in terms of land area), manifested by what is technically termed *urban sprawl*. Such a dispersed growth has subsequently been found to be associated with reduced sense of place and corresponding negative health implications (Ewing, Pendall et al., 2003), notwithstanding the positive health implications of lower density.

This period witnessed a multifold increase in the national wealth of Great Britain, the United States and most Western European countries. Nonetheless, gross inequality in the distribution of wealth became more pronounced. Unemployment and poverty in the sprawling urban communities resulted in the emergence of labour and social ideologies, partly triggered by significant disparities in the health, housing and social conditions that were prevalent. Although the microbiological paradigm dominated research, the sociological paradigm continued to survive, with a marked degree of reorientation of the public health and planning strategy somewhat along the lines of the social reformers of the sanitary movement. Specific importance was associated with the problem of urban areas, with emphasis on housing which promoted clean, sanitary and healthy living. With the objective of overcoming the ills inherent in a typical Victorian industrial city, James Buckingham, the social reformer and architect, proposed the design for the model town of Victoria. The design comprised a series of concentric squares, with industry separated from housing and a green belt buffer of 4000 hectares of agricultural land. He proposed relocating the polluting industries to the outskirts of the city, with the workshops at the centre and houses on the periphery of the land. In another seminal work, *Tomorrow: A Peaceful Path to Social Reform* (reissued as *Garden Cities of Tomorrow* in 1902), Ebenezer Howard wrote an investor's prospectus for the idea of the town and country or garden city. This was an inventor, entrepreneur and amateur political scientist's response to the overcrowding of London, industrial degradation, suburbanization, and building boom. Such a DNA of urban growth would efficiently combine the benefits of town, by way of improved accessibility, organization and financing, with the benefits of country life in a cleaner and altogether more orderly environment. He proposed decentralization of the workers and their workplaces, with a view to transferring the benefits of urban agglomeration to the new settlements, thereby providing them with higher purchasing power and more regular employment (Osborn and Whittick, 1977). In the UK, one of the planning measures employed to negate the effects of urban sprawl was to rehouse thousands of slum dwellers and factory workers to subsidized single-family public housing, generally four to five miles from the city centre. A classic early example of this planning experiment, with due consideration to public health concerns, was the town of Bournville built by the Cadbury brothers in 1894. In their experiment to create a self-sustaining industrial town, the Cadbury brothers transferred their factory from Birmingham city centre to a greenfield site on the outskirts of the city. Intricate attention was paid to house design, provision for suitably sized gardens, landscaped roads, parks and recreational grounds, with a view to alleviating the living conditions of the factory workers. Another successful experiment was Port Sunlight in North-West England, built by the Lever brothers in 1888, again with the aim of balancing industrial production with a model housing development for workers, accompanied with social amenities and facilities (Unilever, 1976).

The focus for healthy city planning had shifted towards devising effective thresholds for the net density of residential areas, creating green belt as buffers around new communities, all-inclusive and aesthetically pleasing urban designs and master plans, and zoning of land uses (Hall, 1975; Peterson, 2003). Howard's concepts of the garden city and social integration were first brought to fruition by architects Raymond Unwin and Barry Parker with the design of Letchworth (with a population of 35 000 people) and Welwyn Garden City (with a population of 10 000), both in the exurban countryside of Hertfordshire, neighbouring county to London. Another classic achievement of this age was the preparation of the New York Regional Plan of the 1920s, wherein Clarence Perry introduced the revolutionary idea of dividing the city into distinct *neighbourhood units* or socially engineered spaces encompassing the existing catchment area of community facilities such as schools and shops (Perry, 1929a, 1929b). These were to be structurally contiguous basic spatial units characterized by a pronounced sense of belonging and social cohesion of residents and were subsequently widely employed as the local planning unit in post-war first- and third-generation Western new towns and later new town planning throughout the urbanizing world. The importance of the neighbourhood as the fundamental spatial unit for studying the contextual effects on health has been subsequently recognized by epidemiologists and public health practitioners, especially the health-promoting and -inhibiting attributes of neighbourhood socio-economic status, built environment configuration, and quality of contained and surrounding natural environment.

In this increasingly automobile-dominated period, many notable architects and planners, including Clarence Stein in New York, Barry Parker in England and Le Corbusier in France, worked on the idea of segregation of local residential areas and pedestrian routes from mass transit routes employed by car owners, with a view to minimizing pollution and congestion. In England, the assistant commissioner of police (traffic) at London's Scotland Yard, H. Alker Tripp, proposed a distinct street typology for post-war Britain. He introduced the idea of British cities reconstructed on the basis of precincts and comprising a hierarchy of roads. He proposed that the high-volume arterial and sub-arterial roads should be void of any direct frontage development and encompass larger block sizes, and would remain sharply isolated from local streets, which would cater to their own shops and service needs (Tripp, 1942). The idea stemmed from the potential health benefits of enabling effective segregation of residential areas from street networks associated with high-density traffic. Public health concerns have subsequently extended to issues related to minimization of traffic-related pollution and the risks of road traffic accidents, particularly those involving injuries and fatalities from vehicle–pedestrian collisions.

In the 1890s the German planner Rudolf Eberstadt argued that high building density in urban centres effectively raised land and property costs, making them unaffordable to the average family. He proposed the creation of zoning laws as an economic solution catering to low-density affordable housing at the fringes of the cities (Logan, 1972). This was the start of modern planned land use zoning, which had both economic and health objectives. According to Logan (1972), the idea was first tested by Franz Adickes, mayor of Frankfurt am Main, in 1891, wherein the city was divided into six zones: single-family residences, factories, banned industrial uses, old inner city and two others for mixed use (comprising residential, commercial and light industrial uses). In 1892 suburban Berlin established two zones. Other German cities followed, formulating their own zoning ordinances that had elements of the Frankfurt and Berlin regulations, including Hamburg in 1896, Stuttgart in 1897, Mannheim in 1901, Hanover in 1902, Nuremberg in 1903, and Munich in 1903 (Logan, 1972). At almost the same time the concept of zoning originated as a land use planning tool in the US, primarily as a borrowed tool from Germany. However, its objectives varied, ranging from overcoming the environmental burdens associated with the industrial land uses and minimizing detrimental health impacts to a discriminatory tool aimed at restricting Chinese laundries from certain neighbourhoods. Over the period between 1909 and 1915, Los Angeles segregated residential and industrial land uses by creating 27 industrial districts and almost 100 residence exception districts solely for heavy and objectionable industries (Pollard, 1931). New York City became the first municipality to pass a comprehensive zoning resolution in 1916 putting constraints on land use, building height, and bulk, as well as lot coverage. It effectively divided the city into three districts or zones: residential, commercial (excluding those listed as noxious trades and industries) and unrestricted zones (New York City Board of Estimate and Apportionment, 1916; McGoldrick et al., 1944). This was the start of a zoning movement that had strong roots in public health, especially in effecting segregation between non-compatible land uses such as polluting industries and residential areas. However, it became somewhat detached from that primary concern over the century, becoming a multi-purpose land-planning tool that was often, to a degree, self-serving.

On another front, community health, with its core principles based on social hygiene and social medicine, re-emerged, adding a new dimension to the discipline of public health. Charles Booth, a social reformer, conducted a detailed survey (1886–91) to measure and map the incidence and causes of poverty in the working-class districts of inner London (the area bounded by Hammersmith in the west and Greenwich in the east, and between Highgate in the north and Clapham in the south), which formed the basis of the contemporary Registrar General's social class scheme (Booth, 1889; Orford et al., 2002). Rowntree in 1899 conducted a similar study for York. Both the studies concluded that, although the general standard of living had improved, a substantial portion of the labouring population had to subsist at extremely low wages well below a level consistent with basic health standards. Unsatisfactory health and social conditions were starkly manifested in the poorer strata of society (Rosen, 1958). Urban poverty resulted in new challenges in the form of high maternal mortality, child mortality, malnutrition and poor health of pre-school and school children. Malnutrition, parental ignorance, contaminated food and, indirectly, poverty were identified as the preventable causes of child mortality. On the public health front, this period saw the emergence of the child and maternity welfare movement in Great Britain, the United States and Western Europe, primarily focusing on preventive approaches, especially improving hygiene, eradication of nutritional deficiency and antepartum care. Pre-maternity services for expectant mothers in hospitals and health services for school children were prioritized. At the same time, proofs of non-microbiological causes of disease began to emerge, thereby somewhat reinforcing the belief in these more holistic preventive practices.

Another important dimension emerged as nutrition science, which had primarily concerned itself with the calorific value of the food intake, reoriented itself to provide rational explanations of the biochemical and metabolic processes. The term *vitamin* was first coined in 1911 by the Polish chemist Casimir Funk, and the subsequent years witnessed the emergence of the concept of *deficiency disease*. A series of accessory dietary factors and vitamins were isolated and subsequently associated with specific diseases (Rosen, 1958). Between 1918 and 1922, vitamins A and E were independently isolated by E. Mellanby in England and E.V. McCollum in the United States. Deficiency of vitamin D provided a logical explanation to the patterns of rickets, and cod liver oil was employed as an effective treatment. In the United States, Joseph Goldberger conducted an extensive study on the role of socio-economic factors in the observed population patterns of deficiency diseases. He identified nutritional deficiency owing to inadequate diet as the primary cause of infection in pellagra (Terris, 1964). Subsequently, along with Edgar Sydenstricker, he conducted one of the classic studies in the social epidemiology of pellagra in the cotton mill villages and among the tenant farmers of rural South Carolina. In addition to dietary deficiency, they observed that enforced poverty arising from crop failures was associated with increased incidences of pellagra (Goldberger et al., 1920; Rosen, 1973). Major Greenwood (1935) introduced the term *crowd diseases* to highlight the role of social environments in disease causation. He used metaphoric terms such as *seed*, *soil* and *animal husbandry*, which were subsequently formalized as *agent*, *host susceptibility* and *environment* by Hampton Frost (1941) within a holistic causal model of disease that is now de rigueur.

2.3 POST-WAR AFTERMATH

Post-war Britain witnessed unparalleled socio-demographic transformations. Immediately after the war, Britain underwent several phases of a waxing and waning of population (see Figure 2.1). The initial baby boom of 1945–47 was followed by an eventual phase of population decline almost to the level of the 1930s. However, this was followed by another unprecedented rise in the national birth rates over the period 1955–64 and a subsequent slight decline. By the late 1960s, the average natural population increase per annum was considerable at approximately 300 000. Social changes such as post-war marriages and economic prosperity in the form of avenues for jobs and education meant that the average household size fell significantly from 3.7 members in 1931 to 2.9 members per home in 1971.

There was strong and continued inter-regional migration, especially from Scotland, Wales and Northern England towards the Midlands and South of England in search of employment. These demographic changes

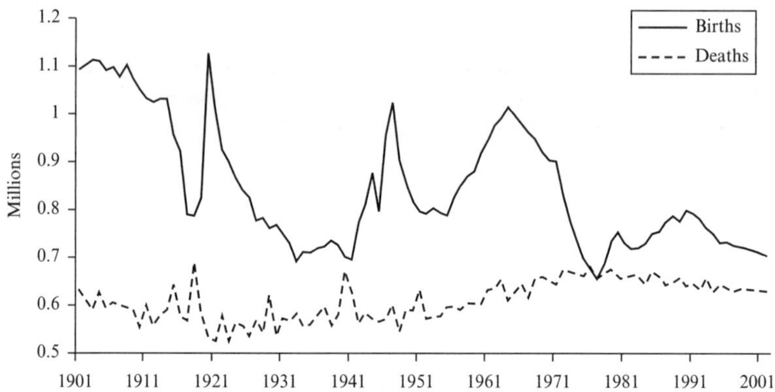

Source: Based on projections of 1996 from the Office of National Statistics and derived from Hicks and Allen (1999). Reprinted by permission of the publisher.

Figure 2.1 Rates of births and deaths in the UK, 1901–2000

created increasing demands for new housing and urban development, especially around the urban cores of the Midlands and the South of England.

To deal with the increasing demands of such a rising population, immediately after the Second World War, the concept of *new towns* was transformed into legislation in the form of the New Towns Act 1946. In the period between 1946 and 1950, 15 first-generation new towns were designated, eight of them established in a ring around London, with an objective of meeting the increasing housing demands. These were conceptualized as satellite towns maintaining the equilibrium between the size and structure of populations and demands for jobs. Each of the towns was designated to cater for a population of around 50 000 people and built on the concept of a neighbourhood that provided easy access to health- and welfare-promoting services. This started a heyday for government-organized city building in pursuit of public goals, including environmental quality and public health. There were separate zones in these settlements for residential and industrial activities surrounding the town centre (Self, 1972). The first-generation new towns laid special emphasis on neighbourhoods with low-density housing with gardens, a balanced mix of employment types, rural-style landscaping and a statutory green belt. However, these were based on the 1947 planning system, which had misestimated the rate of population and economic growth, as well as the capacity of the government to cope with the rate and direction of change. As the population trends continued to be revised upwards, there was far greater demand for housing and public services than had been foreseen. The Town Development Act was passed in 1952 to allow developments in the county districts, thereby relieving the stress on the urban centres. The new towns of Cumbernauld and Hook were designated as a result of this Act (Hook never being built). These were early examples of the evolving *regional cities* characterized by a compact, high-density, multi-level town centre, connected to the *suburban villages* by a system of footpaths. A well-defined hierarchy of roads enabled segregation of walkable roads from mass transit routes. Although the creation of new towns resulted in decentralization from urban cores to beyond the suburban fringes, nonetheless employment and services could not keep pace with the economy's natural urban dynamics. Furthermore, the continuous increase in population, rising affluence and growth of private enterprise in the late 1950s saw a multifold increase in car ownership and the mass motorization of Britain. This brought to a close the idea that planned satellite towns are a kind of quality-of-life intervention substantially different from more general suburban development. The census of 1961 indicated that the population of major conurbations was spilling over beyond the green belt so that rural districts were experiencing a much faster growth than the urban areas. The carefully designed social, economic and public health-conscious environments of the new towns became just another expression of suburban sprawl.

With the aim of overcoming the economic problems associated with such rapid sprawl as well as satisfying the ever-increasing demand for housing and services, planning underwent a paradigm shift, with special emphasis on comprehensive regional-level planning and economic renewal. Several third-generation new towns were designated over the period 1961–66 as multi-growth zones, primarily to act as counter-magnets to the existing urban conurbations, thereby reducing the social and economic burdens of environmental spillovers, congestion and long-distance commuting. The strategy had shifted from the growth of completely new areas (as in the first- and second-generation new towns) to designation for expansion of a pre-existing large town into a regional city, giving due consideration to regional economic and social dynamics and environments. This meant that the third-generation planned towns were much larger in size than their predecessors, with planning targets typically ranging from 100 000 to 250 000 people. Furthermore, older towns in need of retrofitting and regeneration constituted a considerable portion of these. These included: Milton Keynes, Northern Buckinghamshire, Northampton, Peterborough and Southampton, with London as their focal point; Redditch and Dawley–Wellington–Telford in the West Midlands to accommodate the Birmingham overspill; Skelmersdale and Runcorn, designated to receive the Merseyside overspill; Warrington and Central Lancashire for the Manchester spillover; and Washington, south of Newcastle, to receive the spillover from Tyneside and Wearside. House building had risen from a meagre 8100 units in 1944 to 413 700 new dwellings in 1968 (Hicks and Allen, 1999). The trends in urbanization and housing construction are indicated in Figures 2.2a and 2.2b respectively.

The negative impacts of urbanization were more pronounced in the most inner-city areas, often characterized by reduced employment, residential deterioration, overcrowding and socio-economic deprivation. This has been variously and collectively attributed to the policies of dispersal, slum rehabilitation, road building and redevelopment, removal of back-street factories, and zoning constraints, as well as the decline in birth rates. Fundamentally, the deterioration of inner-city neighbourhoods is a problem of inadequate reinvestment, associated with the pattern of land ownership in the UK and the spatial pattern of jobs, housing sub-markets, local taxation revenues and social problems, with considerable adverse impacts upon public health. Over the period between 1969 and 1975, the inner areas of Manchester witnessed a 20 per cent decline in their population, and Liverpool 40 per cent, while Glasgow lost a massive 60 per cent of its population (Department of the Environment, 1977a, 1977b, 1977c).

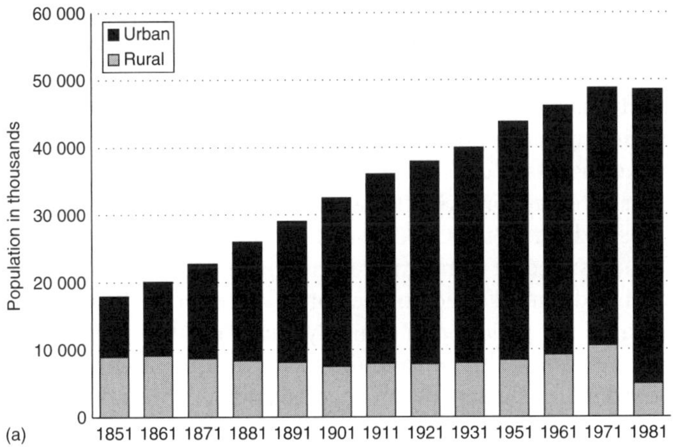

Source: Plotted on data derived from the UK Census summary tables and general tables.

Figure 2.2a Trends of urbanization in England and Wales, 1851–1981

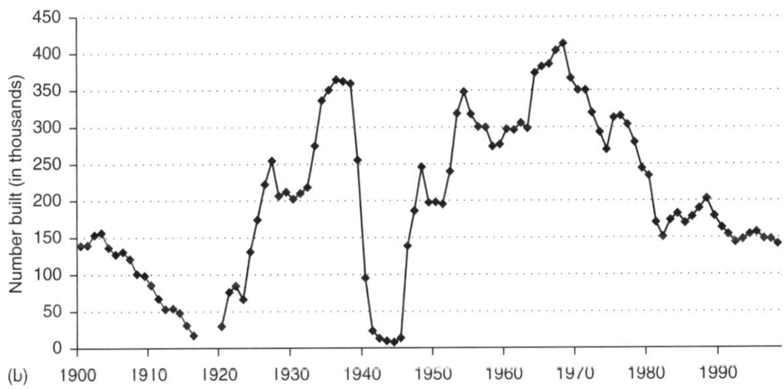

Source: Derived from Hicks and Allen (1999). Reprinted by permission of the publisher.

Figure 2.2b Trends of house construction in Great Britain, 1908–1998

In some ways, planning to address the public welfare challenges in such areas was a more intractable problem than planning for healthy and viable environments in the suburbs and exurbs.

In the US, the impact of post-war urbanization upon social life and health was more detrimental than in the European experience. Immediately after the war, two simultaneous processes of human migration occurred there. While White families migrated outwards from the metropolitan areas to the peripheral suburban rings, Black labourers moved from the rural South towards the Northern cities. In order to cater for the increasing demand for housing and services, urban sprawl became more pronounced. Low-density leapfrogging suburbanization meant development dotted with areas of intervening underdeveloped land, poor accessibility to central services and increased dependence on motorways and private cars. By the early 1960s most major US cities were undergoing a phase of deindustrialization as industries relocated away from the urban cores (S. Lee et al., 2006). This resulted in significant economic and physical decline in inner neighbourhoods manifested in the form of remnant land degraded by noxious waste and pollution in formerly local industrial areas, as well as in loss of jobs, income reduction and the social, health, educational and crime issues attendant on clusters of low-income and 'left-behind' households. In response to such transformations in the labour and real estate markets, pre-existing zoning ordinances were further revamped. Unlike the conventional practice of land use control in Britain, policies in the US relied exclusively upon the strategy of zoning, which had never been the offshoot of a well-conceived comprehensive plan. Although such a policy proved effective in segregating disparate land uses, notably residential and noxious industries, nonetheless they proved to be only semi-effective in controlling the spread of private development into the open countryside. Another drawback of zoning ordinances was their use in pursuit of racial and economic residential segregation. Restrictions on minimum lot size and multi-family dwellings as well as the presence of detailed specifications for allowable housing size and housing materials proved to be exclusionary for low-income and minority families (Branfman et al., 1974; Maantay, 2001).

In the name of general public welfare and environmental (and ultimately individual) health, land use zoning laws became widely experimented with in many if not most sprawling cities of developing countries. In these cases, the joint pressures of an accelerated pace of urbanization and undeveloped or ineffective governance have meant that zoning has largely remained ineffective, often violating the essence of *comprehensive planning* and being associated with externalities that aggravate population health rather than improve it.

The end of the Second World War was also accompanied by a marked transition in the health profile of the developed countries. This was manifested in a significant decline in the rates of infectious diseases and epidemics attributed primarily to the better hygiene, nutrition and living conditions accompanying the economic and social developments, as well as innovations in drug delivery and scientific applications of vaccines, chemotherapy and antibiotics (Rosen, 1958; McKeown, 1979). Two points deserve special mention. Firstly, economic and social developments along with achievements in the fields of epidemiology and public health caused demographic changes. The improvement in life expectancy (which ranged from 70 to 80 years in most developed countries) and the decline in infant and child mortality caused the population distribution to shift towards the middle and older ages. The demographic changes in the UK are shown in Figure 2.3. Secondly, the increasing socio-demographic pressures of urban life manifested themselves in the form of newer and increasingly difficult health issues and challenges, such as stress and mental illness, and complex environmental health risks of non-infectious aetiology, such as those resulting in a rise in incidences of obesity and respiratory and cardiac diseases. The severity and fatality of 'urban' diseases have reduced over the years through innovative medical interventions, but their *chronic* nature introduced new challenges to epidemiology and public health in terms of their eradication on account of their long, insidious latency and multiple causality. In particular, there was an alarming rise in the prevalence of chronic diseases related to exposure to toxic pollutants, sedentary lifestyles, and social, occupational and age-related factors, especially rheumatic heart disease, peptic ulcer, cardiovascular disease and lung cancer (Morris, 1955, 1957). Similarly, higher population density, as well as increased competition for resources and social opportunities, contributed to higher incidences of psychological stress and mental disorders. Currently in Britain (89.9 per cent of which is urbanized), almost 16 per cent of the adult population suffer from one or more mental disorders at any given time (R. Jenkins et al., 2008), while up to 10 per cent of children are prone to learning difficulties such as dyslexia, considerably reducing their ability to achieve good grades at school (Challen et al., 2008).

2.3.1 Chronic Disease Epidemiology

In the United Kingdom, the studies conducted by Richard Doll, Bradford Hill, Jeremy Morris, Donald Reid and Thomas McKeown established chronic disease epidemiology as the new paradigm. The focus was broadened beyond infection to study the role of unknown multiple causes or risk factors. The consideration of multiple risk factors was able to provide logical explanations as to why certain individuals exposed to the disease don't get it, while some of the unexposed get the disease. The objective was to identify single risk factors among the multiple risk factors with the help of the standard 2-by-2 table which compared counts of diseased versus non-diseased, classified by exposure to a specific risk factor. This was made possible through significant advances in epidemiologic survey design and data analysis that occurred almost simultaneously during this period. Cross-sectional surveys, population study of incidence, and repeated cross-sectional surveys paved the way for cohort design and case-controlled

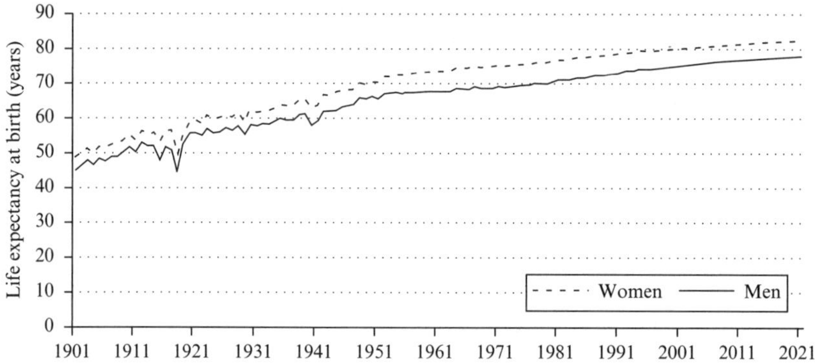

Note: The figures are estimated from 1996.

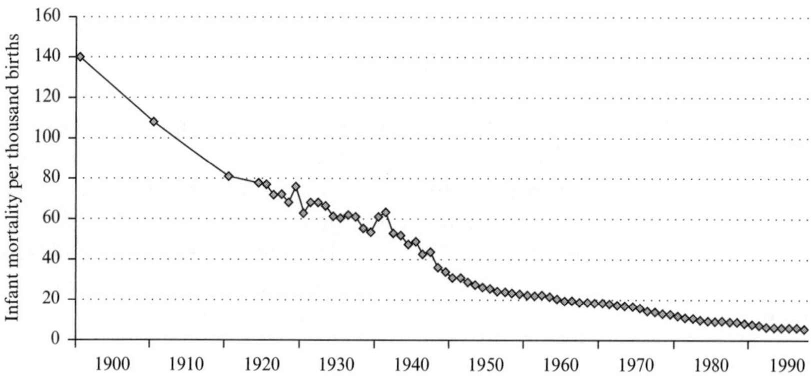

Note: The data is interpolated from 1900 to 1924: it was collected every ten years in 1900, 1910 and 1920. From 1924 an annual record was taken.

Source: Derived from Hicks and Allen (1999). Reprinted by permission of the publisher.

Figure 2.3 Trends of life expectancy and infant mortality in the UK

studies. On the statistical front, odds ratios and relative risk began to be better understood and appreciated, while path-analytic models began to be employed for causal inference. Following the contribution of Mantel and Haenszel in 1959, multivariate relationships began to be extensively employed. Long before, Ryle had observed, in a spirit that anticipated multivariate analysis, that people with specific lifestyles were more vulnerable to stress, which makes them predisposed to peptic ulcer (Ryle, 1948). However, the real fruits of this period were in the form of the classic case-controlled and cohort studies, wherein, for example, Doll and Hill meticulously tested their hypothesis of the association between smoking and lung cancer, thereby espousing the case for an environmental causal model (Doll and Hill, 1950, 1956). In the United States, one of the earliest prototypes of cohort studies was initiated in 1947 to identify the factors influencing the occurrence of heart disease in adults (aged 30–59 years) in the town of Framingham at the outskirts of Boston. The Framingham study started with a representative sample of 6000 respondents and had the ambitious protocol of biennial examination over the subsequent 20 years (Gordon and Kannel, 1970; Dawber, 1980). The term *risk factor* originated from this study, wherein the Framingham study group concluded that cardiovascular disease was a result of a number of contributing causal factors as opposed to a single one. At a later stage, the project was devoted specifically to the study of stroke, cardiovascular diseases and other morbidities associated with ageing as well as the follow-up of the offspring of the original respondents. Morris (1957) conducted another series of classic cohort studies, which identified serum cholesterol and smoking as risk factors in coronary heart disease onset. In another ground-breaking review of the causes of cancer Doll and Peto (1981) concluded that up to 80 per cent of variation in the incidence of malignancies was attributed to differences in environments. These studies provided credibility for risk factor epidemiology, establishing it as the successor to the then fading specific-cause germ theory. The principle of multiple proximate risks for a single disease was more holistic and endeavoured to combine the multiple disciplines of social, biological and statistical sciences. The population-based inferences of risk factor epidemiology had striking similarities with the miasma theory espoused by the hygienists and social reformers of the nineteenth century.

Proponents of risk factor epidemiology popularized it initially as a method of disease prevention through the identification and isolation of risks (Savitz, 1994). Nonetheless it encountered the major criticism of being void of a distinctive theory of disease occurrence at the population level, resulting in the alienation of epidemiology from public health practice (N. Krieger, 1994; N. Pearce, 1996; Susser and Susser, 1996a). Consequently, it effectively became a largely observational science focusing on the identification of risks rather than explanation of causal factors (S. Schwartz et al., 1999). A classic example is that, despite the identification of smoking as a risk factor for lung cancer, intervention strategies largely remained ineffective, primarily on account of overlooking the mediating role of social, behavioural and genetic aspects that may predispose a person to smoking. Risk factor epidemiology had become something of a *black box* paradigm. The black box was a self-contained unit with an opaque interior, a metaphor for an individual whose underlying inner biological processes remained hidden and unexplored (Lakoff and Johnson, 1980). There was a predominant emphasis on the associations between exposure to a maze of proximate environmental risks and diseases while grossly overlooking macro-level contextual social factors as well as the underlying micro-level biological mechanisms involved in disease causation. J.B. McKinlay (1994) termed such an increasing focus on generic methods and risk factor identification and a gross neglect of causality as *biophysical reductionism*. Taubes et al. (1995) stated that such a fervent search for links between lifestyle risks leads to the Catch-22 of modern epidemiology. At a macro level, Vandenbroucke (1988) pointed out the lack of specificity in the definition of environment and the apparent failure to recognize the levels at which the environmental factors operate. The inherent unidimensionality arose on account of these studies being conducted at the individual level, with most of the identified risk factors pertaining to individual lifestyles. Population-level inferences were erroneously conceived on the assumption that population risks were simple aggregations of individual-level risks as mediated by the individuals' lifestyles. Measurements at the individual level, when aggregated, were assumed to be valid at the population level. This overlooked the structural and relational attributes of the organized aggregates at the population level and resulted in a disregard of the social and behavioural models of disease causation (Loomis and Wing, 1990; N. Pearce, 1996; McMichael, 1999). Furthermore, biases of study designs (for example the case-controlled studies) and the existence of multiple confounding factors made it almost impossible to detect weak associations as well as mediating and linking effects in the causal chain (Taubes, 1995; S. Schwartz et al., 1999).

2.3.2 Molecular Epidemiology

By the third quarter of the twentieth century there was a general consensus that individuals manifest varying degrees of vulnerability to exposures from specific environmental agents. The significant technological advances in molecular biology led to studies of the potential role of gene–environment interaction in the disease aetiology (NIEHS, 1993, 1994). Motulsky (1957) was one of the earliest to articulate the idea that genetic mutations affected the nature and rate of drug metabolism and could provide a causal explanation of differential disease susceptibilities. Genetic epidemiology emerged as the study of the reciprocal interactions between the internal genetic characteristics of the body (genetic susceptibilities or predispositions) and the external environmental agents (pollutants, ionizing radiations, etc.) at an individual level (Khoury et al., 1993). Subsequently, in the early 1980s, the term *molecular epidemiology* was first coined by Perera and Weinstein (1982, 2000) and popularized as a framework for the study and understanding of the molecular basis of carcinogenesis. Molecular biological techniques and biomarkers have now been extensively employed for the measurement of internal exposures, detection of biological responses and identification of effect-modifying host characteristics (Hulka et al., 1990). The objective has been to explain between-individual variations in cancer risk through the understanding of the genetic basis of complex interactions between environmental agent and individual susceptibility factors (both inherited and acquired).

However, molecular epidemiology has been viewed by some as the contemporary equivalent of the germ theory of the late nineteenth century on account of its mechanistic view of disease causation at the molecular level. The primary objective has been to conduct randomized clinical trials for the screening of susceptible individuals in the population and thereby perform personalized risk assessments through measuring phenotype, adduct load and acquired mutations (Shields and Harris, 1991; McMichael, 1994). Such a bottom-up reductionist approach overlooks critical factors of disease causation at the population level, especially with respect to the determinants and spatial distribution of disease in populations. Nonetheless, given that chronic disease is multi-factorial in nature and characterized by multiple exposures and variable susceptibilities, it is reasonable to suppose that molecular epidemiology and risk factor epidemiology can act as powerful tools when integrated together, rather than confounding or replacing one other. Such an approach essentially overcomes the weaknesses associated with the 'black box' in risk factor epidemiology by providing deeper insights into the underlying biological mechanisms involved in disease causation by identifying the physiologic responses to internal biochemical exposures to risks (Vandenbroucke, 1988; McMichael, 1994).

This leads to a more powerful paradigm for studying the health performance of cities: individual health is explained by gene–behaviour–environment (natural and built) interactions.

2.3.3 Social Epidemiology

The role of environmental socio-contextual factors in disease causation was deflected in the eras of germ theory and risk factor epidemiology. The shift in emphasis over the course of the century from the environment per se to a set of specific pathogenic, behavioural and lifestyle factors within the environment resulted in unidimensional individualism in epidemiologic research. The predominant focus on individual-centred approaches resulted in relative dissociation from the social factors, which, although operating at population levels, often configure the individual-level determinants of health. The importance of the social determinants of health was reinvigorated following the contributions of Joseph Goldberger, Edgar Sydenstricker, Major Greenwood and Wade Hampton Frost in the early part of the nineteenth century. Increasing consensus towards the restoration of the overlooked social factors responsible for population patterns of health and disease causation led to the evolution of modern social epidemiology (Rosen, 1947; Galdston, 1949). In an investigation of the role of social disparities upon foetal and infant mortality Alfred Yankauer (1950) introduced the term *social epidemiology* in all probability for the first time. Reeder (1972) defined social epidemiology as the study of the role of social factors in the aetiology of disease, while Berkman and Kawachi (2000) defined it as the study of the social distribution and social determinants of the states of health. The social factors or determinants in the definitions tend to pertain to three cardinal strands of stratification – race, gender and class – each of which is thought to play a mediatory role in influencing degree of exposures to risk factors, behaviour, physical constitution and other causes of disease (Rothman, 1992; N. Krieger et al., 1993). They have been termed the 'fundamental social causes' of disease, as they strongly influence an individual's ability to avoid risks or minimize the consequences of disease once it sets in (Link and Phelan, 1995).

The general approach has been to study the pathways by which socio-economic stratifications at the population level contribute to differentials in the health and burden of disease. To elucidate the impact of population-level social transitions upon physiological and psychological health, Cassel et al. compared two contrasting studies. In the first study they compared the health of two population groups of contrasting social class – first-generation industrial workers versus second- and third-generation workers. The second study, on the other hand, assessed the health of stable rural residents of North Carolina counties experiencing varying degrees of urban growth. Both studies concluded that incongruity in demands of the emerging and existing social systems resulted in poorer health outcomes (Cassel et al., 1960; Tyroler and Cassel, 1964). In another of his seminal works, Cassel highlighted the role of *psychosocial factors* of the social environment, including dominance hierarchies, social disorganization, rapid social change, social isolation, bereavement and social support, in altering host susceptibilities to risk factors by affecting neuroendocrine function. According to Cassel, the psychosocial factors in conjunction with the risk factors provided a logical explanation of observed social disease gradients (Cassel, 1976). Subsequently, many studies have found a detrimental association between psychosocial stressors and prevalence of disease (S.A. James and Kleinbaum, 1976; Thoerell, 1981).

Several studies have highlighted the role of social status in the aetiology of a variety of somatic diseases, especially coronary heart disease (CHD).

The general trend has indicated higher levels of incidences of CHD among blue-collar or lower educational groups after controlling for other risk factors (McQueen and Siegrist, 1982; Siegrist et al., 1986). Marmot and Syme (1976) investigated the incidence of CHD amongst Japanese Americans and established that population-level health differentials are not genetic and hence can't be explained in terms of the individual in isolation. Rather, the cumulative socio-economic profile of the individual contributes to such population-level differentials. In a 40-year study of the trends of mortality from heart disease in England and Wales, Marmot et al. (1978) noted a shift in mortality patterns; the risks from heart disease increased progressively in social classes IV and V over 1951–71, in contrast to the higher mortality observed in social classes I and II over the earlier period 1931–51. Marmot and his co-workers conducted two classic cohort studies (popularly called the Whitehall Study of British civil servants) separated by a time gap of 20 years to assess the potential relationship between social class and mortality in a wide range of diseases. A significant inverse association between mortality and grade of employment was observed in both studies, and this relationship persisted over the time period (Marmot et al., 1984, 1991). The Whitehall Study II reported a threefold difference in the prevalence of ischaemic heart disease between the lowest and highest grades of employment. The difference was twofold in the cases of self-reported ill health, cough and sputum. Similar trends in CHD mortality in unskilled workers have been independently documented by Koskenvuo et al. (1980). In another study, Weinblatt et al. (1978) had reported that the risk from sudden cardiac death was more than three times higher in a low-education group compared to the better-educated category. Several other studies have highlighted the racial gradient in health, indicating higher mean blood pressure levels and corresponding mortality and hypertension-related disorders among Black Americans in reference to their White compatriots (Scotch and Gierger, 1963; Stamler, 1967).

Subsequently, Rose (1985, 1992) provided a stronger conceptual basis for the importance of cumulative population-level socio-economic factors in disease causation. He proposed that practically none of the risk–disease relations are exactly binary with a logistic form; the risks are not discrete, but rather are distributed along a continuum. Minor shifts in the risk band of a population can thus result in marked differences in the health of the population. Based on his investigation of the rates of cardiac heart disease, he identified that the different sets of factors act to produce between-population variability and between-individual variability. He strongly espoused a distinct differentiation between the *causes of cases*, which focus on high-risk individuals through an assessment of individual-level susceptibilities, and *causes of incidence*, which study the disease distribution in the population corresponding to the associated risk continuum to which it is exposed.

2.3.4 Contemporary Epidemiologic Paradigms

There is a general consensus that each of the epidemiological paradigms – risk factor, molecular and social – when employed simultaneously but independently cannot on its own explain disease causation. Appreciating the necessity of an integrated approach, Nancy Krieger introduced so-called *eco-social epidemiologic theory*. She defines this as 'a paradigm that embraces population-level thinking and rejects the underlying assumptions of biomedical individualism without discarding biology' (N. Krieger, 1994, p. 896). In her effort to integrate the biologic and social factors of disease causation, she visualized the existing metaphor of the web of causation, but this time with two 'spiders', a social and a biologic. The metaphor of eco-social epidemiology was further refined as a self-replicating fractal object to reflect the interlinked and diverse patterns of susceptibility from the sub-cellular to the societal levels of organization (N. Krieger, 1994, 2001). Such a conceptualization is a manifestation of the fact that health and disease self-evolve in space and time as a result of complex interactions between interlinked multiple and multi-level factors.

Along similar lines, Susser and Susser (1996b, 1998) advocated the necessity of an integrated approach wherein the *universalism of physical sciences* is complemented by the *ecologism of biological sciences*. They proposed a so-called *eco-epidemiologic paradigm* encompassing the macro, meso and micro levels of causal analysis. This has been employed as a comprehensive theory for both the infectious disease of human immunodeficiency virus (HIV) and the chronic disease of peptic ulcer. The black box metaphor was replaced by that of *Chinese boxes* (a sequence of interconnected boxes, each box enveloping a succession of smaller ones), thereby manifesting multiple-level causality. *This implied that the causes of disease should be studied with respect to factors identified at multiple levels of organization from the molecular or cellular level to the individual level and then the population, ecological and societal levels.* Each level is thus construed as a distinct system that interrelates and interacts with the others, the relations within and between the systems being conditioned socially, spatially and biologically.

McMichael (1999) provides a cognitively powerful visual model of modern epidemiology being constrained (imprisoned) by the cube, with axes indicating our overemphasis on proximate risk factors, the individual level of analysis, and the static or modular view of temporal (life-course level as opposed to more static cross-sectional studies) variations in risks, and with limited forecasting ability. He argued that modern epidemiology should follow an integrated approach wherein its range is broadened from proximate to distal factors, individual to population level of analysis, and modular to life course, as well as being fully accustomed to forecasting future health risks from global environmental change.

Such multi-level and all-embracing eco-epidemiological frameworks are pedagogically and philosophically compelling. Nonetheless, their practicality in terms of application via the identification of multi-causal pathway theories, models and studies is still under-researched.

This is the scholarly context in which this book is placed: both the conceptual contribution of the 'urban health niche' (introduced in Chapter 3) and the empirical studies of multiple and multi-scale social–spatial–biological risks of specific morbidities are attempts to explicate, both conceptually and empirically, the multiple causality measurable at different organizational units and spatial scales.

The success of such integrated models depends upon the accuracy of both individual and environmental data (the former have typically been more accurate than the latter) and robust statistical methods for multi-level spatial and temporal analysis aimed at identifying the nature of correlations, variabilities and error distribution at individual, population and intervening levels (Susser, 1998; N. Krieger, 2001).

This is the spirit in which the studies in Chapters 5–8 have been conducted.

2.4 CONCLUSION – RECONNECTING URBAN PLANNING AND PUBLIC HEALTH

It is the advent of advanced statistical methods for multi-level modelling, together with advances in spatial data manipulation technology and statistics, that permits a reunification of urban planning and public health analysis. It may be supposed that this will make possible and encourage a reunification of applied analysis and interventions by the respective professions.

The predominant focus in epidemiology on individual-level risk factors and molecular mechanisms involved in disease causation resulted in a scientific oversight of the effects of the *attributes of place* upon well-being, health and disease. In the UK a distinct chasm appeared over the course of the twentieth century between the disciplines of town planning and public health, with town planning drifting towards a process of controlling land supply and land development, and public health becoming a niche of the therapeutic health services. At the legislative and policy level, this weak structural integration between the disciplines was manifested and reinforced by the organizational restructuring in 1943, wherein the then new Ministry of Town and Country Planning was created, effectively divesting planning from the Ministry of Health (Talbot, 1998). Since the late 1980s, however, there has been a resurgence of interest in this historical link, driven by the greater emphasis among public health scholars and practitioners on the role played by contextual factors, also termed *place effects* or *neighbourhood effects* (Blaxter, 1990; Humphreys and Carr-Hill, 1991; N. Krieger, 1992; Diez Roux, 2001). *Place effects* include neighbourhood-level socio-economic conditions as well as the attributes of the built and physical environments.

Since the turn of the present century, epidemiology, public health and urban planning disciplines have begun to grapple with a revised version of the nineteenth-century idea of *miasma of the built environment*. Three emerging health and demographic patterns consolidate such an argument, namely:

1. the increasing number of epidemiological studies highlighting the impending worldwide obesity epidemic (Y. Claire Wang et al., 2011), including the significant increments in the prevalence rates of childhood obesity (Ebbeling et al., 2002; Lobstein et al., 2004) and the associated direct and indirect health costs (Allender and Rayner, 2007);
2. the significant increases in psychological disorders, accounting for 14 per cent of the global disease burden and 28 per cent of all disability-adjusted life-years (Prince et al., 2007);
3. significant demographic shifts, with almost 3.4 billion people now living in urban areas, a figure that is estimated to rise to 6.3 billion by 2050 (United Nations, 2010), and a projected doubling of the population of those aged 60 years and above from 11 per cent in 2006 to 22 per cent of the global population by 2050 (WHO, 2007).

There has been a growing consensus amongst epidemiologists that built environmental factors, especially those influencing the health of eating behaviour and physical activity, are driving the obesity epidemic. Similarly, the health-promoting and -inhibiting influences of the built and physical environment upon mental health outcomes are becoming better understood, as are the detrimental effects of a declining physical built environment upon geriatric health.

Recently, there has been a trend in urban planning research that focuses on ways to plan a city that is activity friendly and aesthetically pleasing and accessible. This resurgence of a public health agenda in urban planning, where health and well-being sit alongside economic and environmental objectives to be optimized by design, has focused on questions such as:

How do we design an activity-friendly city that promotes walking and cycling? How can urban design optimize aggregate accessibility to service destinations (health promoting capital) in a way that contributes to active living? How can an aesthetically pleasing physical environment contribute to improved mental health outcomes? The state of current scientific knowledge about these and other such questions is discussed in Chapter 4.

A series of high-level policy reports since the late 1980s have highlighted the necessity to incorporate health considerations in urban planning and policy. In 1987, the World Health Organization Regional Office for Europe initiated the WHO European Healthy Cities Network (WHO-EHCN), with a strong commitment to implement and consolidate the principles of Health 21 and Agenda 21, thereby attempting to operationalize principles of health equity. The initiative was grounded upon the five basic tenets of equity, participation and empowerment, working in partnership, solidarity and friendship, and sustainable development, requiring a close collaboration between local governments and community organizations (H. Barton et al., 2009; P. Webster and Lipp, 2009). The project followed a holistic view, defining a healthy city as 'one that is continually creating and improving those physical and social environments and strengthening those community resources that enable people to support each other in performing all the functions of life and achieving their maximum potential' (Hancock and Duhl, 1988). The Zagreb Declaration for Healthy Cities was launched during the fifth phase (2009–13) of the WHO European Healthy Cities Project (WHO Europe, 2009). One of the new concerns and challenges identified related to how the built environment and new technologies affect the health of citizens; and the report emphasized the importance of integrating health and sustainable development considerations in questions of how we plan, design, maintain, improve and manage cities and neighbourhoods and how we use new technologies. Reinforcing the concept of urban health, the core theme of the fifth phase of the WHO European Healthy Cities Project revolved around the following (WHO Europe, 2009):

1. Creating caring and supportive environments: A healthy city is a city for all its citizens, being inclusive, supportive, sensitive and responsive to their diverse needs and expectations.
2. Healthy living: A healthy city provides conditions and opportunities that encourage, enable and support healthy lifestyles for people of all social groups and ages.
3. Healthy urban environment and design: A healthy city offers a physical and built environment that encourages, enables and supports health, recreation and well-being, safety, social interaction, accessibility and mobility, a sense of pride and cultural identity and is responsive to the needs of all its citizens.

A parallel urban health initiative in the US was spearheaded by the Department of Health and Human Services when it launched the Healthy Communities concept in 1989. The National Civic League, with federal support, formally launched the Healthy Communities Initiative. Statewide initiatives, especially Healthy Boston, California Healthy Cities Project and Healthy Cities Indiana, were the pioneers of the US Healthy Communities movement (Norris and Pittman, 2000). A workshop report of the Institute of Medicine (2001, pp. 18–27) had identified the *built environment* as that part of the environment designed and constructed by humans, and which presents as many opportunities as challenges to environmental health. It highlighted the importance of innovative design in *smart growth* (the American equivalent to the British *compact city* doctrine in urban planning), stressing that smart growth has many positive effects on the economy, attracting new businesses, encouraging development, and making health problems easier to address in the local community. Underscoring the increasingly important influence of design and configuration at the community level on individual activity behaviour, the Centers for Disease Control and Prevention (CDC) introduced the term *active community environments* (ACEs) as places where people of all ages can easily participate in physical activity. Several studies have gathered evidence of associations between ACEs and physical health (Frank et al., 2003; Hoehner et al., 2003; S. Doyle et al., 2006). In the United Kingdom, the Department of Health (2005) highlighted two sets of design guidelines aimed at achieving physically active lifestyles. The NICE (2008) guidance stresses the role of environmental factors above and beyond individual-level interventions in influencing physical activity. The environment is defined as: 'any aspect of the physical (natural) environment or the urban or constructed (built) environment that subconsciously or consciously relates to an individual and their physical activity behaviour' (Foster and Hillsdon, 2004). The active design guidance published by Sport England (2007) lays out recommendations from the chief medical officer for active living wherein 'activity' is defined as physical activity (structured exercise, sports), lifestyle activity (climbing stairs, cycling, brisk walking, etc.) or a combination of both. Highlighting the importance of neighbourhood activity space in configuring individual activity behaviour, the Sport England guidelines provide a series of innovative design guidelines for master planning of major housing and mixed-use development schemes, with an aim to promote easy access to a choice of opportunities for sport and physical activity, thereby making new communities more active and healthy. The active design checklist lays out the three active design objectives of improving accessibility, enhancing amenities and increasing awareness to promote the recommended levels of physical activity (Sport

England, 2007). More recently, the Lancet Commission conducted an in-depth study into the potential associations between the role of the *physical fabric of towns and cities* upon health and the role of urban planning in improving health (Rydin et al., 2012). The Commission recommended that:

> improved urban health outcomes will need a concerted effort to create and maintain the so-called urban advantage through reshaping city environments. Furthermore, such urban planning needs to take account of the inequalities between cities across the world and within individual cities when devising policy. Urban planning efforts should be based on a complexity approach that recognises multidirectional causality, feedback loops, and unintended consequences. Such an approach is more capable of producing effective action than are more conventional linear approaches. An integral part of such a complexity approach is an emphasis on project-based experimentation and social learning through discursive and inclusive assessment. (Rydin et al., 2012)

This latest report recognizes that the identification and analysis of the contextual effects on health status and inequalities are complicated and require a complex system approach to delve deep into urban dynamics and the underlying social and environmental processes that constitute and shape a city and the health of its population.

We conclude by advocating the need for a paradigm to guide the science and practice of healthy cities that acknowledges the evolving holistic epidemiological paradigms and aims at a stronger collaboration and integration between the disciplines of city planning and health policy. Such an integrated urban health paradigm should be multi- and interdisciplinary, with the objectives of easing the effective organization of data for empirical research and facilitating multi-sectoral policy interventions. This has been highlighted by Materia and Baglio (2005, p. 534): '"Multidisciplinarity". "Integration". "Context". That these have become key terms in public health vocabulary and core features of the health systems can be seen in the multi-disciplinary approach to biomedical research and clinical medicine and in the increasing interest in "alternative" medicine.' Unlike the holism of some branches of alternative medicine, however, the complexity of causes of health disparities in cities can be modelled, since we now have the technology to create multi-scale population and environment variables that can be investigated in multi-level models of individual health. The empirical studies in Chapters 5–8 show just how far we can extend such analysis with current technology. The models employed in those chapters test hypotheses about health–urban-configuration associations using systemic measures of accessibility, capturing the influence of an individual's proximity to multiple health-enhancing and -detracting environmental resources and to population effects at multiple spatial scales.

3. The urban health niche: a new paradigm in healthy city planning

3.1 INTRODUCTION

With increasing urbanization and the resulting spread of sedentary lifestyles, there has, as we noted in Chapter 2, been a marked transformation in the problematization of health, with a transition from *infectious* to *chronic* disease aetiology. The primary focus of contemporary epidemiology has shifted towards conceptualizing *causality* as well as isolating *causes* (Susser, 1991). This has led to the evolution of more sophisticated and holistic paradigms of epidemiology involving a range of complexities of multiple levels, multiple causal pathways, and non-linear interactions, as well as temporal dynamism. Such paradigms have been based on a bottom-up approach, which strives to understand and influence disease causation from a molecular level, moving upwards towards the population level, as well as the more conventional top-down approach, which starts at the population level and studies disease causation as a result of the processes and mechanisms intrinsic to it. Vandenbroucke (1988) had strongly argued for the former, stating that disease (cancer) incidence rates can best be explained by the interplay between genes and environment. N. Pearce (1996), on the other hand, posited that the bottom-up approach is reductionist and positivistic and the aetiologic framework of a disease should be conceptualized at the population level. The individual-versus-population approach often creates a conceptual disconnect often acting as a bottleneck for effective formulation and implementation of public health intervention strategies. The need for a more integrated approach encompassing multiple epidemiological branches and taking into consideration proximal as well as the distal influences on health outcomes has been highlighted by several authors in recent years (N. Krieger, 1994; Susser and Susser, 1996b; McMichael, 1999). In her eco-social epidemiologic model, N. Krieger (1994) succinctly argues that a health outcome is quite often a result of complex non-linear interactions between the social and biologic factors, so that the *cleavage of the social from the biologic, and the biologic from the social* is not sensible. However, in our view, none of these existing paradigms provide sufficient purchase for simultaneous application in empirical studies as well as being effective in organizing thoughts at the strategic level necessary for healthy city policy and planning debates. One of the problems is that the exacerbating or mitigating role of the characteristics of the city's built environment upon an individual's health tends to be underestimated. Social epidemiologists have tended to place considerable stress solely on social factors as determinants of individual behaviour and lifestyle, often overlooking the triad of contextual built, natural and social environments that configure one another over time to generate corresponding risk factors (dynamically varying with time) and that act in conjunction with the inherent individual-level biologic factors to eventually influence health (Sarkar, 2013).

Furthermore, from a policy perspective the specific attributes of a place (built, natural and social environment characteristics) and hence an urban population's health are formed as a result of decisions across well-defined hierarchies of urban and public health planning systems. The built environment channels, shapes and moderates the distribution of social and environmental influences on health and on health behaviour. This demands an integrated multi-sectoral intervention strategy built on multi-scalar and multidimensional analysis. A well-founded urban health system therefore needs to incorporate contextual environmental considerations more explicitly into existing epidemiological frameworks. An all-encompassing approach will help urban planners and public health planners to work together using a unified language and models to assimilate the kind of evidence-based epidemiological thought reviewed and developed in this book, to more scientifically plan for a healthy city.

In the domain of urban health planning and promotion there is now a similar consensus about the effectiveness of a more systemic and integrated approach (Diez Roux, 2007; Giles-Corti and King, 2009; ICSU, 2012; Rydin et al., 2012). In recent years many socio-ecological models have been developed that endeavour to decipher the relationships between the built environment and health promotion in cities (Whitehead and Dahlgren, 1991; H. Barton and Tsourou, 2000; Hoehner et al., 2003; de Hollander and Staatsen, 2003; Northridge et al., 2003; Galea, Freudenberg et al., 2005; ICSU, 2012). However, it is implausible that the frameworks typically adopted in these studies can act as truly integrative models across the two disciplines, since most overlook the existing processes and paradigms of epidemiology. Some also omit an effective dynamic analysis of the functioning of urban planning systems and their spatial hierarchies. Consequently a biomedical researcher or an urban planner cannot easily relate to such models in terms of practical implementation. Any comprehensive model should in effect help overcome the disconnect which presently exists between evidence-based epidemiological research and normative urban health policy and practice, thereby enabling decision making as well as devising effective intervention strategies (Duhl and Sanchez, 1999).

Section 3.2 conceptualizes the notion of *urban health niche* encompassing the epidemiologic triad of *person*, *place* and *time*, offering a novel paradigm for public health analysis aligned to urban planning. The objective is to effectively integrate the various disciplines of epidemiology within a framework that can guide both public health and urban planning professional interventions. With the aim of demonstrating the effectiveness of such a paradigm, an *urban health niche planning model* is proposed in section 3.3. Such a bottom-up planning model has the potential to incorporate and integrate multiple-level spatio-temporal health determinants existing at the different levels of a city's functional and organizational hierarchies, thereby making it possible to devise intervention strategies at both individual and population levels.

3.2 CONCEPTUALIZING 'URBAN HEALTH NICHES' AS A FRAMEWORK FOR PUBLIC HEALTH-FOCUSED URBAN PLANNING

The importance of a powerful model or metaphor cannot be overestimated (Lakoff and Johnson, 1980; MacCormac, 1985). We introduce the concept of the intrinsic *health niche* as a fundamental model for thinking about, theorizing and conducting urban health research and health-related urban planning and related interventions.

The concept of *ecological niche* has long been a fundamental organizing concept in modern ecology. It has found widespread application in fields such as community ecology, physiological ecology, population biology and biogeography, and is used to identify a set of environmental conditions that influences the distribution and optimized performance and functioning of a set of one or more organisms. The idea was introduced by Grinnell (1917) to describe the multitude of environmental requirements of a species, including microhabitat, abiotic factors, resources and predators, as well as the physiological and behavioural adaptations that allow the species to respond to such factors. C. Elton (1927) defined a 'niche' mainly as a functional concept, describing the organism's place in the biotic environment in terms of its relationships to trophic levels and enemies. A more formal definition was given by Hutchinson (1957), who defined niche as the total range of environmental variables (physical, chemical and biotic) to which the species must adapt itself and live within if it is to replace itself indefinitely.

Assuming that there are *n* environmental variables, then a niche can be described in terms of an *n*-dimensional space or a hypervolume that represents the responses of the species to each of the environmental variables. Hutchinson's *niche* provides a means of conceiving of how species relate to the environment and to one another. We extend the idea of *ecological niche* to the concept of *urban health niche*, represented graphically in Figure 3.1.

In this framework, each individual is surrounded by a hypothetical hypervolume (the *urban health niche*), which encompasses the epidemiologic triad of *person, place* and *time*. The urban health niche of an individual, in essence, is a spatio-temporal manifestation of the causal agents and processes functioning at the micro, meso and macro scales at which the health-defining processes function. As envisaged by McMichael (1999), such a framework is thus able to give due credence to the spatial organization of multiple health-defining processes, including both proximal and distal factors, as opposed to an overwhelming preoccupation with proximate risk factors. The micro scale encompasses *within-individual*-level processes, especially those involving the immunologic and genetic predispositions to microbial agents, antibodies or foreign pollutants within the body. This is essentially the domain of physiologic and genetic epidemiology.

At the meso scale, behavioural and lifestyle-level risk factors, especially those associated with nutritional intake, alcohol consumption, smoking status and so on, dominate, making it the domain of risk factor epidemiology.

The macro scale is the realm of social epidemiology and the epidemiology of built and natural environments wherein neighbourhood-level or city-level processes such as ethnicity, socio-economic status, natural environment (especially air, water, noise pollution, proximity to waste disposal sites, terrain, etc.), accessibility to services, land use mix, street-level design and walkability are the principal health-defining factors. The built environment shapes, channels and moderates the distribution of social and natural environmental effects at this level.

If we consider the classic case of coronary heart disease, at a molecular scale, the presence of serum cholesterol may increase the risk ratio. The presence of serum cholesterol in conjunction with high blood pressure may lead to a multifold increase in the risks (P.W.F. Wilson et al., 1998). At a lifestyle scale, smoking may aggravate the condition (Morris, 1957; J.T. Doyle et al., 1962). Even the presence of a family member in the household who is a smoker may increase the risk ratio on account of passive smoking (He et al., 1999). At a neighbourhood scale, living in areas associated with high deprivation may increase the risks (Diez Roux et al., 2001; Sundquist et al., 2004), while living in a good neighbourhood may reduce the risk (Mujahid, Diez Roux, Morenoff et al., 2008). Similarly, the presence of a green space

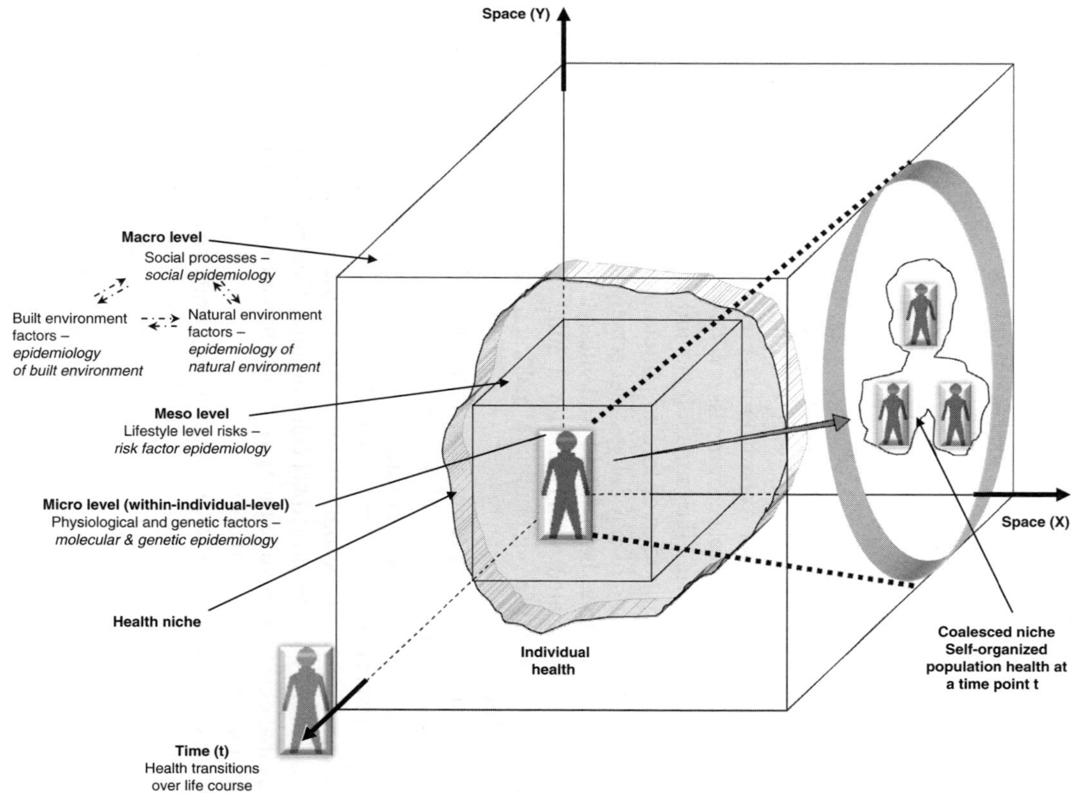

Figure 3.1 Holistic paradigm of the health niche

in the vicinity may reduce the risk ratio (Richard Mitchell and Popham, 2008). Each spatial scale by itself may be considered a subsystem, and the impacts of constituent factors are often synergistic and associated within and between subsystems. The interactions may be non-linear, acting along highly differentiated and specific causal pathways, for many of which there are no well-defined theories. In the above example, residing in a deprived neighbourhood is one of the environmental moderating factors, increasing the risks on account of unhealthy behavioural habits with respect to eating among the deprived. Proximity to green space is another environmental moderating factor, which on the contrary reduces the risks by acting as an incentive for recreational walking and physical activity. All this demands a holistic health planning approach entailing greater collaboration between epidemiological sub-disciplines and associative and cause–effect models functional at each spatial scale. This will facilitate the development of multi-level theory, empirical models and interventions.

The time axis of the health niche paradigm in Figure 3.1 represents the need to take into account temporal progression, phases and hierarchies (from 'life stage' to 'life course') for a more scientifically robust explanation of disease causation. It is now well established that chronic diseases are often characterized by long latency and evolve over a lifetime through cumulative interactive processes. Several studies have highlighted the associations between early-life exposures to risk factors (in the form of unhygienic diets, deprivation and vascular risks) and subsequent higher risks of mortality in adulthood (Forsdahl, 1977; Lauer et al., 1988; Barker, 1994). A temporally dynamic life-course model of disease based on long-term cohort studies can trace disease aetiology over a life course, encompassing in-utero, infancy, childhood, adulthood and geriatric phases (Ben-Shlomo and Kuh, 2002; Kuh and Ben-Shlomo, 2004).

The health of an individual is thus a function of the spatio-temporal variations in the corresponding urban health niche. Epidemiological studies should ideally thus be based not only on cohort data relating to risk factors and health outcome variables, but also on prospective data representative of variations in the triad of social, natural and built environmental causal and moderating factors.

The urban health niche framework also takes into account the multiple levels of aggregation at which health data are produced, distributed and studied. Thus, as one moves from the individual level to a higher level of organization, a collection of individuals may come together to constitute a population. The population may range from a set of individuals living in a city to specific demographic or behavioural groups such as older adults, children, smokers and so on. Each population is characterized by its unique culture, structure, and economic and social form. The subset of individuals residing in a neighbourhood or any other spatial unit is characterized by specific environmental (built and natural), spatial, social, cultural and individual preference structures. Individual health niches self-organize, reconfiguring one another and intertwining together to constitute the *coalesced niche* for the population. As a result of the coalescence of individual spatially explicit urban health niches, diverse individual susceptibilities and exposures are interlinked together to produce universally configured group effects acting upon the constituent individuals' health, which gives rise to overall population-level risk factors and a health *continuum* (Rose, 1985).

Once the coalesced niche for the population is formed, such aggregates configure individual health niches and thereby influence individual health outcomes and vice versa. In other words, the manifested health of individuals and populations is an emergent and self-organizing phenomenon arising from the spatio-temporal variations in individual urban health niches and the corresponding population aggregates. To use an analogy, neighbourhood-level health niches can be assumed to self-organize in relation to each other in the same way that neighbourhood housing markets self-organize, with changes in one neighbourhood spilling over in unpredictable non-linear ways to adjacent sub-markets and affecting changes in distant locations and in the overall systemic urban land economy (a comparison with Nobel economics laureate Thomas Schelling's tipping model of urban social mix would be a worthwhile extension to the idea of urban health niches; Schelling, 1971, 2006).

As a classic example of health niche self-organization, higher prevalence rates of a particular disease observed in populations belonging to a specific ethnic minority may have individual- and population-level causes. The intrinsic individual health niche may comprise biologic factors (such as genetic predispositions and physiologic and immunologic factors) and lifestyle factors, as well as social, natural and built environmental factors working at the neighbourhood level. At a population level, there may be spatial clusters of ethnic minorities, all predisposed to similar lifestyles or occupation and hence exposed to similar behavioural and occupational health hazards. Causative processes may include compounding endogenous effects such as social exclusion, which amplifies income and service poverty, as well as exogenous effects such as quality of governance, prevailing policy measures and historical interventions.

Hence, the coalesced niche of the population or region manifests not only the characteristics of the individual-level niches but also the aggregated effects of occupational hazards, cultural exclusion, social deprivation and neighbourhood physical decline, which often tend to enhance the degree of exposure to risk factors as well as exacerbate their effects on health. In other words there exists a bidirectional and reciprocal association between individual and coalesced urban health niches that configure each other so that their spatio-temporal variations produce corresponding variations in the individual health and population health continuums. It is acknowledged that the boundaries between the upper levels of the hierarchy are often fuzzy, with no standard guidelines to what constitutes the standard size of a population, community or region, and this is therefore a productive research frontier. The exploration of spatial scale in our empirical chapters (Chapters 5–8) contributes to pushing back this frontier and offers a new methodology for such studies.

Such an integrated approach that gives due credence to existing spatial and organizational hierarchies provides urban as well as public health planners with an effective way to assimilate research outputs derived from the various epidemiological sub-disciplines and thereby to devise intervention mechanisms and policy across each of the spatial as well as organizational hierarchies.

Rose (2001) noted that the cause of illness at an individual level may be quite different from that at a population level, wherein it emerges as a result of intrinsic characteristics of the component individual as well as interactions and interdependencies between them. Consequently, different policy and intervention strategies are necessary at the individual and population levels.

3.3 A HEALTHY CITY MODEL BASED ON THE IDEA OF THE URBAN HEALTH NICHE

Studies aiming to explore contextual effects of the built environment upon individual behaviour and health have increasingly pointed to the conceptual and methodological challenges inherent in doing so (Auchincloss and Diez Roux, 2008; Galea et al., 2009, 2010). The risk factors operating at multiple spatial scales and levels of organization are often interdependent, and it is highly unlikely that causality is unidirectional and continuous in nature. The fact that individuals select their neighbourhoods on the basis of personal preference, based on socio-economic constraints, perceived degree of satisfaction and so on, makes causal inference from statistical associations difficult. These so-called *migration effects* confound causal reason and interpretation in cross-sectional and case study investigations. Furthermore, the effects are cumulative in nature. Individuals may adapt their behaviour according to the characteristics of the social cluster or population they belong to or according to the environmental habitat they occupy. Similarly, as we have noted, individuals and population as well as neighbourhoods configure one another, each adapting in response to the others. In order to address these constraints, recent research has promoted the adoption of systemic approaches to healthy city planning (ICSU, 2012; Rydin et al., 2012; Sarkar, 2013). In this section, we conceptualize a systemic healthy city planning model employing the idea of the urban health niche (Figures 3.2 and 3.3 on pp. 50–51). The model conceptualizes the healthy city to be composed of three parallel coexisting systems.

First is the individual–population system, where the health outcomes are manifested. An individual may be construed as comprising tissues, cells and genes, while populations comprise several individuals.

Second is the household–neighbourhood–city system, where health determinants function at distinct spatial, behavioural and organizational scales. The household space may comprise several components, such as floor area, heat, light, amenities and so on, while neighbourhoods comprise multiple households, streets, amenities and so on.

The third type of system is the governance and decision-making systems, ranging from local to regional governance hierarchies and their associated land, services and health planning competences. Thus, the health of an individual is an outcome of the interactive causal processes connecting the components of these three categories of systems. As has been discussed earlier, the causality is non-linear and bidirectional, with feedback loops (N. Pearce and Merletti, 2006). An integrative approach enables us to conceptualize inherent complexities in a healthy city system, and this helps us to unravel the underlying multiple causal pathways connecting the various agents of the component systems (ICSU, 2012).

The existing spatial scales in the model are represented as the *urban hierarchy cone*, comprising a hierarchy of functional spatial aggregates – household space, several households within neighbourhoods, and neighbourhoods clustered into cities – which combine together to form regional aggregates. As we move up the levels, the cones have increasing surface area and yet all originate from the same base, reflecting the idea that individuals form the basic building blocks of the urban system. In an analytic sense, the household–neighbourhood–city (HNC) system comprises two categories of causal factors. The physical environment is constituted by natural and built environment factors, while the social environment is formed by clusters of individuals (populations), forming cohesive networks with well-defined social structures maintained by flows of social capital, economics and information.

Corresponding to the spatial scale, there exists a well-defined hierarchy for devising health-enhancing interventions. This has been represented in the model by a set of concentric *cylinders of integrated planning*. These governance and decision-making systems consist of factors such as policy constraints and interventions at each level which have an impact on the health of an individual and at population levels. In terms of urban theory, they roughly divide into public services, physical infrastructure, regulations and educational interventions aimed at changing behaviour. In the empirical models in Chapters 5–8, physical infrastructure (the urban road grid) is considered to assume a crucial role in health by virtue of its function of distributing to individuals the benefits of collective health-promoting investments.

The model suggests that healthy city planning requires interventions that should be guided by considerations functional at each level of the ecological hierarchy. Thus, regional-level health planning initiatives should originate from the individual level and go on to the household, community and, subsequently, city level, thereby assimilating all the determining factors at each spatial hierarchy. Such an approach will demand more effective multi-agency and interdisciplinary collaborations between the disciplines of biomedicine, epidemiology, public health and urban planning.

Following WHO (2005a), the healthy city model conceptualizes the health of an individual to be a function of three components. Physiological health may be measured in terms of the presence or absence of infectious, chronic and life-threatening diseases. Mental health may be measured in terms of the prevalence of common psychiatric disorders including depression, anxiety and cognitive impairment. Social health is essentially governed by the degree of social support and connectivity enjoyed by individuals, thereby encouraging or prohibiting social interactions that have behavioural and health effects. Social health is dependent upon a number of factors in the social environment such as living arrangements, social bondage and social capital, as well as degree of well-being (efficacy, self-esteem, life satisfaction, positive affects, etc.).

Spatially, an individual occupies the common edge of three enveloping cubes, each successively increasing in area, reflecting the spatial hierarchy of eco-niches in which it is located. The first cube in Figure 3.2 indicates the household/work space, representing the entire household (or office or unit in an industrial building). The second cube, enveloping the building space, is the neighbourhood space, of which the dwelling unit (office or factory) forms a part. The third cube represents the city space, that is, the cityscape of which the neighbourhood forms a component. The health niche is conceptualized this way following a long tradition in urban economic, social and planning theory that consistently identifies the neighbourhood as a distinct unit of functional and behavioural organization linking individuals and households with the wider urban system (C. Webster, 2003). An alternative would be to conceptualize the spatial dimension of the model as a continuum, assuming that neighbourhood and population effects vary continuously rather than discretely. The truth is that both happen: both

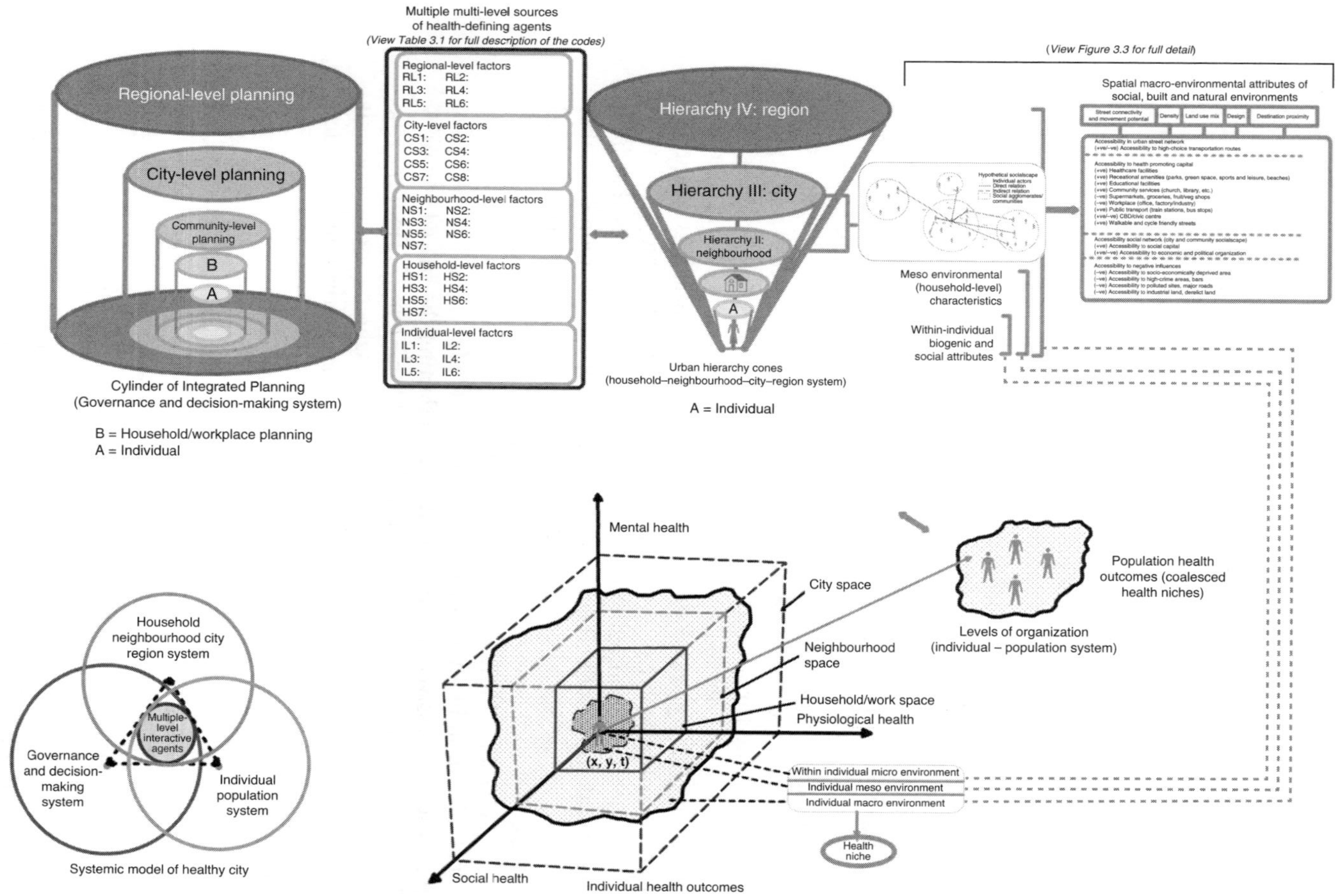

Figure 3.2 Health niche-based model of the healthy city

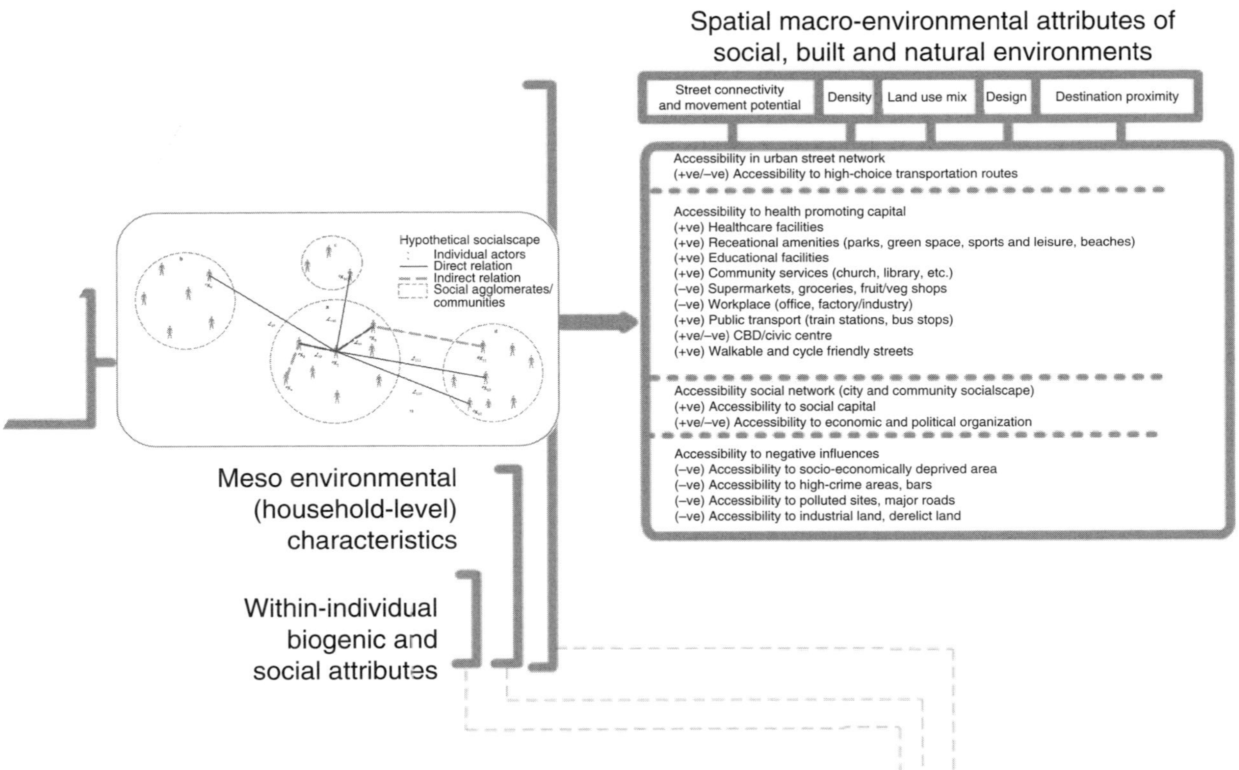

Figure 3.3 Detail of section of Figure 3.2

Table 3.1 Multiple multi-level health-defining factors in the healthy city model

Hierarchy	Determinant code	Health-defining factors
Regional level	RL1	Governance
	RL2	Macroeconomics
	RL3	Social ideologies (democracy, human rights, racism, customs)
	RL4	Urban regeneration
	RL5	Sprawl, suburbanization, immigration
	RL6	Biodiversity, natural habitats, climate stability or change
City level	CS1	Route morphometrics (city-wide network connectivity or accessibility)
	CS2	City-wide land use dynamics (location and density of service destinations)
	CS3	Transport (role of active transport, policies)
	CS4	Governance and enforcement regulations
	CS5	Microeconomic structure
	CS6	Labour market, agricultural market and food network
	CS7	Educational system, health services, welfare benefits, etc.
	CS8	Pollution, waste disposal, aesthetics
Neighbourhood level	NS1	Route morphometrics (network connectivity / accessibility)
	NS2	Land use morphometrics (density and proximity of service destinations)
	NS3	Residential density
	NS4	Design (pedestrian-friendly design)
	NS5	Neighbourhood socio-economic status
	NS6	Social capital, sense of community
	NS7	Safety (crime rates, graffiti, road safety)
Housing space/ workplace	HS1	Household type, tenure, floor level and household overcrowding
	HS2	Household income or wealth, amenities
	HS3	Sanitation and household pollution levels (indoor pollution, noise levels)
	HS4	Physical conditions (lighting, dampness, sunlight hours, average individual space, etc.)
	HS5	Social bonds, social support, living arrangements
	HS6	Nutrition and diet, hygiene

Table 3.1 (continued)

Hierarchy	Determinant code	Health-defining factors
	HS7	Lifestyle (sleep hours, smoking, drinking, addiction, physical activity)
Individual level	IL1	Age, gender, ethnicity
	IL2	Education, employment
	IL3	Physiologic factors (allergic reactions, immunologic competence, drug reactivity, exposure to pathogens, etc.)
	IL4	Genotype
	IL5	Nature of responses to prevailing psychosocial factors
	IL6	Birth defects, accidents and disabling injuries

continuous and discrete functions may best describe the impact of spatially sensitive factors on individual health. In our empirical models, this is captured, for example, by the use of continuous variables within discretely defined neighbourhood buffers.

Each individual is thus enveloped by a hypothetical hypervolume, coined as the *intrinsic health niche* at a given instant of time, which is a composite of all the predictor factors in an urban system that interact synergistically to produce the health of an individual. Variations in the health of individuals are deemed to be a result of spatio-temporal variations in health niches. As has been described earlier in this chapter, individual niches coalesce to constitute population niches, so that we have individual–population systems that co-configure one another. The urban health niche of an individual at a given space–time coordinate (x, y, t) may thus be conceptualized to comprise multiple factors that interact synergistically to produce health outcomes and continuums at individual and population levels respectively.

In sum, we conceptualize a *health niche* as the fundamental component of a *healthy city* model. It is self-emergent, essentially a function of interactions between multiple factors divided into three constituent components, namely intrinsic-individual-, meso-environment- and macro-environment-level factors. The micro-level factors consist of the inherent within-individual biogenic factors that govern the nature and degree to which an individual reacts to the surrounding environment, thereby defining the degree of risk or proneness to a particular health risk. These may include: individual-level health-defining factors that are unique to a particular individual, such as age, gender, ethnicity, genotype; physiological agents such as allergic reaction, immunologic competence, drug reactivity, levels of exposure to pathogens, and so on; psychosocial agents measured by levels of psychological distress, or delinquency; and experience of life events, accidents and disabling injuries.

The meso-environmental factors of the health niche typically consist of the health-defining factors of dwelling place and work space. They may include physical factors associated with sanitation, pollution (indoor, noise), physical conditions (lighting, dampness, sunlight hours, average individual space, floor level, etc.), amenities and heating (Howden-Chapman, 2004), as well as socio-demographic and lifestyle-level factors such as education, income, family bonding and support, nutrition, smoking, and so on.

The factors of the meso environment assume particular importance in high-density and impoverished families. It is common to find several individual family members occupying a single room in high-density suburban and rural neighbourhoods of India, for example, often lacking proper ventilation and without adequate sanitary facilities. The tendency to depend upon biomass and coal as the primal energy source for household needs, especially cooking and heating, further aggravates the situation for many of the world's poor (Smith, 2002). At the onset of respiratory disorder in an individual, such micro-environmental factors may further exacerbate the condition into chronic asthma. Household overcrowding has the potential to make an individual more prone to exposure to the pathogens of infectious diseases if another family member falls ill (Kellett, 1993; Fonseca et al., 1996), as well as cause the stress of enforced involuntary social interactions (G.W. Evans and Lepore, 1993). Set against these increased risks, increased interpersonal contact may result in enhanced social capital and support. Poverty in the West is more likely to be associated with a micro environment such as cold and damp housing infested with spores of fungi (Burr et al., 1981; C.J. Martin et al., 1987; Billings and Howard, 1998). In the work environment, occupational health hazards originate from agents of air, water, noise, thermal and radioactive pollution, and interpersonal contacts. A worker vulnerable to cardiovascular risk factors in the work environment (such as having high blood pressure and spending 40 hours a week working in front of a blast furnace, exposed to thermal and noise pollution) will be more likely to have work-related anxiety, cardiovascular disease and other related chronic disorders (Landsbergis et al., 2003).

An individual spends most of the time in the house or workplace, the spatial location of which determines the attributes of the individual macro environment. The macro-environment factors are active at scales of neighbourhood, city and region. An individual residing in a household located in a spatially well-integrated neighbourhood and city may enjoy the health benefits of:

- an optimized density of health-promoting resources;
- an optimized mix of land uses in the neighbourhood;
- a street configuration conducive to walkability;
- denser social networks and levels of social capital;
- greater density of accessible welfare-enhancing destinations.

All these may together define accessibility within an urban system as well as in the social networks constituted, facilitated and accommodated within it. Their role in influencing health behaviour and eventually individual and population health is reviewed in detail in Chapter 4.

The overall urban health niche enveloping an individual in a city is also shaped by a self-organizing arrangement of people, activities and places. Individuals locate to optimize distances between other individuals with whom they wish to cooperate in pursuit of wealth and welfare, work, daily subsistence and leisure. As individuals populate a built environment niche they change the ecology of a city and affect the location calculus of other individuals. Health care facilities, like other services, locate in certain places because of the accessibility of those places to target users and customers. In turn, a distribution of facilities and services will affect the location and movement behaviour of other individuals. As a result of this iterative process by which individuals respond to accessibility and thereby modify accessibility, a city's accessibility 'surface' (a mathematical model describing various kinds of accessibility at each location or each link in the network – formally defined and implemented empirically in Chapters 5–8) is a rich source of information. Given that the spatial behaviour of individuals, including home, work and other activity locations, is influenced by multiple distance optimization criteria in multiple time periods, there is an a priori reason to view an urban accessibility surface as some kind of aggregate indicator of locational benefits. This is the outworking of Figure 3.2 that we develop in the empirical work of this book.

Other macro-environment factors influencing health may include those associated with the quality of the natural environment such as proximity to highly polluted sites. Residents living adjacent to major roads may be prone to the negative health effects of poor air quality and elevated noise levels from traffic flows (Stansfeld et al., 1996; Kunzli et al., 2000; Brauer et al., 2002; Stansfeld and Matheson, 2003), while residents living in the vicinity of major industrial sites generally have a higher propensity to suffer from chronic disease on account of factors causing pollution of air and water (Ginns and Gatrell, 1996; Elliott et al., 1999; Corcoran et al., 2010; Drechsel et al., 2010). Other health-defining factors include those related to the amount of urban green (de

Vries et al., 2003; Lachowycz and Jones, 2011; Dadvand et al., 2012), electromagnetic fields (Knave, 1994; Röösli, 2008) and urban heat island effects (Tan et al., 2010), as well as those functioning at the regional scale such as climate change (McGeehin and Mirabelli, 2001; Patz et al., 2005; McMichael et al., 2006). Aesthetic neighbourhood quality related to physical manifestations of incivilities and territorial dysfunctioning, defensible space and fear of crime have been shown to influence health (Newman, 1972; R.B. Taylor, 1988; D. Cohen et al., 2000; Weich et al., 2002; Stafford, Chandola et al., 2007). And, of course, the role of neighbourhood-level socio-economic status is, as we noted in Chapter 2, one of the longest-studied macro influences on health-related behaviour and health outcomes (Pickett and Pearl, 2001).

What the model described above adds to this well-founded field is an overarching conceptual framework that recognizes complexity in scales and times of interactions and causation, and provides a theoretical basis for empirical models of multi-scalar, multidimensional and multi-temporal associations between the built environment and health.

3.4 CONCLUSION

The proposed urban health niche paradigm follows a holistic and multidisciplinary approach to studying public health and healthy city dynamics. The objective is to unravel the black box of contextual determinants of health. The potential of such an approach stems from its effectiveness in organizing and integrating prospective data across the multiple subdisciplines encompassing clinical medicine, genetic epidemiology, risk factor epidemiology, social epidemiology, and epidemiology of built and physical environments, as well as urban planning and public health planning. It thereby facilitates multidisciplinary empirical research by specifying a data model across multiple and multi-level health-defining factors and thereby provides a basis for multi-level policies and intervention strategies.

Gene–behaviour–environment (natural and built) interaction models of health recognize the role of genotypic distribution in affecting spatial variations in health behaviour and disease. At the same time, the role of contextual social, built and natural environmental factors in disease causation is determined by an individual's genetic make-up. Only an integrated approach to studying the dual role of genotype as well as context (encompassing micro to macro levels) will enable us to decipher the causal paths of disease causation (Diez Roux, 2007).

The urban health niche is not a static hypothetical space surrounding the individual; it varies in space and time coordinates, in response to the individual's behavioural pattern within urban space. Thus medical geographers may be interested in the spatio-temporal dynamics of personal behavioural patterns, defined by multiple multi-level factors and often unique to each individual. They can be captured by a diurnal space–time activity graph. The minimum convex polygon, the smallest convex polygon consisting of a set of point events, may be employed to examine the association between urban morphology and individual activity patterns (Buliung and Kanaroglou, 2006; Moorcroft and Lewis, 2006). Similarly, kernel density estimation may be employed to conceptualize space–time utilization of health-promoting services as well as spatio-temporal distribution of diseases (Bithell, 2006). Other sophisticated technologies such as network-based space–time prisms or isochrones may enable us to operationalize the diurnal trace of individuals' behavioural niches within a network (Neutens et al., 2008). An effective collaboration between medical geographers and clinical practitioners will enable us to examine the nature of association between health outcomes and context-based behavioural data derived from these technologies. At a longer time scale, an effective multidisciplinary approach will help in examining cumulative contextual health effects through collaborative use of cohort data relating to risk factors and health outcome as well as prospective data pertaining to variations in social, natural and built environment context.

The authors are investigators of a study, funded jointly by the UK Economic and Social Research Council and the UK Biobank, that will create a unique database structured along the lines of the urban health niche model described in this chapter and facilitating models that explicitly analyse health impacts from genetic to macro built environment scales for 500 000 UK residents.

At a macro level, urban and public health planners must strive to formulate evidence-based plans and policies. This can be possible only through effective understanding by epidemiologists of the complex dynamic interactions from micro to macro levels. As an example, city-level health intervention strategies can be devised by urban planners based on prior retrospective epidemiological studies of the long-term health effects of urban regeneration and retrofitting at neighbourhood and city scales. Such informed spatial planning should guide city- and regional-level policies with respect to housing, land use and transport, thereby enabling optimization of health-defining services.

The proposed healthy city model, based on an understanding of health niches, also highlights the inherent complexity involved in the socio-spatial production of health in a city. The risk factors operating at multiple spatial scales and levels of organization are often interdependent, and it is highly unlikely that causality is unidirectional and continuous in nature. Similarly, as we have noted, individuals, populations and neighbourhoods configure one another, each adapting in response to the others. The methodological challenges of developing reliable knowledge about complex dynamic non-linear interactions between causal factors (both at individual and population levels and at multiple spatial scales) have led some epidemiologists to test the potential applicability of more explicitly complex approaches to analysis, such as agent-based complex adaptive systems (CAS) models (Koopman and Lynch, 1999; Materia and Baglio, 2005; N. Pearce and Merletti, 2006; Diez Roux, 2007; Auchincloss and Diez Roux, 2008; Galea et al., 2010). However, this is still an emerging area of research in contemporary spatial epidemiology, and the challenge that lies ahead is to find ways to operationalize an integrated approach – combining the predictive, inferential and explanatory powers of statistical models with the exploratory and emergent powers of CAS models. Our implementation of an urban health niche model in Chapters 5–8 extends the boundary of conventional approaches by improving the quality of the connectivity data linking multiple potentially causal factors across multiple scales. We leave to subsequent studies the exploration of CAS and specific generative algorithms as means of further unravelling the spatial-temporal dynamics of urban health niches.

4. Spatial determinants of health

This chapter comprises a systematic review of epidemiologic literature on the built environment and health, structured by the idea of the urban health niche (Chapter 3). Key determinants of health at housing and neighbourhood levels are discussed in detail.

4.1 FACTORIZING THE HOUSING-LEVEL DETERMINANTS OF PHYSICAL HEALTH

The relationship between residential environment and health is multi-dimensional and complex in nature. Although there has always been a symbolic recognition of this relationship, little deciphered quantitative evidence exists regarding its exact nature. The importance of quality and quantity of housing for urban health has been emphasized by the United Nations Human Settlement Programme (UN-Habitat), which estimates that approximately 1 billion people out of a global population of 6 billion are presently living in slum-like conditions and that this figure is expected to double to 2 billion by 2030. In recognition of this, UN-Habitat holistically defines adequate housing as:

> accommodation associated with attributes of privacy; adequate space; physical accessibility; security; security of tenure; structural stability and durability; adequate lighting, heating and ventilation; adequate basic infrastructure such as water supply, sanitation and waste management facilities; suitable environmental quality and health-related factors; and adequate and accessible location with regard to work and basic facilities: all of which should be available at an affordable cost. (United Nations Commission on Human Settlements, 1996)

The associations between housing, socio-economic conditions and health outcomes are complex. Housing space provides the immediate environment where individuals in urban populations spend more than 80 per cent of their time (Leech et al., 2002). The figure is currently close to 16 hours daily for the developed countries, a figure that is likely to increase in the coming decade with current policies aiming to minimize dependence upon urban transportation and encouraging working from home. A housing unit is characterized by a set of physical conditions, which consists of the health-influencing biochemical factors to which each individual is exposed. Housing units differ in their ability to shield us from exposure to adverse climatic conditions, vectors of pathogens and pollutants. Every house has a unique set of personal and household hygiene-related attributes such as dampness, lighting, indoor pollution, supply of potable water, sanitation, waste disposal, storage, space and methods of food storage and preparation, and so on (WHO, 1990). Houses provide an environment for the household economy: for making things, consuming things and disposing of things. These activities carry various types of health risks that are mitigated or enhanced by the configuration of internal and external space.

Residential units also provide us with the private space for relaxing, interacting and developing social relationships within a family. Housing environments can foster social bonds, support specific living arrangements and alleviate psychological stress processes. There is a plausible connection therefore between a household's micro environment and the mental health of individuals (Halpern, 1995). The amount of space and the levels of comfort available per capita generally depend upon the socio-economic status of residents. The physical structure of housing in terms of building design and quality of materials used, as well as the attributes of the indoor environment, directly influences the health of residents. Poor-quality construction increases risk of accidental injuries, dampness and so on and can reduce protection from natural elements and human-made pollutants. Housing should not be considered in isolation but as building blocks of neighbourhoods, communities and the city as a whole. At this level, the density, the location of a dwelling in the overall emerging urban matrix, and the presence of externalities from proximate land uses all have an indirect influence upon the health of a house's occupants.

Healy (2003) performed an assessment of health-defining housing conditions, levels of energy efficiency, affordability and degree of satisfaction with housing in 14 European countries using longitudinal data sets from the European Community Household Panel over the period 1994–97. Serious housing deficiencies in the form of poor thermal efficiency, high fuel poverty, burdensome housing costs and low housing-satisfaction rates were identified as the key health-inhibiting factors in Southern Europe, while, in Northern Europe, dampness and overcrowding were identified as the health-inhibiting factors, especially in the UK, Ireland, France and Belgium (Tables 4.1 and 4.2). There has been a spate of research over the last two decades identifying the physical and mental health problems associated with inadequate house conditions. These include respiratory tract infection, asthma, pulmonary disease, lung cancer, cardiovascular diseases, anxiety, depression, attention deficit disorders, aggressive behaviour,

Table 4.1 Dwelling type and tenure in Europe – mean percentage, 1994–97

	Percentage detached	Percentage semi-detached/terraced	Percentage small MFDs	Percentage large MFDs	Percentage owner occupier	Percentage tenants	Percentage rent-free
Germany	26.0	13.4	34.3	18.8	42.3	54.4	3.2
Denmark	50.2	12.6	12.7	19.2	62.5	37.0	0.5
Netherlands	13.0	51.8	4.4	18.1	52.1	47.0	1.0
Belgium	33.9	42.0	11.1	7.7	67.7	28.9	3.4
Luxembourg	38.1	30.8	19.1	10.1	72.2	24.7	3.1
France	38.6	21.4	13.3	24.5	56.5	38.1	5.4
UK	22.5	58.8	11.3	3.9	68.4	28.3	1.6
Ireland	51.0	42.9	2.3	0.9	85.8	13.3	1.8
Italy	20.2	12.1	37.3	23.5	74.0	19.1	6.9
Greece	31.8	19.0	29.3	18.4	78.7	17.9	3.4
Spain	17.5	19.2	18.8	43.8	80.7	12.9	6.4
Portugal	51.1	26.7	13.8	4.9	68.5	20.0	11.5
Austria	47.9	4.5	11.8	27.6	58.7	34.6	6.6
Finland	47.2	17.6	2.4	30.0	73.8	16.9	9.2

Source: Healy (2003, p. 414). Reprinted by permission of the publisher.

Table 4.2 Households with housing problems – mean percentage, 1994–97

	Leaky roofs	No hot running water	Objective overcrowding	Subjective overcrowding	Damp	Rot
Germany	4.3	4.6	9.4	15.0	7.9	5.3
Denmark	3.9	0.8	5.0	16.0	6.2	5.6
Netherlands	4.4	0.5	–	9.8	10.8	9.7
Belgium	5.7	3.6	5.0	14.6	14.4	9.1
Luxembourg	5.0	3.1	8.4	11.5	7.5	4.8
France	5.3	2	8.2	13.6	16.3	10.4
UK	3.8	0.2	5.2	18.0	13.0	12.7
Ireland	4.1	4	14.8	12.5	9.6	7.3
Italy	6.3	2.8	24.3	19.9	5.4	6.2
Greece	16.4	70.2	–	26.9	18.8	9.3
Spain	11.4	3.5	15.8	21.6	21.5	7.6
Portugal	18.7	22.6	19.9	27.9	33.4	25.2
Austria	3.6	2.4	–	14.1	8.8	4.6
Finland	2.9	1.8	13.3	15.3	3.8	2.6

Source: Healy (2003, p. 417). Reprinted by permission of the publisher.

substance abuse, obesity and so-called sick building syndrome (Raffestin and Lawrence, 1990; Fullilove and Fullilove, 2000; Fisk, 2001; Howden-Chapman, 2004). We look at particular housing-related causes in the following subsections, denoting the principal hypothesized causes as factors, with notations H1 . . . Hn from the health niche-based healthy city model (described in Figure 3.2).

4.1.1 Factor H1: Cold, Damp Dwellings and Physical Health

Residential units maintained at proper temperatures provide comfort to occupants and foster good health. The optimal temperature for maximum comfort varies between climate zone, individuals, age groups, and levels of fitness and physical activity of occupants. The World Health Organization recommends a minimum indoor temperature of 20°C for the sick, handicapped, very old and very young (WHO, 1987), based on research into the effects of temperatures on expressed and revealed well-being. There is a general consensus that there exists an enhanced chance of respiratory impairment at a temperature below 16°C, cardiovascular strain below 12°C, and hypothermia at temperatures below 6°C (K.J. Collins, 1993). Furthermore, cold and damp domestic environments are often found in conjunction with each other, as insufficient heat encourages condensation, which in turn promotes the growth of pathogens and hence compromises the health of the occupants. In a study conducted on 858 respondents in Western Scotland, Gemmell (2001) highlighted the relationships between socio-economic factors, house conditions, inadequate home heating and poor health in respondents aged 55–60. As mentioned earlier, the associations between poor-quality housing, fuel poverty and disease outcomes have long been identified (Rudge and Nicol, 2000; Healy, 2003). Ireland and the UK exhibit the highest rates of seasonal mortality in Northern Europe on account of inadequately protected and thermally inefficient housing, especially from myocardial infarction, stroke and respiratory conditions (*BMJ*, 1980; Curwen, 1991; Healy, 2003). In Great Britain there is considerable maldistribution of decent housing, often termed the 'inverse housing law', which implies that those areas prone to a colder climate are the ones that tend to have worse housing conditions. An estimated 40000 extra winter deaths occur each year in Great Britain between the months of December and March, primarily attributable to poor housing quality and deprivation (Aylin et al., 2001). Increased rates of morbidity in inadequately heated homes may be attributed to bronchospasm (which in turn has been independently identified as being triggered by smoking), upper respiratory tract infections and cardiovascular diseases (WHO, 1987; Blane et al., 2000; J. Evans et al., 2000; Richard Mitchell et al., 2002).

4.1.2 Factor H2: Damp, Mould and Physical Health

Damp conditions are associated with high moisture levels and can harbour pathogens that can be damaging to health. In most dwellings, dampness results primarily from water leakage. Viral and bacterial infections are long known to be more prevalent in damp houses (Karim et al., 1985). Damp in the form of condensation provides a breeding ground for the germinating spores of mould fungi. They form saprophytic colonies on plugs of mucus-producing lesions in respiratory tissues. They further act as respiratory allergens causing rhinitis, alveolitis and asthma (Hosen, 1978; C.J. Martin et al., 1987; Platt et al., 1989). Burr et al. (1981) in their study conducted on men and women aged 20–44 in South Wales highlighted the associations between coal fires, dampness and respiratory diseases. C.J. Martin et al. (1987) conducted a study on the effect of damp on ill health for one postcode sector of Edinburgh (with over 2000 dwellings). The study defined a 'damp house' in terms of the degree of damp, condensation or fungal mould present. A significant association between living in a damp and, more specifically, 'mouldy' house and ill health was reported among children. In addition to respiratory problems, other symptoms of infection and stress were reported to be more prevalent among children residing in damp houses. The positive relationship between damp and mouldy housing and recurrent headaches, fever, nausea and vomiting, and sore throats is well established (Platt et al., 1989; Institute of Medicine, 2000). Howden-Chapman et al. (2008) reported negative associations between improved home heating and the incidences of asthma among children. Dedman et al. (2001) conducted a life-course study of the association between their five categories of housing variables (crowding index, water supply, toilet facilities, ventilation and cleanliness) during childhood and later-life mortality from all causes and from coronary heart disease, stroke and cancer. The study was carried out in 16 survey areas of England and Scotland and comprised 4301 people. Their evidence suggested that, on the whole, respondents living in better-quality housing had lower odds of age-adjusted mortality. Subsequent to adjustments for childhood and adult socio-economic factors, lack of private indoor tapped water supply was significantly associated with increased mortality from coronary heart disease, while poor ventilation was associated with higher odds of overall mortality. A positive association between damp dwelling and the incidences of asthma has been found in several other studies (Billings and Howard, 1998; Institute of Medicine, 2000).

4.1.3 Factor H3: Overcrowding and Physical Health

Overcrowding is associated with lack of privacy and stress contributing to both physical and mental illness and increased incidences of accidents. Several measures have been developed to quantify overcrowding within a household. Objective overcrowding is measured as the total number of residents in the household divided by the number of habitable rooms in it (excluding kitchens, bathrooms, halls, garages, etc.). According to the standard definition of overcrowding, a value greater than 1 is considered as 'objectively overcrowded' (Eurostat, 1996). A more intricate measure is the Canadian Overcrowding Index (Canada Mortgage and Housing Corporation, 1991). For residential apartments, building density (persons or dwelling units per structure) has been identified as one of three types of population density; it essentially indicates the degree of separation of households from each other by the walls, floors and ceilings they share and is an important measure of overcrowding. It acts as an important predictor of mental strain.

Overcrowding has long been associated with higher premature mortality rates as well as enhanced risk of both infectious and non-infectious diseases (Kellett, 1993). There have been reported associations between overcrowding and enhanced incidences of meningoccocal disease (Baker et al., 2000) and a higher propensity to infections of the respiratory tract, both viral and bacterial (Graham, 1990; Murtagh et al., 1993; Fonseca et al., 1996; Marsh et al., 1999), tuberculosis (Stein, 1950; Coetzee et al., 1988) and hepatitis B (Milne et al., 1987). Overcrowding in conjunction with inadequate ventilation poses more potential risks, as it increases the moisture levels of the indoor environment, thereby providing nurturing grounds for mites, roaches, respiratory viruses and moulds, all of which play a role in respiratory disease pathogenesis (Markus, 1993; Bierman, 1996; Billings and Howard, 1998).

4.1.4 Factor H4: Housing Disrepair, Pest Infestation and Physical Health

Residents of sub-standard housing in impoverished neighbourhoods are disproportionately exposed to allergens, pests and air pollutants and hence are prone to greater health risks. Pest infestation in dilapidated dwellings is a common occurrence and is primarily related to structural defects. Housing disrepair and structural defects contribute to easy admission of pests like mites, cockroaches and rodents. Structural defects in the form of leaking pipes, cracks and holes in ceilings and dead spaces within walls also permit the entry of pests. Dysfunctional food storage and waste disposal facilities provide pests with space and water for sustenance (M. Howard,

1993). Pests have long been known to have an aggravating influence on asthma. Cockroaches may cause allergic sensitization, acting as a trigger for asthma. Studies have shown that exposure to cockroaches especially aggravates the condition of asthmatic children, making them prone to hospitalization (Rosenstreich et al., 1997). Mouse allergen has also been known to act as a clinically important agent of allergy that enhances vulnerability to asthma (Phipatanakul et al., 2000). Several other studies have reported increased risk of developing asthma in the presence of dust mite allergens (Institute of Medicine, 2000; Raw et al., 2001). Furthermore, the use of pesticides in dilapidated houses may pose considerable health risks (Cummins and Jackson, 2001; J. Krieger and Higgins, 2002). Small clinically controlled studies have reported an association between the occurrences of bronchoconstriction and the use of insecticides that contain pyrethrin as well as the use of perfumes (Salome et al., 2000). Another commonly observed characteristic of sub-standard dwellings is the presence of old, damp and dirty carpeting, which often acts as a breeding ground for dust, allergens and toxic chemicals. These agents often act as a trigger to allergic, respiratory, neurological and haematologic illnesses (Roberts and Dickey, 1995; J.W. Vaughan and Platts-Mills, 2000). Some studies have reported that dilapidated housing may in itself act as a stressor that affects the human immune system (Lehmann et al., 2002).

4.1.5 Factor H5: Indoor Air Pollution and Physical Health

Indoor air quality has long been identified as an important determinant of health. Choice of building materials, furnishings and cleaning agents, selection of energy and fuel-efficient devices for indoor heating and cooking needs, operating an effective ventilation system and environmental tobacco smoke all determine the levels of indoor pollution in a dwelling (Hodgson, 2002).

Household combustion products primarily consist of carbon dioxide, carbon monoxide, sulphur dioxide and nitrogen dioxide. Carbon dioxide (CO_2) itself is not considered a pollutant and poses no health concern. However, the CO_2 levels inside an occupied building, in the absence of any combustion, should not exceed 650 parts per million (ppm) above ambient levels; often CO_2 levels are employed as an indicator of the degree of ventilation in a facility (Zhang and Smith, 2003). In addition to the combustion of solid fuels, gaseous fuels used in common household devices also act as sources of pollution, including particulate matter (PM), CO_2, eye-irritating volatile organic compounds (e.g. aldehydes), and carcinogenic compounds such as benzene and 1,3-butadiene and polycyclic aromatic hydrocarbons, although at a comparatively lower concentration. Typically, health risks multiply many-fold in cases of incomplete combustion products of solid fuels burned in poorly designed and maintained stoves. These include carbon monoxide (CO), respirable particulate matter, various categories of volatile organic compounds (VOCs) and semi-volatile organic compounds (SVOCs) and are known to pose many acute and chronic health risks (Zhang and Smith, 1996, 2003; Zhang et al., 2000). Health risks from CO arise in cases of acute exposure to very high concentrations from unvented combustion heaters and charcoal fuel, resulting in poisoning fatalities worldwide. Moderately elevated levels of CO have been associated with headaches (Girman et al., 1998; Walker and Hay, 1999). Cases of carbon monoxide poisoning are further exacerbated by inadequate or faulty ventilation systems. By contrast, sustained contact with nitrogen dioxide (NO_2) emitted from gas- and oil-operated furnaces and stoves is reported to pose only modest risk for respiratory diseases compared to their electric counterparts (Neas et al., 1991; Basu, 1999). In a study conducted by H.S. Jenkins et al. (1999), short exposure to high concentrations of nitrogen dioxide enhanced allergen sensitivity, thereby causing enhanced bronchial responsiveness to inhaled allergens in a dose-sensitized population of asthmatics. There is increasing medical evidence that smoke emanating from solid fuels is a potential culprit for ailments as serious as acute respiratory infections (ARI), chronic obstructive pulmonary disease (COPD) and lung cancer (from coal smoke) (Smith, 2002; Zhang and Smith, 2003). Indoor smoke from solid fuels has been identified as one of the top ten risk factors for the global burden of disease by the World Health Organization (WHO) (see Figure 4.1), accounting for an estimated 2.0 million premature deaths annually (almost 3.3 per cent of the global burden of disease), as well as accounting for 2.7 per cent of the total disability-adjusted life-years (DALYs) (WHO, 2009).

In developing countries, energy for cooking food, heating and other domestic activities comes primarily from the burning of coal and biomass fuel, thereby causing significant levels of indoor air pollution. There are varying degrees of evidence to suggest that the mixture of pollutants (especially oxides of carbon, nitrogen, particulates, polycyclic hydrocarbons, and some toxic metals such as lead and chromium from sulphur-rich coal) emitted from these sources has the potential to cause acute respiratory infections, chronic pulmonary disease including asthma, lung cancer, nasopharyngeal and laryngeal cancers, tuberculosis, and diseases of the eye (Ezzati, 2005). The risks are further compounded by poor ventilation in the housing units (Smith and Mehta, 2003; Zhang and Smith, 2007).

Environmental tobacco smoke (ETS), sometimes referred to as passive or involuntary smoking, is another important indoor health-inhibiting pollutant (USDHHS, 2006). Both the primary smoke exhaled by a smoker

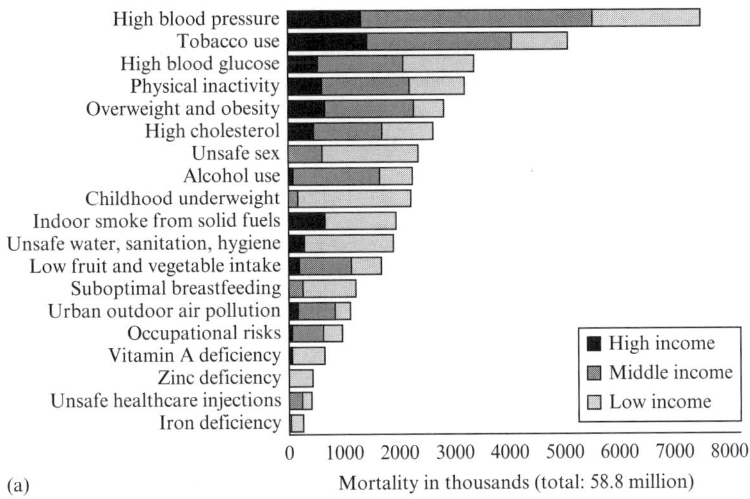

Source: Derived from WHO (2009).

Figure 4.1a *Deaths attributed to 19 leading risk factors, by country income level, 2004*

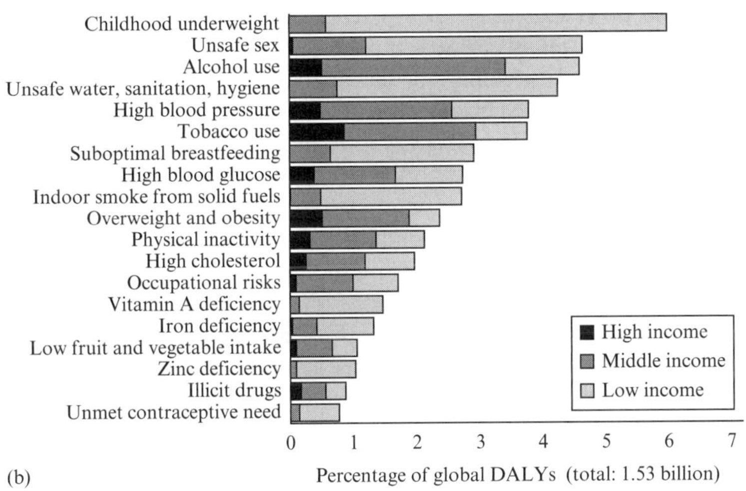

Source: Derived from WHO (2009).

Figure 4.1b *Percentage of disability-adjusted life-years (DALYs) attributed to 19 leading risk factors, by country income level, 2004*

and the secondary smoke generated by the burning tobacco constitute ETS. ETS is the largest source of indoor air pollution, given the fact that 29 per cent of adults worldwide are active smokers (Jha, 1999). An estimated 20–30 per cent increased odds of lung cancer, 25–35 per cent increased odds of coronary artery disease, and potential child health risks in the form of slow lung growth, cough and wheeze, respiratory illness and sudden infant death syndrome have all been associated with living with an active smoker (USDHHS, 2006; Dales et al., 2008). In adults, reported health risks of passive smoking include respiratory disease (USEPA, 1992), lung cancer (Hackshaw et al., 1997), ischaemic heart disease (Thun et al., 1999) and nasal-sinus cancer (Cal/EPA, 1997). Respiratory ailments in children may include lower respiratory tract infection, asthma and recurrent inflammation of the middle ear or otitis media (Cook and Strachan, 1997; Strachan and Cook, 1997, 1998). There is a reported association between prenatal maternity smoking and sudden infant death syndrome (Anderson and Cook, 1997), as well as low birth weight (Windham et al., 1999).

Off-gassing emissions are the gases that are released from indoor materials of a residential dwelling, especially those released from building materials such as wood-based products, synthetic materials, paints, floor finishes, carpets, glues, consumer products, freshly dried clothing, fried food, and so on (Dales et al., 2008). These emissions are highest in new host materials, as well as recently applied paints, but they generally decay with time. Low ventilation may further increase the concentration of these off-gassing emissions, especially VOCs and SVOCs, thereby enhancing the health risks. Off-gassing from wood-based products assembled using urea-formaldehyde resins (plywood, particle board, medium-density fibreboard), as well as certain paints, varnishes and floor finishes, and tobacco smoke, is the main source of formaldehyde in the indoor environment. Concentrations greater than 1230 μg/m have been known to produce acute effects in the form of irritation of the eye, nose and throat (Kulle, 1993). Some studies have reported positive associations between indoor exposure to formaldehyde and respiratory symptoms (Krzyzanowski et al., 1990; Rumchev et al., 2002). VOCs are the carbon-containing compounds present mostly in the gaseous phase. The primary sources are building materials, paints, cigarette smoke, recently dry-cleaned clothes, room deodorizers, showering products, moulds and pesticides. Oil-fried foods are a source of 1,3-butadiene, acrolein and polycyclic aromatic hydrocarbons. The nature of health risks posed by the VOCs generally depends on their type and concentration, the age and surface area of the substrate material, and the depth of VOCs within the substrate material (Ott and Roberts, 1998; Meininghaus et al., 2000). Some VOCs and SVOCs are mutagenic and/or carcinogenic, and sustained exposure increases risks of cancer. Increased incidence of childhood leukaemia has been reported in cases of long-term occupational exposures to VOCs, as well as maternal exposures in pregnant women (Godish, 2000). Respiratory ailments in the form of asthma and bronchial hyper-reactivity have also been reported (Norback et al., 1995; Wieslander et al., 1997; Institute of Medicine, 2000; Zock et al., 2007).

Higher prevalence of bronchial obstruction during the initial couple of years after birth has been associated with living in residences with polyvinyl chloride flooring and textile wallpaper. Jaakkola et al. (1999) conducted an age-matched, case-controlled, 3754 birth cohort study in Oslo and concluded that bronchial obstruction was more common among children living in homes with polyvinyl chloride flooring and textile wallpaper than in homes with wood flooring and painted walls. In another study, plastic wall materials were associated with elevated risk of wheeze, cough and phlegm as well as asthma (Jaakkola et al., 2000). In a study conducted by Hoppin et al. (2004), it was observed that increased levels of monobutyl phthalate were associated with decreased measures of pulmonary function (measured as forced vital capacity, forced expiratory volume at 1 second and peak expiratory flow) in men, but no association was reported in the case of women.

Radon is another carcinogenic radioactive gas and an important indoor pollutant. It originates naturally from the decay of uranium in the rocks. It moves up through the soil pores, primarily driven by convection currents generated as a result of substantial diurnal and seasonal indoor–outdoor temperature and wind pressure gradients. This causes them to accumulate in the indoor environment through the orifices and cracks in the building foundation. It has been estimated that radon concentrations on the first floor of a residence are generally less than half the level in the basement (Committee on Health Risks of Exposure to Radon, 1999). Other sources of radon are domestic groundwater supplies (e.g. well water) and building materials. It has a half-life of 3.8 days during which it decays, producing a series of unstable solid-phase fission products, the reaction eventually terminated by the production of stable lead-210. During the radioactive decay, α, β and γ radiations are also emitted, all of which have the potential to ionize atoms of living cells, thereby causing cell damage. Of these, α radiations are most potent to the respiratory tract. Radon has been primarily identified as the cause of lung cancer, which normally develops subsequent to cumulative exposures of 5–25 years. In the US, an overall 6 per cent of all residences and 30 per cent of residences in Midwestern states have indoor radon levels that exceed the US Environmental Protection Agency (USEPA) prescribed guideline value of 4 pCi/l (Zhang and Smith,

2003). The USEPA has estimated residential radon causes about 21 000 deaths from lung cancer annually in the United States, second only as a cause of lung cancer to smoking. Data on surveys of radon concentration in dwellings summarized by the United Nations Scientific Committee on the Effects of Atomic Radiation for over 20 European countries indicate that average concentrations vary widely between countries. It ranged from 25 Bq m^{-3} in the Netherlands, the United Kingdom and Cyprus to over 100 Bq m^{-3} in Estonia, Finland, Sweden, Luxembourg, the Czech Republic, Hungary and Albania (United Nations Scientific Committee on the Effects of Atomic Radiation, 2000; Darby and Hill, 2003). One of the lowest average indoor concentrations of radon within Europe was reported in the UK (with an average annual dose of 2600 μSv). Even at this low level, it constitutes one of the primary causes of lung cancer, responsible for nearly 35 000 annual fatalities in a population of 59 million. Darby et al. (2001) combined the average residential radon concentration in the UK with data on UK smoking habits and data on lung cancer risks in lifelong non-smokers and interpolated that active smoking constitutes the primary cause, accounting for 89.4 per cent of UK lung cancer deaths. They concluded that residential radon can be held accountable for 6.5 per cent of fatalities, approximately 2275 deaths annually. Interestingly, they identified that, of the 6.5 per cent of lung cancer deaths attributable to radon, 5.5 per cent are caused by radon and smoking acting jointly. The association of lung cancer with smoking and high indoor radon levels is often synergistic in nature. Radon contamination, being naturally derived, is imperceptible to our senses and so is all the more veiled in its risk potency.

Asbestos fibres were extensively employed as a primary construction material in the twentieth century, especially for floors, tiles, insulation, pipes and pipe covers, and their accumulation in indoor environments poses a significant health risk. Continued exposure to asbestos has been identified to be a cause of lung cancer, mesothelioma and lung fibrosis (Ohar et al., 2004). Although the use of asbestos has been banned in most developed countries, it is still being mined in huge quantities, especially in Russia, and asbestos-based products continue to be exported to less developed and developing countries as an affordable housing material. In developed countries, synthetic vitreous fibres (also referred to as man-made mineral fibres, or glass fibres) have popularly emerged as a replacement for asbestos. They are used in spray-applied fireproofing, ceiling tiles, thermal insulation, sound insulation, fabrics, filtration components, plasters and acoustic surface treatments (Zhang and Smith, 2003). Although the cancer risks associated with vitreous fibres are low, health risks magnify when, after considerable use, they get eroded from the parent material, finding their way into the air stream of a building. Potential health risks may involve certain sick building syndrome symptoms, as well as irritation to mucous membranes, the respiratory tract and membranes of the eyes and skin (Vallarino, 2001).

Other notable pollutants found in indoor environments may include lead and inorganic gases like ozone (O_3), hydrogen chloride (HCl), nitrous acid (HNO_2) and nitric acid (HNO_3) vapour.

Lead poisoning is another important health hazard in the indoor environment. The main sources are lead-contaminated water pipes and those originating from the remodelling or demolition of lead-painted surfaces. There is evidence of association between sustained long-term exposure to lead in a domestic environment and impairment of neuro-behavioural functions (Needleman et al., 1990) and hypertension (J. Schwartz, 1988). Children are mostly prone to lead poisoning (Ryan et al., 1999), and a number of studies have reported the detrimental effects of lead exposure in poorly maintained housing. Chronic neurologic damage, and damage to kidneys and reproductive organs, as well as inhibition of early cognitive development, have all been attributed to lead (Bellinger et al., 1988; Sargent et al., 1995; Sharfstein et al., 2001).

Ozone in indoor environments presents another health risk. It originates from its use as an oxidizing agent in purification systems and its use in photocopiers and laser printers. Exposure to high levels of O_3 has the potential to cause difficulty in breathing on account of reduced lung function, to aggravate asthma, to irritate the eyes and nose, to decrease immune resistance to colds and other infections, and to hasten the ageing of pulmonary tissue (Zhang and Smith, 2003). More potent are the indirect risks posed by ozone, especially in initiating a chain of reactions resulting in the generation of secondary pollutants which may act as strong airway irritants producing respiratory and cardiovascular effects (Wolkoff, 2000). Terpenes, often present in indoor environments primarily as solvents in lemon-scented detergents, pine-scented paints, and so on, can react with O_3 to produce a chain of secondary pollutants, especially micro respirable particulates, aldehydes, hydrogen peroxide, carboxylic acids, reactive intermediates, and free radicals including the hydroxyl radical (Zhang and Smith, 2003). The hydroxyl radical thus generated has the capacity to react with virtually all the organic compounds of the indoor environment to produce a series of tertiary pollutants (Weschler and Shields, 1996; Weschler, 2004).

Acidic gas such as hydrogen chloride may be produced in an indoor environment through thermal breakdown of polyvinyl chloride, as well as through transportation from an outdoor environment. Similarly, photochemical smog is the primary source of outdoor HNO_3, which may subsequently be transported indoors. Within residences, HNO_3 may be formed through reactions between O_3, NO_2 and water vapour. Again, indoor HNO_2 may originate from a series of reactions between NO_2 and water films on indoor surfaces. These acidic gases are irritant and corrosive to living tissues.

4.1.6 Factor H6: Lighting and Physical Health

There has been considerable evidence stressing the role of natural lighting in promoting comfort and performance (Boyce, 1981; Lowry, 1989). The direct health consequences arise especially for people undertaking demanding work requiring greater concentration and focus, such as reading or sewing, and lack of natural light causes problems of increased stress, headaches and a feeling of tiredness. Indirect consequences of lack of light are the risk of accidents, especially in badly lit kitchens and stairwells. The Chartered Institution of Building Services Engineers and the Illuminating Engineering Society have recommended a level of illumination of 100 lux at the bottom of a flight of stairs.

Scientific studies have mostly focused on photo-epilepsy and the possibility that fluorescent lights can cause skin cancer, but no direct relationship has yet been established (Whillock et al., 1988). Not enough is known more generally about the potential physiological effects of various forms of domestic lighting. A.F. McKinlay et al. (1989) studied the impact of the ultraviolet emissions from tungsten halogen spotlights on bare skin. They reported the development of erythema after a few hours of exposure on the bare skin on hands.

There is a lack of clear and consistent evidence of the effect of light on mood, emotion and psychological well-being. Lack of exposure to natural lighting may act as an instigating factor in seasonal affective disorder (SAD). The syndrome is characterized by the occurrence of cyclical phases of depression, which usually develops during the autumn or winter months and subsequently remits in the spring or summer for at least two consecutive years (Partonen and Lönnqvist, 1998). Furthermore, patients prone to SAD have been known to exhibit depressive symptoms including bipolar disorder. Generally, two subtypes of SAD have been encountered, winter SAD and summer SAD, of which the former is far more frequent. Exposure to a shorter duration of daylight has been associated with sadness, fatigue and, for some, clinical depression (Rosenthal et al., 1985). The actual aetiology of SAD is however unknown, but the duration of day has been identified to be the contributing factor. Indoor household environments are characterized by a light intensity of 100 lux or less, while in the workplaces it varies from 300 to 500 lux. The outdoor light intensity differs according to the latitude, season, time of day and prevalent local weather.

It may range between 2000 lux or less on a rainy winter day and 10000 lux or more in direct sunshine. Some studies have established that diurnal exposure to bright light for at least three hours during winter may offset the incidence of SAD symptoms (Rosenthal et al., 1985; Lowry, 1989). It is of interest to note that bright-light treatment in the form of exposure to visible light of at least 2500 lux is recommended as the primary option for winter SAD. The impacts of such treatment are thought to be mediated exclusively through the eyes, not the skin (Partonen and Lönnqvist, 1998). In their study, Beauchemin and Hays (1996) reported the positive role of bright-light therapy in the recuperation of patients suffering from severe depression. The average recovery period was significantly less for patients in sunny rooms as compared to dimly lit rooms.

4.1.7 Factor H7: Noise and Physical Health

Involuntary exposure to ambient noise may directly result in impairment of the ear organ and noise-induced hearing loss (NIHL). In addition, indirect non-auditory or extra-aural effects are often reflected in the form of various types of psychosocial and physiologic symptoms and related problems. Even ear-safe sound levels have been known to produce psychological impacts, often manifested in the form of annoyance, reduced performance quality, and increased levels of aggressive behaviour (Passchier-Vermeer and Passchier, 2000; Stansfeld et al., 2000; Stansfeld and Matheson, 2003). Exposure to both traffic and aircraft noise has been reported to be associated with higher odds of annoyance in dose–response relationships. It has been said that noise-induced annoyance in most cases originates as a result of intrusion in day-to-day activities (S.M. Taylor, 1984). Another impact of noise is the disturbance caused to the restorative functions of sleep and relaxation. In the presence of ambient noise, external stimuli are generated that continue to be processed by the sleeper's sensory functions, and such non-conscious perception causes sleep deprivation (Muzet, 2007). Excessive community noise in overcrowded residences, as well as from neighbouring residences and traffic, has the potential to cause sleep deprivation, resulting in impaired concentration and irritability (BMA, 2003). Another study has corroborated the association between microarousal and/or insomnia and elevated levels of metabolic rate, which may further cause health impairments (Raschke, 2004). Indirectly, sleep deprivation has been associated with an enhanced risk of injury and accidents. Exposure to ambient noise also disturbs communication and speech intelligibility, and interferes with mental tasks that require concentration. Chronic noise has been associated with elevated cardiovascular functioning among children (S. Cohen et al., 1986). In another study, Babisch (2000) highlighted the potential associations between noise-induced stress and elevated levels of blood pressure and cardiovascular risks. Several studies have suggested that cumulative occupational exposure to persistent noise at levels in excess of 85 dB have the propensity to increase blood pressure (Y. Zhao et al., 1991; Lang et al., 1992).

Research results have highlighted somewhat confounding relationships between noise sensitivity and psychological disorders (Stansfeld et al., 2000). Traffic noise has been associated with a higher prevalence of depression (Song et al., 2007). In a cross-sectional study conducted by Stansfeld et al. (1996) looking at 1725 adults of Caerphilly, South Wales, aged 50–64, the authors concluded that traffic noise was not an independent cause of overall psychiatric disorder, subsequent to controlling for sociodemographic factors and baseline psychiatric disorder of the respondents. Nevertheless, noise has been shown in other studies to be related to anxiety and depression. In children, noise has considerable negative cognitive performance effects on reading, attention, and long-term and working memory. Chronic exposure to noise and to crowding has been associated with increased vulnerability to negative motivational effects, also called *learned helplessness*. This refers to a syndrome in which individuals exposed to an undesirable and uncontrollable stimulus (noise pollution in this case) learn to adapt themselves to the fact that their efforts to control or escape from it are futile (Seligman, 1975; Rodin, 1977; S. Cohen et al., 1986). G.W. Evans et al. (1995) concluded from their studies that psychophysiological stress originating from chronic exposure to aircraft noise was related to: coronary heart disease; cognitive functioning, including speech perception, memory and basic reading skills; motivation; and emotional affects among children. They reported higher-than-normal baseline levels of adrenomedullary neuroendocrine, as well as marginally elevated levels of systolic blood pressure, in children chronically exposed to community noise. Differential cardiovascular reactivity in response to task demands was observed among noise-exposed children, indicating chronic environmental stress. Among the cognitive processes affected, they reported slight reductions in working memory, poorer long-term recall ability, reading deficits, poorer motivation levels, and higher annoyance levels. G.W. Evans et al. (1995) further observed that, in reference to children from quieter environments, those chronically exposed to noise exhibited reduced sensitivity to distracting and background noise during a speech perception task. In another study, Lercher et al. (2002) considered the relationships between ambient noise levels and multiple mental health indices among 1280 elementary school children after controlling for individual-level confounders of age, sex, education, house type and household density. They reported a linear dose–response function. Early biological risks, especially low birth weight and pre-term delivery, aggravated the psychological impacts of noise exposure. More specifically, exposure to community noise was associated with psychological symptoms and quality of life primarily in those children with a pre-existing biological risk (such as low birth weight). Exposure to aircraft and road traffic noise at home and in school has also been found to have negative implications on the health and cognitive development of children. Exposure to aircraft noise has been associated with the impairment of children's cognition, negatively affecting tasks involving central processing and language comprehension, such as reading, giving attention, problem solving, reading comprehension, long-term memory and motivation (G.W. Evans and Maxwell, 1997; Haines et al., 2001a, 2001b; Hygge et al., 2002; Stansfeld et al., 2005). In their study of 2844 school children aged 9–10 years in the Netherlands, Spain and the UK, Stansfeld et al. (2005) found linear associations between exposure to chronic aircraft noise and impairment of reading comprehension and recognition memory. On the contrary, a non-linear association was established between aircraft noise exposure and annoyance, both in their uncontrolled models and subsequent to adjustments for mother's education, socio-economic status, long-standing illness and extent of classroom insulation against noise. Exposure to road traffic noise was linearly associated with levels of annoyance and impairment of quality of life. Interestingly they also observed that exposure to road traffic noise was associated with improved episodic memory scores, in terms of conceptual recall and information recall.

4.2 FACTORIZING THE HOUSING-LEVEL DETERMINANTS OF MENTAL HEALTH

The housing environment may be viewed as the private, psychosocial space that facilitates and constrains the desired activities of its occupants. Good-quality housing tends to minimize stress and aid the accomplishment of sound health. Furthermore, each individual dwelling unit helps construct the form and structure of its larger neighbourhood, and it is wrong, therefore, to view issues of housing quality as disjointed from the overall neighbourhood context of which they form a part. The physical and socio-economic characteristics of the surrounding neighbourhood play a significant and consistent role in defining the health of residents. For example, at the community level, one of the factors that often results in health inequity is the disparity in the distribution of good standard housing. Sub-standard, overcrowded homes are generally associated with neighbourhoods characterized by low socio-economic status and other indicators of urban decay (Wandersman and Nation, 1998).

4.2.1 Factor H8: Housing Type, Floor Level and Mental Health

Several studies have suggested that multi-unit dwellings and multi-storeyed housing have adverse implications on the mental health of inhabitants. The hypothesis is typically framed in terms of social withdrawal and confinement: the levels of communication between families living in such dwellings are much reduced compared to the levels for those living in landed houses, resulting in isolation and loneliness. In enclosed multi-storeyed residential environments, the physical proximity to other living units, doorway orientation to common access ways and interaction nodes, and the presence of porches, balconies, terraces and patios govern the level of visual exposure and access to neighbours, and all may have implications for mental health. Lack of lobbies, lounges and other communal gathering spaces results in reduced residential control, lack of a sense of ownership or territoriality, and difficulty in developing and maintaining social networks (Festinger, 1963).

In a pioneering study, Fanning (1967) performed an assessment of the health status of families of members of the armed services personnel stationed in Germany, comparing those living in flats with those residing in houses. In a sample of 558 families, he reported a 57 per cent higher morbidity among inhabitants of the flats compared to house dwellers, especially with respect to the incidence of respiratory infections in young women and children, and that of psychoneurotic disorders in women. Psychological strain among apartment dwellers varied directly with the floor level on which their dwelling units were located. The odds of incidence of psychoneuroses in women living in the top (third) floor were reported to be twice as high in reference to those who lived on the ground floor. Furthermore, there was a steady increase in incidence as the height of the residence increased. Robert E. Mitchell (1971) also highlighted the higher degree of segregation and corresponding emotional strain in residents of multi-family buildings living in upper-floor levels of high-density housing in Hong Kong. He observed a positive association between floor level and emotional illness and hostility, but only for residents living with non-related people in one dwelling. Gillis (1977) investigated the relationship between the various facets of high-density design (shared walls, shared floors, shared ceilings, floor level of dwelling unit), internal density (persons per room) and external density (persons per acre), and psychological strain, with sex as an interacting variable, in 442 residents of the Canadian cities of Edmonton and Calgary. Gillis (1977) observed a positive correlation between floor level and psychological strain among women and an inverse relationship in men. Also, a negative relationship between shared floor and strain among women existed, pointing to the insecurity experienced by women living on the ground floor. Hannay (1981) tried to measure the mental symptoms among 964 adult Scots living in mixed dwelling types. He observed that the residents of the fifth floor of high-rise dwellings exhibited twice the number of mental symptoms compared to those living on lower floors of high-rise buildings or other housing types. J.N. Edwards et al. (1982) studied marital relationships and psychiatric problems among 560 family members with dependent children, living in single-family detached and multi-family housing. They reported more psychiatric and parental problems among men living in multi-family housing, whereas the difference was minimal in the case of women. Both men and women living in multi-family housing had more marital problems in the form of arguments, threats to leave, and so on. In another study, conducted on 674 English adults living in diverse housing, P. McCarthy et al. (1985) reported higher levels of psychological distress among residents of high-rise housing within neighbourhoods of low socio-economic status. In well-off neighbourhoods, the effect of housing type was non-significant. In a study conducted upon 600 African American elderly residents living in high-rise buildings and detached homes, Husaini et al. (1991) observed higher rates of depression and psychiatric disorders and social isolation among the high-rise-dwelling elderly people.

Enhanced rates of behavioural ailments in children living in high-rise and multiple-dwelling complexes in comparison to those residing in single-family homes or smaller, low-rise buildings have been highlighted in many studies (Ineichen and Hooper, 1974; Richman, 1977; Saegert, 1982a; Oda et al., 1989). Rates of juvenile delinquency are also higher among adolescents in multiple-dwelling units relative to those in single-family detached homes (Gillis, 1974). In large apartments and other multi-dwelling residences, absence of adequate play spaces, gardens and greenery constrains children into smaller places with limited social contacts as well as opportunities for play and physical activity. Such restrained outdoor play behaviour has been associated with pre-school distress (Bartlett, 1998). Parental practices in enclosed high-rise residential environments tend to be more rigid and restrictive, and these, it is believed, manifest themselves in the form of impaired or undeveloped emotional and social adaptation and associated behavioural problems (W.F.R. Stewart, 1970).

Generally, multi-family dwellings tend to be more proximate to busy streets and have exposure to higher levels of traffic volume and pollution, and residents tend to be more socially withdrawn, with a lesser likelihood of knowing their neighbours (Appleyard and Lintell, 1972; Mueller et al., 1990). Housing tenure or the occupancy status is another important factor that has been found to influence the health of residents. A dwelling may be either occupied by the owner or rented (Howden-Chapman, 2004). In the case of owner-occupied homes, they may be owned outright, share-owned or owned with a mortgage. Rented dwellings may be rented from the local council, housing association or registered social landlord, outright from a private landlord or through a letting agent. Generally, home owners, outright or with a mortgage, tend to report a greater sense of satisfaction, security and control and consequently a better health status than those who rent their house. A few British studies have highlighted such variations in health status between owners and tenants (Ellaway and Macintyre, 1998; Macintyre et al., 1998, 2001). They observed that, in addition to being a marker of income, which is a direct predictor of health, housing tenure may have an independent effect on health on account of its association with housing stressors and types of area, which may themselves be directly health damaging.

4.2.2 Factor H9: Housing Quality and Mental Health

The overall quality of housing, often parameterized by the existence of structural deficiencies, presence of cold, damp and mouldy interiors, pest infestation, level of indoor air quality and noise, level of housing dissatisfaction, and so on, has a considerable influence on psychological processes and thereby affects mental health. Most cross-sectional studies indicate that poor housing quality is associated with elevated levels of psychological stress among residents. This may be attributed to the negative perception of stigma and neglect associated with people living in poorly maintained houses in impoverished neighbourhoods. They feel disjointed from the larger community, resulting in poor social capital and support, enhanced stress and dissatisfaction, poor self-esteem and self-efficacy, and a general lack of well-being (Halpern, 1995). Another source of anxiety and worry may originate from insecurity related to structural hazards and lack of proper hygiene in poor-quality housing. Physical hazards posed to elderly residents owing to step design, flooring material, lighting and so on may have an aggravating effect on their physical and mental health (van Rossum et al., 1993).

Hyndman (1990) reported significant associations between damp, mouldy and cold indoor environments and elevated levels of anxiety and depression. Gabe and Williams (1993) reported a J-shaped relationship between household density and psychological distress in women. Furthermore, the women were more prone to the detrimental effects of overcrowding compared to men, often manifested in sleep deprivation, dissatisfaction with housing repairs and cleanliness, and the stress of unwanted rehousing. Platt et al. (1990), in their study that controlled for social class, employment status and household income, reported significant levels of association between damp housing conditions and female scoring on a General Health Questionnaire (GHQ). In another study, conducted by Packer et al. (1994), damp housing conditions were found to be associated with a significantly greater likelihood of reported problems related to lack of energy, sleep and social isolation after adjusting for age, sex and social class. A study conducted on 451 Glasgow residents aged 17–65 demonstrated that household dampness resulted in higher odds of mental health disorders among its residents subsequent to statistical adjustment for socio-economic status. A potential cause of social isolation of residents of sub-standard housing may be the occupants' reluctance to invite guests into their homes (Hopton and Hunt, 1996). On the contrary, K.J. Collins (1993) reported a linkage between excessive indoor temperature and higher degrees of irritability and social intolerance. In another study, conducted by Weich and Lewis (1998), data on 9064 UK adults aged 16–75 years from the British Household Panel Survey reported that common mental disorders measured by the 12-item General Health Questionnaire were significantly associated with a poor material standard of living. One of the standard-of-living indicators of the study included the presence and number of structural housing problems, namely damp, condensation, leaking roof, and/or rot in wood. Zahner et al. (1985) performed a longitudinal study on 337 Black and Latino US women, controlling for income, and reported that rat infestation was consistently associated with increased psychological symptoms.

Other studies have focused on the relationships between overall housing quality indices and the state of the mental health of residents. Obasanjo (1999) studied housing quality of 680 urban African American adolescents aged 13–19 years based on eight self-reported parameters of housing maintenance. After statistically controlling for socio-economic status, race, age and gender, housing quality was a significant predictor of social support, directed attention fatigue and psychosomatic illness. G.W. Evans et al. (2000) employed trained raters to evaluate the quality of residence and its immediate environment and developed a three-point rating scale using psychometric scaling procedures consisting of six sub-scales: structural quality, privacy, indoor climatic condition, hazards, cleanliness and clutter, and neighbourhood quality. They evaluated psychological distress with the Demoralization Index of the Psychiatric Epidemiological Research Instrument (PERI). Their cross-sectional study of low- and middle-income, White, rural mothers reported that good housing quality was independently associated with lower odds of psychological distress subsequent to adjustments for income. Another longitudinal study assessed the levels of psychological distress before and after moving to better-quality housing. The pre- and post-move psychological distress among low-income African American and White women residing in an urban area was measured using PERI scores. The study reported a significant relationship between changes in housing quality and residualized psychological distress. In another study, Galea, Ahern et al. (2005) examined the impact of internal and external quality of housing and adjoining built environment upon depression in 59 neighbourhoods of New York City. They observed that the residents of neighbourhoods distinguished by poorer physical built environment features were associated with 29–58 per cent greater odds of reporting depression in the preceding six months and 36–64 per cent greater odds of reporting lifetime depression in reference to residents of better-quality neighbourhoods.

Insecurity from crime contributes to psychological stress, and there exists a complementary relationship between poorly maintained dwellings, crime and mental health. It is generally considered that, when a building has more than 50 apartments, residents tend to treat one another as strangers, making them more vulnerable to crime (D.A. Cohen et al., 2003). Territoriality is a characteristic of the physical environment and pertains to the ability to supervise and control use of neighbouring space. Generally, extensive building structures, long interior hallways and lobbies, lack of group spaces, and poor visual surveillance capability (e.g. inability to monitor entrances and places of concealment) have all been associated with reduced supervision, surveillance and sense of ownership (Newman, 1972; R.B. Taylor, 1988; Sampson et al., 1997). Houses located in areas with high traffic speed limits and characterized by fewer fences and barriers, insecure entryways, poor lighting, and fewer signs of being occupied or with low visual access to neighbours (reducing territorial control) are more likely to be burgled (Newman, 1972; Rand, 1984; R.B. Taylor and Harrell, 1996). The presence of vacant or boarded-up housing in a neighbourhood generates increased fear of crime amongst the residents and outsiders and is associated with reduced accessibility to business, markets and community services, thereby contributing to social exclusion and poorer health outcomes (Sampson et al., 1997). Chandola (2001) employed the 1996 British Crime Survey data and reported that the fear of crime was independently associated with poorer self-rated health, subsequent to statistical controls for individual- and household-level socio-economic factors, as well as individual health behaviour. In another study, D.A. Cohen et al. (2003) highlighted the positive association between the number of boarded-up dwellings and rates of gonorrhoea, as well as mortality due to neoplasms, diabetes, homicide and suicide. Some studies have tried to focus on the potential relationships between subsidized public sector housing, often called council housing or affordable housing, and health; however, no conclusive evidence has been demonstrated. In another large-scale study, of 10000 London-based civil servants, Stafford, Chandola et al. (2007) found that the respondents reporting greater fear had 1.93 times higher odds of depression, reported lower mental health scores and were less likely to be physically active.

Several studies have highlighted positive effects of relocating from low-income neighbourhoods in terms of improvements in mental health of both adults and children (P. Elton and Packer, 1986; Delgard and Tambs, 1997; Johnson et al., 2002). On the contrary, low-income residents of sub-standard housing have to deal with the inconveniences of maintenance and are often subjected to higher rates of involuntary relocations (G.W. Evans and Kantrowitz, 2002). Involuntary or uncontrolled housing relocations have been known to produce negative impacts on the psychological health of older adults (Lawton, 1980), in addition to causing socio-emotional stress in children (Adam and Chase-Lansdale, 2002).

4.2.3 Factor H10: Overcrowding and Mental Health

Household overcrowding is synonymous with high-density living and congestion of land, liveable space and facilities. Loss of control over inter-personal relationships and increasing unwanted social interactions have been identified as causes of adverse effects on psychological well-being (D. McCarthy and Saegert, 1979; Saegert, 1982b). Enforced involuntary interactions and loss of privacy result in higher instances of intrusion or unwanted inputs from other residents. This causes potential interferences in individuals' activities. Another potential negative impact of crowding is the impairment of development and maintenance of socially supportive relationships and subsequent social withdrawal (G.W. Evans and Lepore, 1993). Research has increasingly highlighted the association between higher levels of interior residential density (people per room) and elevated levels of psychological distress among adults (Marsella et al., 1970; Hassen, 1977; Gove and Hughes, 1983; Gabe and Williams, 1987; Jain, 1987; G.W. Evans et al., 1989; Lepore et al., 1991). Gove et al. (1979) reported that domestic overcrowding was negatively associated with psychological health subsequent to adjustments for socio-demographic factors and social class. They observed that the subjective perception of crowding was more potent to psychological health than objective crowding. Duckitt (1983) studied the nature of relationships between household crowding and psychological well-being among 433 Coloured South African residents. After controlling for potentially confounding demographic and socio-economic variables, he reported that crowding showed a statistically significant association with negative psychological effects. The nature of variation of the negative effects was non-linear: an initial spike followed by a flattening phase. He explained that crowding introduces psychological discomfort, which creates motivational pressures on individuals resulting in reduction or reorientation of the time spent at home. In a comparative study of differential effects of household crowding across gender, Gove and Hughes (1979) reported that married women had greater reactivity to crowding than their male counterparts. Fuller et al. (1996) studied the nature of the relationship between crowding and five indices of psychological well-being (measured in terms of psychological distress, unhappiness, irritability, 'losing your mind' and 'contemplating suicide') among 2017 randomly selected households in Bangkok. Crowding was operationalized in terms of both objective and subjective components. Objective crowding was measured with the help of three indicators, namely persons per room, persons per hundred-square-metre area in the dwelling unit, and others per room. Subjective crowding was associated with the experience of crowding originating from inability to achieve desired levels of privacy, and was measured using a 'lack of privacy' scale. Subsequent to statistical adjustments for sex of respondents, socio-economic status, household structure, stage in the family life cycle and household control, they reported that objective crowding was mediated by subjective crowding, and was non-beneficially associated with well-being. The study could not identify any gender differences. Furthermore, the effects of both objective and subjective crowding were identical in both two- and three-generation households, as well as in one- and multiple-couple households. Zlunick and Altman (1972) made a distinction between residential crowding and community or urban crowding, with the former referring to the interior density or the number of people per house or room, and the latter to exterior density or number of people or houses in the neighbourhood. The nature of configuration of the two types of density in an urban setting governs the degree of interpersonal contacts and the stimulation produced in a person both inside and outside the residence. Stokols (1976, 1978) identifies a two-level hierarchy of social environments: primary and secondary environments. The primary environments (especially our homes and offices) are where the personal interferences originate as a result of the individual staying in them over long periods of time, maintaining close social relations, and behaving appropriately in a manner well recognized by the fellow members. Secondary environments are more of a source of neutral interferences as a result of encounters that are often transient, casual and intermittent, having minimal effects on the relationships established. Crowding caused by personal interferences in primary environments has stronger and more persistent impacts upon mental health as compared to crowding produced by neutral interferences in secondary environments.

Wachs and Gruen (1982) highlighted the delayed cognitive development evidenced in pre-school children dwelling in overcrowded homes. G.W. Evans, Lercher et al. (2002) have studied the potential role of built environment design in exacerbating or improving the deleterious impacts of overcrowding upon the mental health of children. They observed positive correlations between residential density (people per room), housing type (single-family, row house, multiple-dwelling unit) and a standardized self-reported index of psychological health (KINDL), as well as teacher ratings of behavioural conduct among 1236 third- and fourth-grade Austrian children. They concluded that the relations between residential density and psychological well-being are moderated by housing type. Children residing in multiple-family residences exhibited greater reactivity to high-density environments than those living in either single-family or row houses.

A better-designed inner residential environment has the potential to foster better regulation of interpersonal contacts. A. Baum and Valins (1979) conducted a series of studies showing that long-corridor dormitory designs caused elevated crowding and greater problems with respect to the regulation of social interaction in comparison with either suites or short-corridor designs. In a follow-up study, the negative effects of crowding were further exacerbated in a redesigned environment, wherein long-corridor dormitories were remodelled in order to reduce the number of residents sharing a common corridor (A. Baum and Davis, 1980). G.W. Evans et al. (1996) employed space syntax analysis to measure the degree of integration (connectivity) of residential floor plan configuration among off-campus student housing units. Floor plans with greater 'depth' (more spaces that are less connected) indicated a higher level of separation and lower integration, thereby acting as buffers to the crowding–distress relationship. The existence of an array of niches for social contact, such as intimate private spaces, group spaces for close-knit small network interactions, community spaces such as parks, and community centres for large-scale interactions, has been associated with greater perceived control and comfort in residential settings. The size, location and permeability of interior rooms govern the level of social control afforded and hence the interactions among residents (Zimring, 1983; G.W. Evans et al., 1996).

Gómez-Jacinto and Hombrados-Mendieta (2002) conducted two cross-sectional studies on 191 and 259 residents of Malaga, Spain, to identify the multiple effects of interaction between community and household crowding, reporting similar results. A strong interaction between both kinds of density was thought to intensify the negative effects of both stressors on residential satisfaction. On employing an interactive model for both densities, high community density was reported to have strong negative effects on psychological stress only when household density was also high. In other words, community density effects are cancelled out by an optimal density within the household. Furthermore, in low-density communities, increments in household density resulted in a slight reduction in psychological stress, emphasizing the role played by increased levels of social support in high-density households.

On the contrary, research has pointed to the fact that high-density neighbourhoods are generally associated with more walking. Ross and Dunning (1997) analysed the results of the National Personal Transportation Survey, 1995, and observed that, in the densest neighbourhoods with over 3000 dwelling units per square mile, 14.9 per cent of the trips were made on foot or bicycle, while, in the least dense areas with fewer than 100 dwelling units per square mile, trips made on foot or bicycle formed only 3.3 per cent, indicating an almost fivefold reduction. Thus planning at the neighbourhood level should envisage an appropriate mix of the different categories of housing, in terms of housing type, affordability and tenure. The availability of diverse housing options arms the households with an opportunity to find a dwelling consonant with their income and needs, thereby reducing housing stress and consequent ill health. The policy of housing diversity tends to facilitate a diverse social mix, thereby inhibiting social exclusion, and promotes a sense of community, which can have positive health effects.

4.3 NEIGHBOURHOOD-LEVEL DETERMINANTS OF HEALTH

In the United Kingdom, the publication of the Black Report in 1980 by the Working Group on Health Inequalities was a significant landmark, reorienting interest towards neighbourhood-level determinants of health. It initiated developments in the empirical measurement of socio-economic status, health inequalities and premature deaths, as well as longitudinal designs and linkages with census-level data (Department of Health and Social Security, 1980; Macintyre, 1997). With the increasing consensus among epidemiologists that risk factors operate at population levels and that there is a need to assess cumulative population-level socio-economic factors, the importance of contextual factors gained predominance (Rose, 1985; Susser, 1994a, 1994b; McMichael, 1999). It has been hypothesized that, in addition to individual predispositions, the specific socio-economic, cultural, physical and built environment attributes of a place influence our health-related behaviours and exposure to risk factors, and thereby configure the health outcomes and mortality. The case for due consideration to place effects was seminally articulated by Townsend et al. (1992) by stressing the importance of the local neighbourhood. Based on the UK

Health and Lifestyle data, Blaxter (1990) highlighted the role of the external living environment in the significant geographical variations in lifestyle. Macintyre et al. (1993) discuss whether the origins of area-level differences in health outcomes are compositional or contextual in nature.

Most of the initial research tended to concentrate on large-scale ecological studies involving aggregated area-level measures of exposures to specific socio-economic variables such as income, educational attainment, occupational levels and indices of deprivation, while health has typically been expressed in terms of aggregated mortality and morbidity. Lack of data at the individual level meant that aggregate measures merely acted as surrogates for individual-level data. Through the aggregation effects of selection, distribution, interaction, adaptation and so on, ecological models have generally been argued to be successful in capturing contextual effects that cannot be analysed at an individual level. Proponents of these studies highlighted their effectiveness in identifying population patterns and studying the emerging public health impact of policies, as illustrated by this 1992 quote:

> Although ecological studies are clearly inferior when the purpose of research is to isolate 'independent' risk factor–disease associations, they are essential for addressing population characteristics such as epidemic cycles or economic relations. The ecological design is chosen here not as a substitute for a 'superior' individual study, but as a tool for investigating population-level determinants of disease that cannot be addressed with individual-level study designs. (Wing et al. 1992, p. 204)

Most studies employ data aggregated at the levels of census-defined regional and local geographies. The Office of Population Censuses and Surveys (OPCS) longitudinal survey of England and Wales followed up 1 per cent of the population of the 1971 census to link them to subsequent censuses and vital statistics. Significant variations in mortality were observed across the 36 types of places (Fox and Goldblatt, 1982; Fox et al., 1984). Another study employed the same survey data to classify local authority districts into 30 socio-residential clusters based on housing tenure and social class and reported significant differences in mortality between the areas or clusters (Britton et al., 1990). Eames et al. (1993) conducted an ecological study of the association between premature mortality and social deprivation, operationalized in terms of a Carstairs index, Townsend index, and underprivileged area score across 14 regional health authorities covering 8464 electoral wards of England. Higher mortality from all causes, coronary heart disease and smoking-related diseases was found to be significantly associated with increasing area-level deprivation scores. Another decadal English study noted significant differences in life expectancies across 105 district health authorities (DHAs) in relation to the Jarman deprivation scores of the DHAs, with deprived areas manifesting lesser longevity and higher gender differentiation (Raleigh and Kiri, 1997). A comparable study identified area-level educational attainment and deprivation as significant predictors of all-cause, coronary and infant mortality in 107 local educational authorities of England (Morris et al., 1996). Shouls et al. (1996) developed an area typology based on the clustering of a set of variables pertaining to life stage, ethnic composition and socio-economic status for 278 sample of anonymized records (SAR) districts of England from the 1991 census, and studied the association with mortality and morbidity. Limiting long-term illness and premature mortality were found to be significantly associated with area-level socio-economic conditions and the urban–rural divide. The study also highlighted the prevalent North–South divide in health. Results along similar lines were reported in many of the simultaneous large-scale US studies. In one of the earliest studies employing census tract data for Houston, Briggs and Leonard (1977) observed that the mortality differentials were significantly associated with socio-economic disadvantage. Wing et al. (1987) studied the relationship between the population-weighted age-adjusted rates of ischaemic heart disease (IHD) and occupational structure across 3102 counties of the US. A lower IHD mortality was associated with communities having higher fractions of white-collar employment for both men and women. A subsequent study conducted exclusively for White women in the US identified that the structural economic parameters of the state economic areas (SEAs), especially average income, educational attainment and occupational levels, determined the shape of the CHD epidemic curve (Wing et al., 1992). In another study, Logue and Jarjoura (1990) found that the risks of age- and sex-adjusted census tract specific heart disease mortality among the lower-middle-class and the working-poor category were respectively 1.9 and 4.5 times the rate observed in the referent upper-middle- and middle-class category.

Much of these well-intentioned epidemiological studies, however, are deemed less meaningful on the grounds of a long-standing critique (Thorndike, 1939; Robinson, 2011) that the relationships observed at the aggregate level cannot provide an accurate manifestation of individual-level relationships. Selvin (1958) coined the term *ecological fallacy* to illustrate the bias associated with attempts to extrapolate data from area-level analysis to make inferences at an individual level (a fundamental inferential fallacy). More precisely, there exists a bidirectional inferential fallacy (Alker, 1969; Susser, 1994a; Diez-Roux, 1998; N. Pearce, 2000). In individual risk factor analysis, the failure to statistically control for the effects of population context leads to the *atomistic/individualistic fallacy*, wherein a predominantly individualistic approach overlooks the contextual aggregation effects and may also be prone to specification bias. On the other hand, large-scale ecological studies are prone to bias from aggregation effects as well as specification errors.

Sociologists point out that social processes are operationalized at population levels and are manifested over spatial aggregates within which the social groups function, and these aggregate effects configure an individual's exposure and vulnerability to risks. Hence, the aggregated area-level factors pertaining to variables relating to demographics, lifestyle, socio-economics and deprivation reflect how the cumulative health-defining characteristics of individuals such as education, employment, income, deprivation, socio-economic status, social capital, and so on are distributed in a specific place and over a specific population. It has been highlighted that these contextual macro-level factors have an independent effect upon an individual's health outcome (Blalock and Wilken, 1979). It is also noteworthy that almost simultaneously, over the same period, there has been a substantial development in statistical techniques that has led to the proliferation of models and software that have the capability to handle hierarchical data structures (C. Duncan et al., 1998; Diez Roux, 2001). All these developments have led to the evolution of a new epidemiological approach aimed at minimizing the bidirectional inferential fallacies wherein, in addition to the micro-level compositional (individual) variables, a set of macro-level group or area variables are used to simultaneously capture the myriad social processes considered important in the causation of disease. Such modelling approaches that incorporate area-level ecological measures of socio-economic context into the individual-level risk equations are termed multi-level or contextual analysis (Von Korff et al., 1992; Diez-Roux, 1998). Two categories of group-level variables are typically included in such models: the derived variables, which are aggregated analogues of individual-level variables within the group or area; and the integral variables, which pertain to the intrinsic characteristics of the group or area as a whole. Such models are operationalized by using a regression equation in which the variances and errors are partitioned into individual- and aggregate- (or spatial-)level factors, thereby being able to deal with the ecological fallacy problem as well as overcoming the issue of the lack of contextualization in earlier individual-based models.

In recent years an increasing number of studies have reported a variety of area aggregated measures of poverty and socio-economic deprivation to be significantly associated with health outcomes after adjustments for individual-level variables (Pickett and Pearl, 2001). In a nine-year prospective study of the impact of socio-physical environment in Alameda County, Haan et al. (1987) observed significantly higher rates of mortality among the residents of poverty areas as compared to non-poverty areas, the differences persisting even after subsequent statistical adjustments for individual-level socio-demographic, lifestyle and health factors (age, sex, race, baseline physical health status, low income, lack of medical care, smoking, unemployment, education, health practices, social isolation and psychological uncertainty). Diehr et al. (1993) reported significant areal variations in the four lifestyle behaviours of smoking, consumption of alcohol, consumption of dietary fat and use of seatbelts, independent of individual characteristics; and the magnitude of area effects was reported to be less than 1 per cent. Waitzman and Smith (1998) conducted another national-level study employing the data from National Health and Nutrition Examination Survey (NHANES) I and observed significantly higher risks of all-cause, cardiovascular and cancer mortality among those aged 25–54 years subsequent to adjustments for a number of individual and household characteristics. In another study in four US communities, Diez Roux et al. (1997) concluded that neighbourhood context shaped the population distribution of coronary heart disease such that living in deprived neighbourhoods was associated with increased odds of coronary heart disease and exposures to risk factors, with the associations persisting after adjustments for individual-level variables. From their studies conducted in the towns of Renfrew and Paisley in West Scotland, Davey Smith et al. (1998) observed that both individual social class and area-level deprivation were independently and inversely associated with all-cause and cardiovascular disease mortality. They advocated that socio-economic measures in epidemiological studies should be operationalized at both individual and neighbourhood levels to overcome any residual confounding. Along similar lines, J.W. Lynch et al. (2000) argued for the necessity to employ measures of income distribution as well as individual income to identify the multi-level health differentials across individuals and aggregated spatial units. Another multi-level Swedish study identified higher hazards of coronary heart disease among individuals living in neighbourhoods associated with lower area-level income and education independent of individual-level variables (Sundquist et al., 2004).

Some studies, though, have reported negligible contextual effects. In a nine-year follow-up study of 300 000 respondents of the Office of Population Censuses and Surveys, Sloggett and Joshi (1994) found that all-cause mortality was significantly associated with ward-level deprivation for both men and women. However, adjustments for the regional zone and wide range of individual socio-economic circumstances (economic activity, social class, presence of spouse, car access and housing tenure) progressively minimized and explained away the effect of ward deprivation in men, while it was strongly attenuated in the case of women. The study thus could find no evidence of social miasma whereby living within deprived areas was independently associated with higher rates of mortality. Another subsequent study conducted by the same team similarly found no evidence of area-level deprivation upon adverse fertility events in women (Sloggett and Joshi, 1998). Another comparative study of mortality differences between West Scotland and South England concluded that the regional variations originated on account of differences in the distribution of deprivation among individuals in the two areas rather than differences between the places per se (Davey Smith et al., 1995).

A number of multi-level studies have attempted to evaluate the magnitude of place effects by partitioning the variances into *between-individual (within-area)* and *between-area* effects in addition to adjustments for individual- and area-level variables. Stressing the significance of within-area correlations in a social epidemiologic context, Merlo (2003) points out that a higher correlation is synonymous with a greater homogeneity in the health outcomes of individuals within a neighbourhood, which in turn reflects the potential effects of neighbourhood context upon the determinants of individual health. Humphreys and Carr-Hill (1991) employed data from the Health and Lifestyle survey data to construct a series of two-level models with significant ward-level variability in health outcomes after controlling for individual socio-economic characteristics and health-related behaviour. K. Jones and Duncan (1995) employed a similar study design on a larger sample size, also allowing for complex interactions, and reported similar findings. C. Duncan et al. (1993) constructed a three-level model upon the Health and Lifestyle survey data to study the geographical variations in lifestyle behaviour with respect to smoking and alcohol consumption across the UK. They reported a predominantly individual-level effect, with negligible place effects across wards and regions. A similar subsequent study observed no significant variations in psychiatric morbidity at the ward and regional levels of the UK. Furthermore, the study demonstrated that compositional attributes were a predominant determinant of mental health, with no neighbourhood effects (C. Duncan et al., 1995).

Several conceptual and methodological challenges still remain to be overcome in multi-level epidemiological studies. Several authors have highlighted the issues with respect to causal inference and the lack of theory on the mechanisms as to how neighbourhood-level factors configure the risks and thereby health outcomes (O'Campo, 2003; Oakes, 2004). The second point pertains to the choice of optimized definition of areal units or neighbourhoods with respect to size and degree of heterogeneity so that it can accurately capture the population-level socio-economic, political, cultural, environmental and institutional processes within it (Diez Roux, 2001; O'Campo, 2003). It may be noted that this is all the more difficult without well-formed theory about the causal process resulting in the alleged area or aggregate effects. Thirdly, these models are sensitive to the choice of individual- and area-level variables, and hence due care should be given so as to avoid misspecification of models at the more important individual level and to avoid psychologistic and sociologistic fallacies (Riley, 1963; Diez Roux, 2001).

Since the early 2000s, in addition to neighbourhood-level socio-demographic and deprivation variables, urban planners, epidemiologists and public health scientists have conducted extensive research into the role of the neighbourhood built environment. They have attempted to unravel Macintyre's *black box* of *contextual determinants of health*. The independent association of both objective and subjective built environment factors (as neighbourhood-level factors) with individual health outcomes after adjustments for individual-level covariates has become an important field of research.

The remaining chapters of this book continue in a similar tradition by asking the basic question: is there a *miasma* of urban built environment factors that influence health and behaviour? The book both reviews the research evidence in the field and goes on to add new evidence using a new method of capturing more accurate objective built environment contextual data (employing methods from graph theory to measure network accessibility effects).

We conclude this section by quoting Sally Macintyre's following remark, which highlights the importance of studying the contextual determinants of health:

> 'Context' is thus often treated as a residual category, containing those factors influencing human health behaviours or health, which remains once every imaginable individual characteristic is taken into account. It is indeed a black box, an unspecified 'miasma' which somehow, but we don't know how, influences some aspect of health, health related behaviour or health risks in some population groups. (Macintyre et al. 2002, p. 129)

4.3.1 Factorizing Neighbourhood-Level Determinants of Health

There has been a growing consensus amongst epidemiologists that built environmental factors, especially those influencing healthy eating, physical activity behaviour and social interactions, are independent predictors of health outcomes. The defensive role of physical activity in offsetting a number of chronic diseases, both independently and via its inhibitory effects on weight gain and obesity, has been long acknowledged. Similarly, the health-promoting and -inhibiting influences of the neighbourhood built environment upon mental health outcomes is well established. The projected worldwide increase in the older adult population further exacerbates the problem. With reduced physical capacity, the aged tend to be more vulnerable to the inhibiting influences of their immediate activity space, tending to lead more sedentary lifestyles and thereby be prone to health risks.

Given the positive health implications of physical activity, recent decades have witnessed considerable community-based initiatives to achieve appropriate levels of physical activity. A strong research agenda has emerged that poses the question: what attributes of the neighbourhood built environment promote physical activity and health? Neighbourhood streets have been recognized as the most obvious sites for engaging in physically active behaviour, and this has led to the emergence of the popular concept of *neighbourhood walkability*.

Neighbourhood walkability may be conceptualized as the degree to which the physical characteristics of the built environment may be conducive to or inhibitive of facilitating local residents to walk or cycle for leisure and recreation, exercise or transport to services or workplace destinations. Aspects of land use, transportation, and community design have been identified as governing factors, influencing the extent to which residents are physically active, with reduced dependence on automobiles. Handy (1992) stressed the importance of accessibility in this context, as she tried to assess the impact of alternative urban forms upon shopping travel patterns. She considered two components of accessibility, namely micro-level local accessibility, which calculated the closeness to local opportunities of activity, and macro-level regional accessibility, associated with the degree of connectivity to large regional service destinations. Comparing the levels of local and regional accessibility of the Santa Clara and Santa Rosa valleys of the San Francisco Bay Area, Handy found that residents of high-local-accessibility areas generally reported significantly higher-than-average walking trips to local commercial destinations. Furthermore, in higher-regional-accessibility areas, the downtown shopping trips did not appear to substitute for trips to regional shopping centres. On the contrary, in low-regional-accessibility areas, the downtown shopping trips acted as a substitute for regional trips to some extent. In a subsequent study conducted on the San Francisco Bay Area, Handy (1996) highlighted the role of urban form, concluding that residents of traditional neighbourhoods with higher physical accessibility to community resources are generally associated with a higher proportion of walking trips. Another important study was conducted by Frank and Pivo (1994) on the relationships between urban land use configuration and travel mode choice in terms of use of single-occupant vehicles (SOVs), mass transit, and walking for shopping and work trips. They employed data from the Puget Sound

Transportation Panel, the US Census Bureau and three local agencies in Washington State and reported that configuration indices of both density and land use mix were significantly associated with travel mode choice. In a pioneering work, Cervero and Kockelman (1997) employed travel and socio-economic data derived from the 1990–91 Bay Area Travel Survey (BATS), and data on land use design and configuration collected through field surveys of 50 sampled neighbourhoods in the San Francisco area, and introduced the concept of the 3Ds – density, diversity and pedestrian-oriented designs – as the dimensions of the built environment that have statistically significant influences on active transport. Subsequently, two more Ds, in the form of destination accessibility and distance to transit stops, were added to the list to make it 5Ds (Ewing and Cervero, 2001; Ewing et al., 2009). Lee and Moudon (2006b) highlighted the importance of the availability of fine-grained data and GIS analysis at intricate spatial levels in walkability research. They considered a set of objectively measured micro-scale built environment variables in their study. Identification of variables involved initial screening, iterative grouping, weighing and statistical modelling to obtain a parsimonious model fit. They were able to isolate a small subset of built environment correlates of walking, which were grouped as destination, distance, density and route, i.e. 3D + R.

Researchers have therefore considered various groups of measures to assess the degree of walkability of urban neighbourhood environments. The identification of a reliable cluster of measures, as well as the relative importance of each, is still in contention, however. One of the major bottlenecks is the scarcity of micro-scale data on built environmental variables as well as those related to non-motorized activity. Another complication stems from the nature of the measures, with some aspects of the built environment being easily captured through objectively measured variables (subject to availability of fine-scale data), while others are more subjective in nature. A review of studies suggests that a mix of quantitatively measured objective variables and surveyed subjective measures has typically been employed. There has been an increasing inclination to employ GIS-based objective measures, however, to operationalize the physical constructs of the microenvironment. Definitions of 'neighbourhood' have ranged from a 0.25 mile street network buffer around a respondent's house to an entire census tract. Another inherent oversimplification originates from the fact that the definition of neighbourhood is fuzzy in nature. The question 'How local is local?' is difficult to answer, as no clear-cut quantitative definition exists and the answer is essentially based on the assumptions and purpose of the study. A study defining a neighbourhood in terms of a network buffer of a 0.25 mile radius around a respondent's household is basically assuming that the built environment within the defined environment influences the health outcomes and that this influence is uniform across demographic scales. In reality, health-defining behaviour such as physical activity is often determined by individual preferences, which may depend on factors such as age, race, gender, social class and so on. However, current definitions of neighbourhood in health studies can seldom take into account the attenuations produced on account of overlooking such individual characteristics. Furthermore, the characteristics of the urban built environment vary at the national, regional and global scales, which further hinders the use of a set of standardized measures. Most of the studies conducted in this field are cross-sectional in nature, which has been criticized for not addressing the issue of selective migration and self-selection. There is therefore a need to construct longitudinal designs for future studies. In reviewing the evidence from published studies, six principal determinants of public health at the neighbourhood level seem to be important, namely: density; diversity; destination accessibility (retail, green space, physical activity facilities, food environments); route connectivity; distance to transit stops; and pedestrian-oriented design (presence of pedestrian and cycling infrastructure, aesthetics, perception of safety). Composite measures of the built environment in the form of indices consisting of more than one of the above-mentioned six determinants as component sub-indices have also been employed. The evidence for each of these is reviewed in the following sections, with hypothesized causes denoted as factors, with notations N1 . . . Nn.

Factor N1: density/intensity

Density, one of the most widely used measures in urban planning, refers to the quantity of people, dwelling units, jobs or specific service destinations distributed per unit of land area such as acre, square kilometre or square mile. This can be expressed as a net or gross measure. Population density and residential density are one of the most commonly employed measures used in studies trying to correlate specific features of the built environment with activity behaviour including walking (and thereby with health). Another synonymous measure often employed in built environment–health correlations is land use intensity. Land use intensity is often expressed in terms of counts or densities of specific service destinations in a defined neighbourhood. In GIS terminology, neighbourhoods are defined by drawing an airline or network buffer of a predefined radius around a dwelling unit. The proportion of the area occupied by different categories of land uses or services is measured, or the number of different facilities is simply counted. Density and intensity reflect the degree of mixed use in an area. The popularity of these measures originates from the ease of data availability at appropriate aggregated geographical scales and inherent computational simplicity. As the land use density increases, trip origins and destinations are brought into greater proximity to one another, resulting in greater accessibility to service destinations. Consequently, high-density compact neighbourhoods tend to shorten trip lengths, while increasing the number of trips. In contrast, the number of motorized trips reduces, resulting in higher demand for walking and cycling. High density has been associated with greater land use mix, reduced impervious surfaces in the form of car parks, and a greater fraction of low socio-economic status (SES) population, all of which discourage car dependence. Furthermore, higher demographic heterogeneity and cultural integration create a physical sense of community, contributing to greater community participation and social capital.

Studies examining the associations between attributes of the built environment, health behaviour (such as physical activity or walkability) and health outcomes have employed diverse measures of density and intensity over the years. Ewing et al. (2004) considered measures of overall density (residents + jobs)/area), while Frank et al. (2004, 2006) enumerated net residential density as the number of persons per residential acre in the census block group containing the household. Rutt and Coleman (2005) considered the number of individuals per square mile and operationalized land use as the percentage of non-residential buildings within a person's surrounding neighbourhood. M. Duncan and Mummery (2005) evaluated the number of physically active people in a 1 kilometre radius of the respondent's residence. Li, Fisher, Brownson et al. (2005) used variables for density of places of employment and density of households in their study. Norman et al. (2006) and Kligerman et al. (2007) also included measures of residential density in their study, while Rundle et al. (2007) included population density. C. Lee and Moudon (2006a) calculated both the net residential density within a 1 kilometre catchment area and the number of residential units in the household parcel. Wells and Yang (2008) considered four categories of density in their neighbourhood design–walking correlation study: population density, employment density, housing density and service-job density. B.B. Brown et al. (2009) considered the population density, proportion of residents walking to work, and square kilometres of each of the six land use categories present within the 1 kilometre street network catchment. In their study, Pouliou and Elliott (2010) evaluated both residential density and the density of opportunities. Wood et al. (2010) operationalized their net residential density as the number of residential units per residential acre within a 1 kilometre road network catchment of a household. Yan et al. (2010) considered census tract population density, 3D population density, and the number of housing units in the tract, while Troped et al. (2010) calculated the residential population density as well as housing unit density. Several other studies have tried to focus upon the health implications of urban sprawl based on a sprawl index whose primary components are the population density and residential density (Ewing, Schmid et al., 2003; R. Lopez, 2004; Garden and Jalaludin, 2009; I.M. Lee et al., 2009).

Factor N2: diversity

Diversity or land use mix measures the number of different land uses as well as their spatial arrangement for a given land area, floor area or employment unit. They have been expressed in terms of the degree of mix, typically quantified as measures of entropy, mean entropy, floor area ratio, balance indices, Herfindahl–Hirschman Index (HHI), dissimilarity index and similar.

Cervero (1988) characterized mixed land use developments as being composed of a multiplicity of offices, shops, restaurants, banks and other activities all amalgamated together. Studies have pointed to the fact that compact dense neighbourhoods are synonymous with not only high degrees of land use intensity, but also heterogeneous mix patterns and integration, resulting in an agglomeration of services like retail businesses, offices, schools, churches, health care facilities and so on. The resulting urban form thus consists of fine-grained neighbourhood blocks with enhanced permeability, connectivity and accessibility, thereby reducing the necessity for longer trips. Indirectly, this may be beneficial to active travel and physical activity by reducing the impervious surfaces in the neighbourhood in the form of motorways and parking space for the space-intensive automobiles. By maintaining an optimized neighbourhood land use balance, the diverse yet essential uses are localized at relative proximity, and furthermore this supports and sustains a better integration of diverse services within the community. Increased accessibility to services and shortened trip lengths within a neighbourhood have been known to diversify transit options. Cervero (1988) explained the advantages of mixed-use urban settings in terms of the economies of travel mode – in the form of lower vehicular trip generation rates and higher non-motorized (e.g. walking, bicycling) modal splits, a more even distribution of trips throughout the day and week, and new opportunities for shared parking arrangements. He reported a 3 per cent increment in active travel in the form of transit and ride-sharing commutes with every 10 per cent increase in commercial floor area. In a separate study of shopping trips of residents from four neighbourhoods in the San Francisco Bay Area, Handy (1992) established that residents of traditional, mixed-use neighbourhoods on an average made two to four more walk and cycle trips per week to their neighbourhood retail stores than those living in close proximity to areas that were served primarily by automobile-oriented, strip retail establishments. In another study of six communities of Palm Beach County, Ewing et al. (1994) found that residents of suburban sprawling areas characterized by homogeneous land uses reported approximately 66 per cent more per capita vehicle hours of travel (VHT) in reference to residents of mixed traditional neighbourhoods served by internal community services in the form of shopping, recreation and school facilities. In a subsequent study, Cervero (1996) was able to establish significant levels of association between the presence of community services including grocery stores within 300 feet of a respondent's residence and increased propensity for active travel, after adjusting for residential densities and vehicle ownership levels. Nonetheless, their presence between 300 feet and 1 mile of residences was associated with higher levels of auto-commuting. This was attributed to the relative ease of efficiently linking work and shopping trips through vehicular trips, beyond the threshold of 300 feet. However, they had employed a relatively simple binary measure of land use mixture ranging from 0 to 1, indicating the presence or absence of non-residential uses within some predefined neighbourhood.

At a different level, enhanced land use mix is expected to foster a sense of community and is associated with increments in social capital and resulting positive health outcomes. Compact neighbourhoods with considerable heterogeneity are able to combine diverse uses – dwellings, shops, supermarkets and food stores, offices, recreational facilities, green or open spaces, schools, places of worship and other uses, thereby encouraging walking, which in turn promotes casual social contacts and a sense of community. Nasar and Julian (1995) conducted a series of 25 interviews in four neighbourhoods of Upper Arlington, Ohio, each of which differs with respect to land use mix (having one, two, three and four categories of land uses). They concluded that single-use residential neighbourhoods were associated with a reduced sense of community as compared with those having multiple uses. In another study, Lund (2002) reported a similar trend, wherein increased sense of community was observed in traditional neighbourhoods, manifested by a distinctively accessible road network and an enhanced mix of diverse land use categories.

A quantitative approach to land use mix calculations was first operationalized as a land use balance measurement by Cervero (1989) in a pioneering study of the proportion of suburban employment centres. This originated from the concept of entropy, one of the fundamental principles of statistical thermodynamics. The theory of information entropy owes its origin to the pioneering works by Shannon and Weaver (1949) and employs probability and numerical statistics to express the degree of disorder in a system. The concept has since been expanded to find widespread cross-disciplinary applications in enumerating information entropies of social, economic, ecological systems, especially in assessing the degree of heterogeneity in the distribution of a certain attribute across *many* spatial units of analysis. Following this, Frank and Pivo (1994) employed cohort travel behaviour data from Puget Sound Transportation Panel to study the impacts of urban form on travel mode choice at the level of census tracts. In addition to density, the entropy index was employed as one of the variables of urban form. They employed the following adapted version (normalized between 0 and 0.845) to measure land use mix:

Level of land use mix (entropy value) = −[single-family • $\log_{10}$ (single-family)] + [multifamily • $\log_{10}$ (multifamily)] + [retail and services • $\log_{10}$ (retail and services)] + [office • $\log_{10}$ (office)] + [entertainment • $\log_{10}$ (entertainment)] + [institutional • $\log_{10}$ (institutional)] + [industrial/manufacturing • $\log_{10}$ (industrial/manufacturing)]. (Frank and Pivo, 1994, p. 48)

They concluded that density (both employment and population) and land use mix were beneficially associated with transit usage and walking to work and shopping trips. In a similar vein, increases in density and land use mix resulted in decline in the usage of single-occupant vehicles for work and shopping trips. Furthermore, a recent study examining the impact of transportation, land use and the built environment variables upon individual health outcomes reported that every percentage decrease in auto use would result in reductions in the odds of obesity (0.4 per cent), high blood pressure (0.3 per cent), high blood cholesterol (1.3 per cent) and heart attack (1 per cent) (Samimi and Mohammadian, 2009).

Sometimes a mean entropy index is used instead of just entropy. This is computed as the average of neighbourhood entropies for all developed hectares within each census tract, where the neighbourhood is defined to include all the developed areas within half a mile of each relevant active hectare (Kockelman, 1997). Effectively this enables the overcoming of any bias originating in smaller tracts with relatively little area to accommodate a variety of land use types, as well as ensures a more adequate representation of the concept of 'neighbourhood'. A 'mean entropy' is also used to overcome such biases, as indicated below:

$$\text{Mean Entropy} = \sum_{k} \frac{\Sigma_j \frac{P_{jk} \ln(j)}{\ln(j)}}{K}$$

where K is the number of actively developed hectares in the census tract, j is the number of land use categories, and P_{jk} is the proportion of land use category j within a half-mile radius of the developed area surrounding hectare grid-cell k.

In studies endeavouring to measure associations between built environment and health outcomes, the measure of land use mix (LUM) pioneered by Frank et al. (2004, 2006) is widely employed. It is quantified as follows:

$$\text{LUM} = \left(- \frac{\Sigma_{i=1}^{n} p_i . \ln p_i}{\ln N} \right)$$

where p_i is the proportion of estimated square footage of land use i and N is the number of land uses. The land use mix values normally range from 0 to 1, with 0 representing a homogeneous, single land use environment, while 1 represents a perfectly heterogeneous neighbourhood comprising all possible permutations and combinations of land use categories. In most studies, non-walkable land use destinations are excluded from the LUM scores. Land use mix may have both vertical and horizontal components. Vertical mixing, more common in most of the European cities and the older parts of American cities, consists of different land uses stacked together in a single building, usually retail on the ground floor and housing on top. Horizontal mixing is characterized by the presence of different types of land uses on adjacent or near-adjacent parcels of land. Frank et al. (2004) measured a four-category LUM, calculating the proportion of estimated square footage of residential, commercial, office and institutional uses within a 1 kilometre network buffer from each participant's household. They concluded that land use mix had a strong association with obesity, reporting a 12.2 per cent reduction in the likelihood of obesity across gender and ethnicity with each quartile increase in land uses mix. Frank et al. (2006) employed a similar approach to that of their earlier study, to evaluate a six-category-score (single-family residential, multi-family residential, education, entertainment, retail and office uses) land use mix. Mobley et al. (2006) used an additional category for rural land in their LUM calculations and reported that body mass index (BMI) was lower by 2.60 kg/m^2 and cardiac heart disease risk was lower by 20 per cent in women living in an environment of maximum mixed land use as compared to those living in single-use uniform environments. Cerin, Macfarlane et al. (2007) employed objective measures of land use mix in their study and reported no significant associations between land use mix and weekly minutes of walking for transport. Nonetheless, significant correlations were observed between land use profiles and walking for transport. F. Li et al. (2008) reported a 25 per cent reduction in the prevalence of overweight and obesity with 10 per cent increases in land use mix.

Forsyth et al. (2008) considered a range of parameters to reflect land use mix: entropy index, dissimilarity index and Herfindahl–Hirschman Index; however, interestingly, they reported statistically significant but negative correlations with physical activity outcomes. This points to the need for more probing theory for interpreting the kind of LUM–health correlations reported in this kind of study.

B.B. Brown et al. (2009) discussed some of the limitations associated with land use entropy measurements, especially the insensitivity of entropy measures to particular land use profiles. Two different categories of land use mix equations may produce the same mix scores; and the absence of a particular land use type may modify the walkability of the neighbourhood considerably, but may not alter the entropy score. Furthermore, the entropy score may sometimes confound the degree of walkability of neighbourhoods, so that it may emerge that the mix of a walkable neighbourhood may score the equivalent of that of a less walkable, car-dependent neighbourhood. To partially overcome these issues, B.B. Brown et al. (2009) employed two-, three- and six-category land use mix scores and calculated the number of each of the six land uses within the defined neighbourhood in their study. They reported that the six-category land use mix score was the best predictor of BMI and overweight and obesity outcomes. Troped et al. (2010) estimated the land use mix across four categories (residential, commercial, recreational and urban public) and reported a significant beneficial association between land use mix and moderate to vigorous physical activity within a 1 kilometre home buffer. Pouliou and Elliott (2010) employed measures of a five-category land use mix index for the two metropolitan cities of Toronto and Vancouver and concluded that residents of areas with mixed land uses exhibited improved weight outcomes compared to those living in areas with single or fewer land use types for Vancouver. However, no significant association could be established in the case of Toronto. Wood et al. (2010) considered measures of three-category land use mixes of residential, commercial and office land uses within a 1 kilometre network buffer, as well as the commercial floor area ratio in their study, and reported significant associations with their sense of community (SofC) score. However, contrary to the general trend, land use mix was inversely associated with SofC – those living in low mixed land use areas were 23.27 per cent more likely to have a higher SofC score than respondents in a high mixed land use area. Expectedly, SofC was also positively correlated with higher commercial floor space to land area ratios. In another study, Saarloos et al. (2011) reported similar results. A higher land use mix was independently associated with higher odds of depression among older men. On the contrary, Leslie and Cerin (2008) reported that a more heterogeneous land use mix was beneficially associated with four of the five domains of neighbourhood satisfaction, namely safety and walkability, access to destinations, social network and travel network, which in turn acted as independent predictors of mental health.

Several indices of balance have also been employed to reflect the diversity of the urban neighbourhoods. In their studies, Cervero and Duncan (2003) used an employed residents-to-jobs balance index, and employed residents-to-retail/services balance index within 1 mile of the trip origins and destinations:

Employed residents-to-jobs balance index (within 1 mile of origin) = 1 − {|ABS(ER − JOBS)| /(ER + JOBS)}

Employed residents-to-retail/services balance index (within 1 mile of origin) = 1 − {(|ABS(ER − RS)| / (ER + RS)}. (Cervero and Duncan, 2003, p. 1480)

where ABS = absolute value, ER = number of employed residents, JOBS = number of workers, and RS = number of retail/service jobs.

In another study, Ewing et al. (2004) employed measures of jobs–residence balance and job mix, each index ranging from 0 to 1. Jobs–residence balance reflected the degree of land use balance between jobs and residents within proxy neighbourhoods of traffic analysis zones (TAZs), while job mix quantified the degree of homogeneity of distribution of jobs among the various employment sectors and indicated the degree of land use mixing at the TAZs level, and was defined as:

Job mix = −[commercial jobs × ln(commercial jobs) + industrial jobs × ln(industrial jobs) + service jobs × ln(service jobs)]/ln(3). (Ewing et al., 2004, p. 58)

Wells and Yang (2008) used land use mix measures of jobs-per-resident ratio and service-worker-to-resident ratio, which reflect the prevalence of non-residential land uses in the neighbourhood. In contrast to the general trend, they reported that increases in service-worker-to-resident ratio (increased non-residential uses) were associated with less walking. Norman et al. (2006) calculated land use mix within each 1 mile street network buffer as the geometric mean of residential, institutional, entertainment, retail and office acreage. A higher land use mix score indicated a more diverse land use. However, they could not establish any significant association between mix score and adolescent physical activity or BMI. Rundle et al. (2007) considered the balance of commercial and residential uses in their study of the impact of urban form on obesity in New York City.

They calculated the ratio of building area devoted to commercial use and residential use for each census tract. The two ratios were multiplied by one another and then scaled by a factor of 4 to arrive at an index that ranged from 0 to 1. Thus, for a perfectly mixed area, containing equal proportions of residential and commercial space, the index returns a value of 1, while, whenever either type of use dominates, the index moves towards 0. They found that land use mix scores are inversely and significantly associated with BMI outcomes. Boer et al. (2007) considered the number of different types of businesses in a neighbourhood to parameterize their mix measures. They reported that moving from two different business types to three types significantly improved the probability of walking. Similar improvements in walk propensity were reported when moving from three to four different business types in the neighbourhood.

The Herfindahl–Hirschman Index has usually been employed to study market concentrations, especially to identify potential monopolies, but has also been used for the characterization of land use mix (Forsyth et al., 2008; Yan et al., 2010). It is expressed as the sum of squares of the percentages of each type of land use in the user-defined neighbourhood. A higher HHI score indicates a lower level of land use mix.

Another indicator of land use heterogeneity is the extent to which the diverse land uses are in contact with one another, often parameterized as the dissimilarity index (Kockelman, 1997). It may be expressed as:

$$\text{Dissimilarity Index} = \sum_{k} \frac{1}{K} \sum_{i}^{8} \frac{X_{ik}}{8}$$

where K is the number of actively developed hectares in the census tract and $X_{ik} = 1$ if the central active hectare's use type differs from that of a neighbouring hectare and $X_{ik} = 0$ otherwise. This index has also been employed in the study conducted by Forsyth et al. (2008).

Generally, what may be concluded from these diverse approaches to measuring the association between land use mix and physical activity and health outcomes is that higher mix is generally synonymous with the presence of diverse destinations, shorter trips lengths, and hence a more permeable and walkable neighbourhood. Many of the studies have reported expected positive association of land use mix and physical activity and body mass index. Nonetheless, some of the studies have reported counterintuitive findings, for example those conducted by Wood et al. (2010), who found a negative association between land use mix and sense of community in metropolitan Atlanta. Thus, although a high land use mix may represent a walkable community, nonetheless it is also a manifestation of high density, high economic activity, and impervious surfaces and hence may be associated with micro-level deterrents to health (such as overcrowded streets, traffic pollution, lack of safety from traffic, etc.), more so in purely urbanized areas. This has perhaps been captured in the study conducted by Saarloos et al. (2011), who report a positive association between land use mix and prevalence of depression in older adults in metropolitan Perth.

Factor N3: destination accessibility

A healthy neighbourhood should strive towards optimized clustering of health-promoting community services at a local level. Destination accessibility measures the degree of residential proximity to community facilities and services. The location of key local infrastructure (retail, healthy food provision, health care facilities, educational institutions, green space, etc.) in the spatial matrix relative to the residential units has been known to have an impact on health. Besides promoting a range of viable job opportunities or attractive destinations, easier destination access implies multi-purpose short trips, thereby encouraging residents to walk and cycle as well as reducing dependence on cars. Indirectly, with more destinations closer to one another, there are more people on the streets, fostering a sense of community. Thus, healthy urban planning will entail clustering of the facilities along the local high streets and town centres, with equal impetus on maintaining a mix of appropriate housing density. Most studies looking at these issues have sought to measure the proximity to and density of various community resources.

Factor N3.1: retail Retail in the form of shops and commercial establishments acts as a choice destination, and its density has been extensively employed in several studies of physical activity behaviour and related health. In their study, Giles-Corti et al. (2003) reported a positive association between obesity and the perception of no shops within a walking distance. Handy et al. (2006) used objective neighbourhood characteristics including number and types of service establishments within a distance of 400, 800 and 1600 metres and concluded that close proximity to potential amenities such as shops and service destinations acted as the most important predictors of walking. C. Lee and Moudon (2006b) considered the log count of the number of retail stores within a 1 kilometre buffer, but found no significant association with recreational walking. Forsyth et al. (2008) evaluated GIS-based measures of the percentage of total land area occupied by major land uses, employment per unit land area, retail employment per unit area and density of employees in the various retail sub-categories, but did not report any significant findings. In their study, Cerin, Leslie et al. (2007) performed a two-step cluster analysis to aggregate similar census collection districts (CCDs) into three groups: residential, recreational and commercial/industrial. They reported that the residents of neighbourhoods with commercial/industrial LUM had significantly higher transport-related walking as compared to the residents of neighbourhoods with a recreational profile. However, in another Australian study, Saarloos et al. (2011) considered the retail availability within CCDs as proxy neighbourhoods. They reported higher prevalence of depression among older adults in neighbourhoods with retail. Nagel et al. (2008) considered the number of commercial and select establishments within a 0.25 and 0.5 mile buffer and reported a beneficial association with the total walk time. Similarly, Sallis, Bowles et al. (2009) reported a beneficial association between physical activity prevalence and presence of shops within a 10- to 15-minute walk distance.

Retail floor area ratio (FAR) is another variable of importance in built environment health correlation studies. High commercial FAR in the neighbourhood indicates that a major fraction of the land parcel is occupied by built-up construction, while leaving the rest for open impervious surfaces such as parking space and landscaping. Such a configuration implies that the built-up retail outlets are accessible to pedestrians, being more or less adjacent and in close proximity to sidewalks. On the other hand, a low value is reflective of only a fraction of the parcel being taken up by buildings, the rest usually being allotted to parking. High commercial FAR has been found to be a manifestation of pedestrian-oriented design, while a low FAR value is indicative of automobile-oriented design. Norman et al. (2006) computed the average retail FAR for commercial land parcels within a 1-mile network buffer. They reported a positive association between retail floor area and physical activity of adolescent boys. Wood et al. (2010) considered the commercial FAR within a 1 kilometre street network buffer and reported a beneficial association between high commercial FAR and sense of community. Several other studies evaluated commercial FAR and employed it as one of the components of their composite walkability index (Frank et al., 2006; Kligerman et al., 2007; Sallis, Saelens et al., 2009; Owen et al., 2010). In another study a positive association was reported between walkability and smaller size of closest office complex (<36 659 square metres), as well as longer distance to closest office or mixed-use complex (>544 metres), for King County, Washington. The composite walkability score developed comprised eight components, including the aforementioned, and was beneficially associated with walking and lower odds of depression (Berke, Gottlieb et al., 2007; Berke, Koepsell et al., 2007).

In conclusion, there is almost unambiguous evidence of a positive association between the presence of retail on the one hand and physical activity and improved weight and mental health outcomes on the other. This is attributed to retail being an attractive destination and hence encouraging walking and social interaction. Only one study, conducted by Saarloos et al. (2011), reports evidence to the contrary. This may be attributed to the fact that the study focused on the psychological health of older adults in a metropolitan area.

Factor N3.2: accessibility to green space The role of green spaces (in the form of green parks, squares, pocket parks, playgrounds, etc.) in promoting community health is a multiple one. Green spaces provide natural pollution-free environments and hence are associated with many possible direct positive health outcomes. They act as natural sieves that absorb and dilute urban pollution, act as catchment areas for water harvesting, improve drainage and groundwater quality, maintain species biodiversity, help in CO_2 sequestration, and can lessen the heat island effect in an urban setting. Green spaces provide habitats in which individuals can relax in a serene natural environment and hence are associated with recreational and aesthetic value, with potential mental and physical health-related outcomes. The presence of green space in a neighbourhood has been associated with enhanced recreational walking and cycling. Residents tend to spend more of their spare time outdoors, thereby contributing to greater physical activity. The presence of green spaces in compact, high-mix neighbourhoods tends to provide an incentive for walking to work and shops, thereby resulting in lower vehicle hours travelled. In addition, they act as the places where local residents tend to assemble and thus can foster a sense of community, with associated health benefits. With more than 50 per cent of the world's population presently residing in urban settlements, daily exposure to green spaces is fast becoming rarer, thereby underscoring the importance of access to neighbourhood green space for promoting healthy behaviour and enhancing the quality of life (Chiesura, 2004; UNFPA, 2007). A survey of cities participating in the WHO European Healthy Cities Network has highlighted the stark cross-country disparity in accessibility to green space. In an international study of selected cities, almost all of the Northern European residents of Brussels, Copenhagen and Glasgow could access neighbourhood green space within 15 minutes, while only 47 per cent of those in the cities of Bratislava and Kiev could do so (Tsourou, 1998). In a study conducted in Dutch cities, de Vries et al. (2003) reported a decrease in the number of symptoms comparable with a decrease in age by five years with every 10 per cent increase in green space in the neighbouring environment. In a study of the physical activity of 1281 residents of Rockhampton, Queensland, M. Duncan and Mummery (2005) reported that the respondents having the nearest parkland beyond a network distance of 0.6 kilometre had 41 per cent higher odds of achieving recommended levels of physical activity as compared to those with parkland within the distance. Again, the respondents with direct route connectivity to the nearest parkland were 41 per cent less likely to achieve sufficient levels of physical activity than those who resided in areas having indirect route connectivity to parkland. In another study, J. Maas et al. (2006) noted that people with a greener environment (both agricultural and natural green) within a 1 kilometre or 3 kilometre radius enjoyed better self-perceived general health. The relationship between green space and health was observed to be stronger for people with a low socio-economic status, as well as for youth and the elderly. Nielsen and Hansen (2007) employed self-reported measures of distance to eight categories of green areas, as well as frequency of visits to them. They reported that proximity to publicly accessible green areas, as well as access to a private garden or a shared green area at the dwelling, was associated with less stress and lower likelihood of obesity. However, the frequency of utilization of green areas in the study could not explain the association between green areas and health. Kaczynski et al. (2010) studied the relationship between the potential likelihood of a park being used for physical activity and adjacent land use diversity and highlighted that land use mix may act as a disincentive to park use. They reported that parks located in neighbourhoods with low land use diversity but with a higher number of facilities were significantly more likely to have been used for physical activity as compared to those having high adjacent land use diversity and high facilities. In another study, Troped et al. (2010) measured the landscape greenness within a 1 kilometre buffer of a respondent's home in terms of the average Normalized Difference Vegetation Index (NDVI) score calculated from the Landsat ETM+ satellite imagery. Interestingly, their greenness score was inversely associated with physical activity. The relative influence of green space upon physical activity was perhaps subordinated in this study by the presence of highly dense and intricately connected urban form. In another study, Tilt et al. (2007) examined the impact of both objectively measured and self-reported destination accessibility and vegetation upon walking trips and body mass index. Objective measurement of greenness was based on the NDVI index. Both objective accessibility and subjective greenness were positively associated with walking trips per month. Respondents residing in areas of high accessibility and high NDVI measured greenness reported lower BMI. In another longitudinal study, conducted over a period of eight years on 3173 children aged 9–10 from 12 communities in Southern California, Wolch et al. (2011) reported that both park space (in acres) within a 500 metre buffer and the number of recreation programmes within a 10 kilometre buffer of children's homes were beneficially associated with weight outcomes.

Besides promoting physical activity, evidence also suggests that exposure to green spaces also contributes to improved mental health outcomes via diminishing stress and providing opportunities for recovery as well as enhanced levels of physical activity and social cohesion (Ulrich, 1984; Hartig et al., 2003; Pretty et al., 2005). In a study of the relationship between green public areas and longevity among 3114 senior citizens, Takano (2002) reported that living in areas with walkable green spaces was positively associated with longevity over the subsequent five-year period. In another study, comprising 953 randomly sampled respondents from nine Swedish cities, Grahn and Stigsdotter (2003) reported independent association between the utilization of urban open green spaces and self-reported experiences of stress after adjusting for the respondent's age, sex and socio-economic status. The distance to public urban open green spaces and access to a garden were identified as the key factors in the study. Pretty et al. (2005) highlighted the importance of green exercise, reporting that exercise in pleasant environments has a greater effect on cardiovascular health measures of blood pressure and measures of mental health than exercising elsewhere. In another study, conducted on 1895 adults in Adelaide, Australia, Sugiyama et al. (2008) reported that better perception of neighbourhood greenness was associated with 1.37 and 1.60 times higher odds of reporting improved physical and mental health respectively in reference to respondents having poorer perception of neighbourhood green. Furthermore, perceived greenness was independently associated with walking for recreation, social capital and local sense of community. Another large-scale study, conducted by Richard Mitchell and Popham (2008) in England, reported that the populations exposed to greener environments exhibited lower levels of income-deprivation-related health inequalities in all-cause mortality and mortality from circulatory diseases. The incidence rate ratio for all-cause mortality for the most income-deprived quartile was 1.93 times higher as compared to the least deprived in least green areas, while the same ratio was relatively low, only 1.43 times higher, in the most green areas. In another study of older adults conducted in Bogotá, Colombia, Parra et al. (2010) reported a beneficial association between self-rated health and more than 8 per cent of the land being covered by public park spaces. In a meta-analysis of ten UK studies involving 1252 respondents, J. Barton and Pretty (2010) reported that acute short-term exposures to facilitated green exercise had a significant beneficial effect on both self-esteem and mood independent of duration, intensity, location, gender, age and health status.

In a nutshell, there is fairly conclusive evidence of positive associations between neighbourhood accessibility to (expressed as either proximity to or density of) green and open spaces and physical activity, general health and mental health. Besides being attractive destinations where people can walk to, they also provide therapeutic stress-relieving environments as well as environments for social interaction and bonding.

Factor N3.3: accessibility to recreational facilities and physical activity resources The presence of accessible recreational or physical activity (PA) facilities in the local neighbourhood complements an individual's effort to stay physically active and healthy, and a mounting body of evidence has highlighted the beneficial association between availability of and improved access to recreational or PA resources and PA levels. Most of these studies have endeavoured to objectively measure the number of the selected types of recreational or PA facilities as well as enumerate the shortest distance to such facilities, while other studies have depended upon perceived proximity to facilities. In a study conducted by Sallis et al. (1990), individuals' perceptions of the convenience of physical activity facilities were not associated with objectively measured density of physical activity facilities. Giles-Corti et al. (2003) used GIS-based measures of the proximity of key categories of recreational facilities (sport and recreation centres, gyms, golf courses, tennis courts, swimming pools, public open space, and the beach or river foreshores) from a respondent's dwelling location. They reported that reduced access to four or more recreational facilities was associated with 68 per cent higher odds of being obese in reference to those with improved access. In another study, Rutt and Coleman (2005) considered the number of physical activity facilities in the form of parks, gyms, schools and biking or walking paths within a 2.5 mile radius catchment around each subject's home, as well as the proximity (shortest distance) to each of the nearest physical activity facilities. They reported significant associations between walking frequency and number of physical activity facilities. In a study of inequalities in physical activity among the 78 neighbourhoods of Eindhoven, van Lenthe et al. (2005) tried to characterize the general attractiveness of the neighbourhood, proximity to neighbourhood facilities, and neighbourhood safety, using survey questionnaires and scale measurements of 1–5. Quality of green facilities and availability of sport and recreational facilities were also considered. Residents of neighbourhoods with the poorest proximity to sports facilities reported higher odds of almost never participating in sports and physical activity. In a study of neighbourhood-level environmental correlates of adolescent physical activity and BMI outcomes, Norman et al. (2006) enumerated the number of private and public recreational facilities and parks within a 1-mile network catchment of each respondent's dwelling. They reported significant associations between moderate to vigorous physical activity (MVPA) and the number of recreation facilities, as well as number of parks, but only for girls. However, neither community design nor access to recreation variables was observed to be significantly related to BMI outcomes. Jilcott et al. (2007) considered both perceived and objectively measured proximity to physical activity resources. Perceived proximity to PA resources was based on proximity to the nearest school, gym, recreation centre or park and the presence of the school, gym, recreation centre or park within a ten-minute driving distance from home. Objectively measured proximity was parameterized as road network distance of the participant's home to the closest PA resource and the number of each type of PA resource in a 1- and 2-mile crow-fly buffer. The study found no significant relationship between physical activity and proximity to parks, in cases of both perceived and objectively measured predictors. Nonetheless, counter-intuitively, the number of resources within the buffer was negatively associated with MVPA. Both the predictors of perceived distance to gyms and objectively measured number of schools within 1-mile buffers were also negatively associated with physical activity. In another study, Gordon-Larsen et al. (2006) calculated the number of physical activity facilities per census block and reported higher odds of achieving MVPA in census blocks with a higher number of facilities relative to those with zero facilities per block group. Kligerman et al. (2007) employed two recreation-based environmental variables of shortest distance to the nearest public or private recreation facility, and the total number of recreation facilities within the street network buffers of 0.25, 0.5 and 1 mile. They could not find any association between their measures of proximity and intensity of recreation facilities and physical activity or BMI. Boehmer et al. (2007) evaluated the number of recreational facilities and non-residential destinations within a 400 metre radius surrounding each respondent's residence as an objective measure of the availability of recreational facilities; no significant association with obesity could be determined. Diez Roux et al. (2007) considered the density of recreational resources (team sports, dual sports, running areas, water activities, tai-chi, Pilates, yoga, martial arts, aerobics, cardiovascular equipment weight training, gymnastics, dancing, skating, skiing, golf and others), as well as the number of parks, in windows of varying radii (0.5, 1, 2 and 5 miles) around each participant's residence. They reported that the density of physical activity resources within neighbourhoods of 1 mile to 5 miles was beneficially associated with higher odds of achieving recommended physical activity levels. These associations were observed to be slightly stronger among minority and low-income residents. In another large-scale study, based on large public health surveys in suburban and rural areas of southern Sweden, Björk et al. (2008) reported that the number of recreational values of the natural environment (expressed in terms of serene, wild, lush, spacious and culture) in the neighbourhood of the residence was beneficially associated with neighbourhood satisfaction and physical activity. The association was significantly higher among tenants. Furthermore, tenants residing in areas with higher recreational values exhibited higher odds of reporting a low or normal body mass index. Pan et al. (2009) characterized the availability of physical activity facilities in terms of the number of sites to safely walk, or ride a bike safely, number of publicly owned multi-purpose recreation trails, number of facilities, places and programmes designed specifically for physical activity and sports, and number of other places that could be used for physical activity. Physical activity facility availability was observed to be more strongly associated with higher levels of physical activity among respondents with a university degree in reference to those with a lower level of educational attainment. In another cross-continental study encompassing 11 countries, Sallis, Bowles et al. (2009) considered the presence of a free or low-cost recreational service as one of the components of a neighbourhood environment index. Higher levels of physical activity were reported in neighbourhoods having more low-cost recreational facilities.

According to the underlying hypothesis in this book, studies have consistently reported evidence of positive health benefits from the presence of sports and physical activity facilities. In these studies the health-promoting benefits operate via physical-activity-related mechanisms. Nonetheless, a few studies have reported null findings. An explanation may be that the use of a particular sports or recreational facility is governed by individual affinities rather than by availability within a defined neighbourhood. In other words, the presence of a facility may not imply its usage if it is not the type of facility that an individual chooses to use. In terms of the economics of service provision and planning, this implies that such services are not perfectly substitutable for each other, meaning that people cannot therefore be expected necessarily to use the nearest. Thus, models capturing choice may further refine these studies, as will studies that use a finer classification of service or facility type.

Factor N3.4: accessibility to local food environments Unhealthy, high-calorific food consumption has long been known to be one of the contributory causes of obesity. Food environments, especially the availability of and access to healthy food, have been one of the research domains within the contextual determinants of physical activity and healthy weight outcomes. Several studies have tried to establish associations between access to supermarkets, restaurants, fast-food outlets, groceries and so on and obesity outcomes. Mobley et al. (2006) considered facilities per capita, for example the number of fitness facilities, full-sized grocery stores, fast-food establishments, restaurants and minimarts per 1000 residents for each zip code of residence. They also considered the percentage of the workforce commuting outside the county. Increments in fitness facility per 1000 residents were associated with lower odds of BMI and CHD risk outcomes; however, none of the food environment variables were significant. In another study, Inagami et al. (2006) reported that respondents residing in socially deprived areas and shopping from grocery stores located in deprived areas exhibited a higher BMI. Furthermore, car owners travelling farther to shop also had higher BMI levels. The Atherosclerosis Risk in Communities (ARIC) Study conducted by Morland el al. (2006) examined the association between the local food environment and the prevalence of cardiovascular disease risk factors. They considered all types of food stores and food service places including supermarkets, grocery stores, convenience stores, full-service restaurants, and franchised fast-food and other limited-service restaurants per census tract. The availability of supermarkets was associated with lower odds of obesity and being overweight; however, the availability of grocery stores and convenience stores was associated with an increased prevalence of overweight and obesity. Another large-scale study of 714054 adults based on the data from the 2002–06 Behavioural Risk Factor Surveillance System reported that the density of fast-food restaurants and a higher ratio of fast-food to full-service restaurants were associated with higher BMI and obesity outcomes (Mehta and Chang, 2008). However, reduced odds of obesity were observed in areas having a higher density of full-service restaurants. In the study, the restaurant density was measured in terms of the number of restaurants per 10000 residents, and the restaurants were further classified into fast-food and full-service categories. F. Li et al. (2008) operationalized the local food environment in terms of the number of fast-food outlets per unit area of census block groups and reported a 7 per cent increment in overweight and obesity with every 1 standard deviation (SD) increase in the density of fast-food outlets. In a subsequent short-term longitudinal study conducted over a period of one year, F. Li, Harmer, Cardinal, Bosworth et al. (2009) reported a similar trend. Residents of neighbourhoods with a high density of fast-food outlets who utilized such facilities more frequently reported increments of 1.40 kilograms in weight and 2.04 centimetres in waist circumference. In contrast, the residents of high-walkability neighbourhoods participating in vigorous physical activity were associated with decreases of 1.2 kilograms in weight and 1.57 centimetres in waist circumference. Dengel et al. (2009) studied the association between metabolic syndrome (METS) and neighbourhood environment in adolescents. The density of food and physical environment resources (convenience stores and gas stations, grocery stores, and large grocery stores) was calculated within a 1600 metre network buffer of a respondent's dwelling. The proximity to the nearest facilities, especially the nearest parks, gym, recreation centre, walking/biking trail and school, was also calculated in reference to the respondent's dwelling location. Higher distance to convenience stores was significantly associated with a lower METS score (indicating lower odds of development of METS). Black et al. (2010) considered the number of supermarkets, restaurants, emergency food providers, small grocers, fast-food outlets, beverage and snacks stores and physical activity facilities per 100 000, as well as the percentage residential and commercial land use in 34 New York City neighbourhoods. They reported a significantly reduced risk of obesity with increasing availability of large supermarkets, restaurants and fast-food outlets and beverage and snack food bars. Also, there was a reduced risk of obesity with increasing access to fitness facilities and commercial land use. In another study, conducted by Burgoine et al. (2011), the number of food outlets was population-standardized for each census-defined middle super output area (MSOA) level and expressed in terms of food outlets per thousand population in the MSOA. Quintile scores were calculated at the MSOA level and subsequently converted to the lower super output area (LSOA) level, which acted as proxy neighbourhoods. However, the study did not report any significant relationship between food availability and BMI levels.

Some studies have been able to establish a direct positive association between the availability of unhealthy food (fast-food outlets, etc.) and the prevalence of obesity, while the presence of healthy alternatives (supermarkets) has been associated with lower odds of obesity. Future potential studies need to find a standardized classification system for categorizing food environments. To have clearer and more robust evidence, in addition to the measures of density and network distance to the food environments, survey data on actual visits to various categories of food environments need to be employed in epidemiological models. Furthermore, there is a necessity to develop more intricate objective measures of physical activity–obesity–heath models taking into account the highly individualized routines people follow in their daily lives, for example differentiating between physical activity associated with walking (for both transport and leisure) and exercise versus physical activity from within-household chores through accelerometry, so as not to underestimate the total effect of context on individuals (Michael and Yen, 2009).

Factor N4: street network morphology and connectivity

Street network morphology influences street-level accessibility, thereby shaping individual travel and physical activity behaviour. Typically, dense urban grids comprising highly interconnected straight streets crisscrossing at right angles are manifestations of archetypal highly connected networks.

This gives rise to fine-grained urban blocks with a high degree of permeability, connectivity and accessibility. In contrast, sparse suburban grids tend to comprise 'loops and lollipops' formed by narrow curving residential streets that feed into fewer arterial roads. The characteristics of street networks can be used to indicate the ease with which various service destinations can be reached, because they influence trip route choice and mode of transportation. US national data point toward the fact that journeys within walkable catchments of half a mile and a mile constitute up to 14 per cent and 27 per cent of total journeys respectively, while those within bikeable distances of 5 miles constitute 63 per cent of all journeys made (Federal Highway Administration, 1994; Sallis et al., 2004). In another study, Ross and Dunning (1997) highlighted the fact that 83 per cent of all journeys are inherently short and for non-work purposes, occurring in the relative vicinity of home locations and well within walkable and bikeable distances.

Connectivity or route directness indicates the ease of travel between trip origins (home location) and various destinations (workplace, community centre, park, recreational centre, supermarket, etc.) following the configuration of the urban network. A street network with high road intersection density shortens the access distance and thereby provides more routeing options. In studies assessing the effects of urban morphology and street network accessibility upon activity behaviour and health, the various attributes of street network morphology have been enumerated by objectively measured GIS variables, often parameterized in the form of intersection density, percentage of four-way intersections, and number of intersections per unit length of street network, as well as block-based measures such as block perimeter, block size and so on.

Frank et al. (2004) quantified connectivity in their study as the density of intersections with more than three legs within a 1 kilometre household network catchment, but reported non-significant associations with BMI outcomes. They attributed this to the spatial collinearity between the land use diversity and street connectivity measures in high-density urban areas. Rutt and Coleman (2005) measured intersection density in terms of the total number of intersections within a 0.25 mile radius. They also included the percentage of cul-de-sacs and four-way intersections in their analysis. However, they found no significant association with BMI or physical activity outcomes. In their study, Nelson et al. (2006) employed street connectivity as one of the attributes to classify neighbourhoods into six distinct cluster classes, namely rural working class, exurban, newer suburban, upper-middle class and older suburban, mixed-race urban and low-socio-economic-status inner-city areas. Their connectivity measure was operationalized within a 3 kilometre buffer and had the following components: density of three-way and four-way intersections; an γ index, which is the ratio of observed to maximum possible route alternatives between nodes; a γ index, which is the ratio of observed node linkages to the maximum possible links in the network; and a cyclomatic index, which is the number of route alternatives between nodes. They also considered road type expressed in terms of the proportion and total length of A1 and A4 roads within a 3 kilometre buffer. The study reported that the adolescent residents of rural working-class, exurban neighbourhoods had higher odds of being overweight compared to those in newer suburbs. Adolescent residents of older suburban areas reported a higher propensity to be physically active in reference to those of newer suburbs, while adolescents living in low-SES inner-city neighbourhoods were also reported to be more active, though it was not significant. Rundle et al. (2007) expressed intersection density as the number of street intersections per census tract and reported no significant association between intersection density and individual BMI. Forsyth et al. (2008) considered several variables as quantitative representations of street patterns. These included average and median census block area, number of access points, road length per unit area, intersections per unit area, ratio of four-way intersections to all intersections, four-way intersections per unit land area, ratio of three-way intersections to all intersections, connected node ratio, median perimeter of the block, and ratio of the area within X street distance to area within X distance radius. However, the study reported a negative association between travel and leisure walking and street pattern expressed in terms of intersections per unit area. B.B. Brown et al. (2009) considered the intersection density of three or more local streets within a 1 kilometre network catchment (excluding street intersections involving interstate highways) in their study. They reported non-significant associations with BMI, overweight and obesity outcomes. In their study of neighbourhood-level correlates of the sense of community, Wood et al. (2010) considered density of intersections with more than three legs contained within the household buffer as the measure of street connectivity and reported non-significant association. In another study, Burgoine et al. (2011) parameterized connectivity by summing up the number of street intersections within each census-defined proxy neighbourhood (lower super output areas) and thereafter standardized by the size of the respective neighbourhood. However, the study did not find a significant association with BMI. Recently, Ball et al. (2012) employed a connectivity index of each data zone for the city of Glasgow comprising seven component measures: direction density, intersection density (for three or more directions of travel), density of cul-de-sacs, street density, length density, beta index (ratio between links and intersections) and eta index (average length per link). However, no significant association was reported between street connectivity and BMI or BMI categories.

In a multi-level study, F. Li, Fisher, Bauman et al. (2005) reported a positive association between the number of street intersections per unit area of neighbourhood and walking activity at the neighbourhood level. Norman et al. (2006) measured intersection density as the number of street intersections per acre of a 1 mile street network buffer around the participants' dwellings. They reported that intersection density was negatively associated with propensity for moderate to vigorous physical activity only in the case of adolescent girls, while no association was observed in the case of boys. Boer et al. (2007) reported significant associations between measures of the fraction of four-way intersections and average length of the long side of a city block in a neighbourhood with observed walk propensity in ten US metropolitan areas. Moving from areas with 0–24 per cent four-way intersections to areas with 25–49 per cent resulted in a 36 per cent increase in propensity to walk, while moving further up from 25–49 per cent to the level of 50–74 per cent four-way intersections resulted in an increase of 38 per cent. Neighbourhoods with 75–99.9 per cent of four-way intersections promoted more walking compared to the level of 50–74 per cent. However, the association between block length and walk propensity was somewhat contrary to expectations. It was observed that moving from block lengths less than 600 feet to 600–804 feet resulted in an increase in the probability of walking. F. Li et al. (2008) took the number of street intersections divided by the area of the census block in square miles as their measure of density of street connectivity and found that neighbourhoods with high street connectivity were significantly related to higher prevalence of walking activity and meeting physical activity recommendations. Wells and Yang (2008) characterized the street network by the total linear length of streets, number of street intersections and number of cul-de-sacs within a 0.25 mile street network buffer. In their longitudinal analysis of walking levels prior to and after relocation to new neighbourhoods in four towns of the South-East US states of Georgia, Alabama and Florida, they reported that relocation to neighbourhoods with fewer cul-de-sacs was associated with increments of 5303 steps per week (or 757 more steps per day) after controlling for demographic variables. Gómez et al. (2010) operationalized street connectivity in terms of the number of street links divided by the number of street nodes within a 500 metre buffer of the neighbourhood centroid. They observed that, in reference to the residents of low-connectivity neighbourhoods, those residing in high-connectivity neighbourhoods exhibited lower odds of walking for at least 60 minutes. In another study, Troped et al. (2010) operationalized intersection density as the number of intersections within a 1 kilometre network buffer divided by the total street segment length. They reported a positive significant relationship between their calculated intersection density and levels of MVPA within a 1 kilometre home buffer. Contrastingly, intersection density was inversely associated with MVPA within a 1 kilometre work buffer, and the relation was non-significant.

In sum, the evidence of association between street-level configuration and health is mixed, and it is hard to draw general conclusions. A majority of studies have reported null results, while a fraction have established significant associations. However, the direction of association depends upon the overall city structure and is also related to the availability of facilities. On the one hand, enhanced connectivity can encourage physical activity and social interaction on account of improved accessibility to choice destinations, as in the studies reported by F. Li et al. (2008) and Troped et al. (2010). On the other hand, increasing intersection density may equally well be a manifestation of higher transit congestion, increasing levels of pollution and overcrowding, and reduced perception of street-level safety. Furthermore, the effects may be different in high-density urban areas and low-density suburban areas.

Two weaknesses may be noted in the studies discussed above. One weakness of the connectivity metrics employed in this field thus far stems from the fact that they are disjointed from land use and other socio-economic processes and, hence, may not be a realistic representation of degree of usability of a particular street link. It is, after all, the land use and the socio-economic processes that exist adjacent to streets that are the primary determinants of pedestrian and transit behaviour. Secondly, studies have rarely taken into account the impact of street-level morphology upon behaviour and thereby on patterns of physical activity and health. Network accessibility and movement potential at multiple spatial scales need to be assessed. For example, in a suburban area, higher accessibility and movement potential at a local scale may be synonymous with higher social interaction and cohesion. On the contrary, parts of the network with higher transit-level accessibility tend to be more motorized and less pedestrian-friendly, with the potential to produce detrimental effects upon individual health outcomes. In the subsequent chapters, we have employed a street network modelling technique to overcome these deficiencies.

Factor N5: access to public transit stops and stations and active transport

The use of public transportation options reduces reliance on private vehicles and has been associated with enhanced levels of physical activity in the form of exercise through walking and subsequent health benefits. The presence of public transport services at walkable distances tends to encourage residents to walk to and from the bus stops or the light rail stops. In

Europe, the threshold distance is around 400 metres, beyond which the proportion of residents opting to walk declines progressively and the corresponding car dependence rate increases. Physically active commuting to work (PACW) has been associated with several direct health benefits in the form of reduced HDL cholesterol (Vuori and Oja, 1999) and reduced cardiovascular risk factors (G. Hu et al., 2002). Besser and Dannenberg (2005) estimated that, in a sample of 3312 public transit users from the 2001 US National Household Travel Survey (NHTS), a median of 19 minutes daily were spent walking to and from stops, with approximately 29 per cent of the respondents exceeding 30 minutes of daily physical activity. Cerin, Macfarlane et al. (2007) considered perceived proximity to bus or train stops in their study, but did not report any significant association with walking. In a study of the associations between built environmental variables and BMI outcomes in New York City, Rundle et al. (2007) considered access to public transit as one of their measures. They measured the availability of public transit in terms of density of bus stops and subway stations per square kilometre in each census tract. They reported that availability of public transit showed inversely significant association with BMI after statistically controlling for individual- and neighbourhood-level sociodemographic attributes. Wener and Evans (2007) found that train commuters on average walked 30 per cent more steps per day, equivalent to ten minutes or more walking, than the automobile commuters and were four times more likely to meet the standard recommendation of 10 000 steps per day. In a study employing the NHTS data, R.D. Edwards (2008) reported that using public transport was associated with an average of 8.3 additional minutes of walking time per day, equivalent to expending 25.7–39.0 kcal/day. He estimated that obesity generated an annual $34 200 in health costs per person, and an additional 8.3 minutes' walking is equivalent to saving $4800, $5500 and $6600 per person, depending on the intensity of walking, as well as considerable savings in quality-adjusted life-years. F. Li et al. (2008) expressed density of public transit stations as the number of bus and transit stations divided by the area of the census block group in square kilometres. They observed that the density of the transit stations was significantly associated with both walking for transport and meeting the physical activity recommendations. B.B. Brown and Werner (2008) studied ridership behaviour among 51 residents of a traditional, mixed-use neighbourhood of Salt Lake City, Utah, after it had been invigorated with the newly laid TRAX light rail network. They classified their subjects into three categories: non-riders; new riders, who reported undertaking recent rail rides only after the stop opened; and continuing riders, who reported recent rail rides both before and after the new stop opened. They reported that the prevalence of obesity was comparatively higher among non-riders

(65 per cent) in reference to new riders (26 per cent) and continuing riders (15 per cent). In a separate study, B.B. Brown et al. (2009) measured the proximity to bus stops and rail stops and reported that being farther away from a rail stop was significantly associated with higher BMI and increased risk of obesity, albeit only among females.

Cycling as a mode of active travel has also been reported to make significant contributions to health-promoting physical activity (Oja et al., 1998). Within Europe, Denmark, the Netherlands and Belgium have emerged as the top three countries for cycling rates (http://dataservice.eea.europa.eu). Regional-level comparisons indicate that, over the years, European cities have emerged as more walkable and cycle-friendly, promoting higher levels of walking and cycling, compared to those in Australia and North America. In a regional study employing national surveys of travel behaviour and health indicators in Europe, North America and Australia, Bassett et al. (2008) reported that the residents of Europe walked more than their counterparts in the United States (382 versus 140 kilometres per person per year) as well as bicycled more (188 versus 40 kilometres per person per year) for the year 2000. Countries with the highest levels of active transportation reported the lowest prevalence of obesity. Pucher et al. (2010) studied cross-sectional health and travel data across 14 countries and reported statistically significant relationships between walking, cycling and health (in terms of a lower prevalence of obesity) at the country, state and city levels. Data from Denmark indicated that a 20 per cent increase in cycling levels in the period 1996–2002 has been associated with a corresponding five-month increment in life expectancy in the case of males.

To summarize, in the majority of the studies the presence of public transit facilities within a walkable range has been found to reduce reliance on cars and enhance physical activity. It has been reported that the presence of a nearby bus stop or light rail stop enhances the propensity to walk to them en route to the final destinations, thereby reducing the odds of obesity.

Factor N6: pedestrian-oriented design

Design features of streets and the building structures adjacent to them such as the nature of sidewalks or pavements, presence of traffic-calming features, safety provision, speed impediments, and aesthetic aspects all influence the walkability of a neighbourhood. Road design features which encourage pedestrian walking include sidewalk coverage measured by the proportion of block faces with sidewalks, ratio of sidewalk length to road length, sidewalk width, average street width, number of pedestrian crossings, and so on. Other features include clearer traffic signs, the presence of buffer zones between busy routes and footways, enclosed bus shelters with seats, frequently located public benches, and clearly marked slope changes with hand-rails. Building setback is another important parameter supporting pedestrian movement. Road safety provisions include limits on traffic speed and volume and traffic-calming provisions. Achieving optimum traffic speed limits reduces the risk of accidents, and this may be achieved by advocating appropriate impediments through narrow road width, tighter bends, reduced sightlines, the presence of junction platforms and rough surfaces, the addition of traffic circles or roundabouts and the installation of pavement treatments. Several studies on physical activity behaviour have employed measures of the presence of pedestrian infrastructures and degree of road safety (Giles-Corti et al., 2003; Saelens, Sallis, Black et al., 2003; Hoehner et al., 2005; F. Li, Fisher, Brownson et al., 2005; Boehmer et al., 2007; Cerin, Macfarlane et al., 2007; Forsyth et al., 2008; Nagel et al., 2008; Santana et al., 2009; Gómez et al., 2010; Yan et al., 2010). Giles-Corti et al. (2003) reported a significant association between absence of sidewalks as well as perception of no sidewalks with the outcomes of overweight and obesity. Ewing et al. (2004) reported that roads with sidewalks along them as well as sidewalk coverage were significantly associated with higher walk propensity. M. Duncan and Mummery (2005) reported a negative association between walking for recreation and not having a footpath network within a 400 metre buffer. At the same time, a good perception of footpath condition was beneficially associated with recreational walking. Boehmer et al. (2007) established a positive association between obesity and the perceived and objective measures of sidewalk quality. In their study, Forsyth et al. (2008) reported a significant positive association between sidewalk length per unit area and travel walking. Nagel et al. (2008) reported that the presence of a greater proportion of high-volume streets was beneficially associated with minutes walked per week, while a greater proportion of low-volume streets was negatively associated. Another study reported a beneficial association between walking for at least 60 minutes and subjective feeling of safety from traffic (Gómez et al., 2010).

Designing cycling networks with a modest degree of safety, comfort and route convenience encourages cycling and thereby results in increased levels of physical activity of residents. In the UK, the average cycling trip is 3 kilometres, with a cut-off limit at 5 kilometres, beyond which there is a sharp reduction in the propensity to cycle. Several studies have considered the presence of cycling infrastructure (presence of cycling paths) and its potential impacts on travel behaviour (Giles-Corti et al., 2003; Saelens, Sallis, Black et al., 2003; Ewing et al., 2004; Hoehner et al., 2005). Owen et al. (2010) reported a positive association between bicycle use and degree of neighbourhood walkability for the cities of Ghent and Adelaide.

Aesthetic factors in the form of an increased number of street trees, squares, pocket parks, and wider pavements adjacent to retail services and bus stops provide a pleasant pedestrian walking and cycling environment. On the contrary, the presence of signs of physical decline and incivilities in the form of littering, garbage, vandalism and graffiti may have a negative influence on walkability and psychological health. Besides, such environments have generally been related to higher prevalent rates of crime, as well as fear of it, and hence a reduced sense of security (Perkins et al., 1992, 1993; D. Cohen et al., 2000). A number of studies have employed various indicators of neighbourhood aesthetics (Saelens, Sallis, Black et al., 2003; M. Duncan and Mummery, 2005; Ellaway et al., 2005; Hoehner et al., 2005; van Lenthe et al., 2005; Boehmer et al., 2007; Stafford, Cummins et al., 2007; Leslie and Cerin, 2008; Mujahid, Diez Roux, Shen et al., 2008). Balfour and Kaplan (2002) considered six urban neighbourhood problems, namely crime, lighting at night, traffic, excessive noise, trash and litter, and access to public transportation, and reported that older adults residing in multiple-problem neighbourhoods were associated with higher odds of functional loss. M. Duncan and Mummery (2005) employed a perceived measure of neighbourhood cleanliness and reported a beneficial association between clean neighbourhoods and physical activity. In another study, Ellaway et al. (2005) considered the amount of graffiti, litter and dog mess in the immediate residential environment and reported a negative association between the levels of incivilities and physical activity, while the associations were positive for being overweight or obese. Van Lenthe et al. (2005) reported negative associations between perceived measures of general neighbourhood design and noise pollution from traffic. Boehmer et al. (2007) reported that being obese was significantly associated with perceptions of an unpleasant community, as well as observed indicators of physical disorder and presence of garbage. Stafford, Cummins et al. (2007) considered the number of special constables and police officers, the presence of vacant or derelict land, and the violent crime rate, as well as the number of missed waste collections, as the indicator of neighbourhood disorder, and reported the first three to be significant. In their path model, neighbourhood disorder was significantly associated with sports participation rate. Leslie and Cerin (2008) reported a positive association between their perceived measure of aesthetics and greenery and the neighbourhood satisfaction domains of safety and walkability, access to destinations, social network and travel network.

Several studies have considered indicators of neighbourhood crime (Saelens, Sallis, Black et al., 2003; Burdette and Whitaker, 2004; M. Duncan and Mummery, 2005; Hoehner et al., 2005; Mobley et al., 2006; Black et al., 2010; Wood et al., 2010; Yan et al., 2010). Van Lenthe et al. (2005)

had reported a negative association between sports participation and neighbourhoods requiring police attention. Santana et al. (2009) established a positive association between BMI and crimes against property. In another study, Guite et al. (2006) reported that a perceived unsafe daytime environment was negatively associated with mental health and vitality.

Visual outlook and complexity are another factor that influences the environmental psychology of a place. Ewing et al. (2006) and Ewing and Handy (2009) hypothesized that qualitative urban design attributes of street environments define the individual perceptions of streetscapes and thereby influence people's willingness to walk and be active in them. Their study considered nine perceptual qualities of built environment, including imageability, complexity, visual enclosure, human scale, transparency, linkage, legibility, coherence and tidiness, and developed operational definitions and objective measurement protocols for the first five.

There is evidence to suggest, therefore, that neighbourhoods with pedestrian-friendly design – those with pedestrian and cycling infrastructure, better aesthetics and safety from traffic and crime – promote physical activity, with potential benefits to physical and mental health.

4.4 FACTOR N7: COMPOSITE MEASURES OF WALKABILITY AND ENVIRONMENTAL QUALITY

One of the problems associated with assessing the nature of the relationship between a health outcome and a set of individual built environmental variables is that the built environmental variables often come as a parcel of highly correlated measures, which often leads to multicollinearity problems, resulting in inaccurate model estimation. It may be that, because of interaction effects therefore, the core dimensions of the built environment cannot be captured by any single individual variable. Several studies have conducted research on various composite neighbourhood-level indicators of active living (Craig et al., 2002; Ramirez et al., 2006). A group of studies have resulted in the development of indices of walkability, which are composites of density, diversity, design and route variables. Such compact indices reflect the interrelatedness of the individual-level built environmental variables more effectively and have often been employed as a planning and policy tool. At the same time, a major criticism associated with such an approach is that we are able to get the overall picture, but at the cost of a loss of resolution and loss of purchase in terms of designing interventions: the impact of specific neighbourhood attributes upon health cannot be ascertained per se in this method.

A number of studies have reported the development of a composite walkability index. Cervero and Duncan (2003) employed factor analysis to combine a number of determining built environment variables, including an employed residents-to-retail/services balance index, an employed residents-to-job balance index, mixed-use entropy, average square metres per block within 1 mile, proportion of three-way, four-way, five-way or more intersections, and dead-end proportions within 1 mile of origins and destinations, and eventually reduced them to four factors – the pedestrian- and bicycle-friendliness of trip origins, pedestrian- and bicycle-friendliness of trip destinations, land use diversity of trip origins and land use diversity of trip destinations. The study reported that land use diversity at the origin was beneficially associated with walking. Saelens, Sallis, Black et al. (2003) developed a survey tool called the Neighbourhood Environment Walkability Scale (NEWS) to assess the key built environment characteristics theorized to be associated with physical activity. It was based upon built environment measures of residential density, proximity and ease of access to non-residential destinations (expressed as land use mix–diversity and land use mix–access), street connectivity, walking and cycling facilities, aesthetics, traffic safety, and crime safety. Residential density was expressed in terms of the frequency of various types of neighbourhood residences and was weighted relative to the average density of single-family detached residences. Mix was evaluated in terms of walk proximity from home to various types of services. The responses ranged from 1–5 minutes' walking distance (coded as 5) to ≥30 minutes' walking distance (coded as 1). A Likert-type scale was employed to put the responses in one of the four categories, ranging from 'strongly disagree' to 'strongly agree', with higher scores indicating a more favourable value of the built environment characteristics. Subsequently, an Australian version of this instrument was developed (Cerin et al., 2008). Frank et al. (2006) conducted the Neighbourhood Quality of Life Study (NQLS) in King County and Seattle, Washington and in the Baltimore–Washington, DC region, to assess the nature of the relationship between urban form and physical activity and obesity. They developed a walkability index which reflected the composite measure of built environment design expressed as the sum of the z-scores of residential density, intersection density, land use mix and retail floor area ratio. An Australian study modelled on the NQLS study was the Physical Activity in Localities and Community Environments (PLACE), conducted by Leslie et al. (2007) at the level of Australian Bureau of Statistics census collection districts, which included 156 CCDs representing households from 32 communities. The walkability index had four similar components – dwelling density, intersection density, land use entropy and net retail area. A 1–10 score was employed for each of the components, which were summed to produce walkability scores ranging from 4 to 40. The walkability index scores for each of the CCDs were classified into quartiles, the first quartile representing low-walkability CCDs and the fourth quartile high-walkability CCDs. Another large-scale European study, equivalent to the NQLS and PLACE, was the Belgian Environmental Physical Activity Study (BEPAS) conducted by Van Dyck et al. (2010) in 24 neighbourhoods from 201 statistical sectors of Ghent. The study aimed to examine the nature of association between neighbourhood walkability, SES and physical activity among Belgian adults. Their neighbourhood walkability index comprised three components of objectively measured residential density, intersection density and land use mix, which were normalized and converted to z-scores. Walkability was expressed as:

$$\text{Walkability} = (2\text{z-connectivity}) + (\text{z-residential density}) + (\text{z-land use mix})$$

The impact of urban sprawl on physical activity and weight outcomes has been an active area of research. In another study, S. Doyle et al. (2006) developed a composite measure of walkability which was the summation of the z-scores of the negative average block size, the percentage of all blocks having areas of less than 0.01 square mile, and the number of three-, four- and five-way intersections divided by the total number of road miles. They reported a higher propensity to walk and improved weight outcomes in respondents residing in counties that were more walkable and had lower crime rates in reference to those that were less walkable and more crime-prone. Under the Walkable and Bikeable Communities Project, data on approximately 200 directly observable neighbourhood attributes within 1 kilometre and 3 kilometre circular buffers were captured, and measured distance to destinations up to 3 kilometres from a respondent's home were enumerated. Of the Euclidean and network buffer models developed, eight of the built environment variables were found to have a significant association with walkability in the Euclidean buffer model. They included: shorter distance to closest grocery store; more dwelling units per acre; more grocery stores, more restaurants, or higher retail density; fewer educational parcels; fewer grocery stores or markets within a 1 kilometre buffer; smaller size of closest office complex; longer distance to closest office or mixed-use complex; and smaller size of block where residence is located. They were combined to compute composite walkability scores within 100, 500 and 1000 metre buffers (C. Lee and Moudon, 2006a; Berke, Koepsell et al., 2007). High walkability scores were reported to be beneficially associated with walking for exercise but not with weight outcomes (Berke, Koepsell et al., 2007). In another study Berke, Gottlieb et al. (2007) reported that walkability scores at 100, 500 and 1000 metres were associated with lower odds of depression among men, but not among women.

Several studies have reported beneficial associations between mental health and improvements in built environment (Halpern, 1995; Delgard and Tambs, 1997). In recent years, several studies have investigated the role of composite micro-level local neighbourhood environmental quality and design clearly in determining individual behaviour as well as psychological health. These studies are mostly based on detailed environmental audits and surveys conducted by trained individuals reporting objective measures as well as subjective perceptions of the built environment.

Weich et al. (2001, 2002) reported the 27-item observer-rated instrument called the Built Environment Site Survey Checklist (BESSC), which was developed to assess the built environment across 11 housing areas in two electoral wards of North London. The component items included questions with respect to the predominant characteristics of buildings, audit of the immediate space around the buildings, neighbourhood facilities and accessibility as well as perception of safety and security. The instrument was employed as a psychometric tool to study the association between environmental quality and depression and reported higher odds of depression in properties characterized by predominantly deck access and those more recently (post-1969) constructed. Dunstan et al. (2005) reported the development of the survey instrument known as the Residential Environment Assessment Tool (REAT), used to assess the contextual physical aspects as well as the extent to which residents establish territoriality over their neighbourhood. The composite REAT index comprised 28 items measured at the postcode level in the Neath Port Talbot borough of South Wales. Each item was scored between 0 and 1 and subsequently multiplied by an assigned integer weight ranging from 1 to 3. It comprised component sub-indices for physical incivilities, territorial functioning, defensible space, natural environment and a miscellaneous component. It relies on the subjective evaluation of surveyors. H. Thomas et al. (2007) employed REAT as a psychometric tool to study the contextual variations of mental health but found no significant association between REAT measures and psychological health. Araya et al. (2007) developed a similar instrument, called the Built Environment Assessment Tool (BEAT), for the city of Santiago, Chile. It comprised 25 items across four factor-analysis-derived components representing: general quality of the area; facilities, noise and traffic in the area; public green areas; and empty sites. Their study reported a significant association between the quality of the built environment and the prevalence of common mental disorders. S.C. Brown et al. (2009) employed the University of Miami Built Environment Coding

System (UMBECS) to assess 3857 property lots in East Little Havana, Florida. They considered seven building-level indicators representing the *eye on the street*, including above-grade front entrance (i.e. a building whose base lies at least 12 inches above the level of the adjacent sidewalk), stoop, porch, ground-floor parking, window area, window sill height and building setback. The study reported that architectural features of the front entrance that promote visibility of the building's exterior were beneficially associated with perceived social support, while those promoting visibility from the building's interior were negatively associated. Structural equation path models indicated a positive association between perceived social support and reduced psychological distress among the elderly.

4.5 WHAT NEXT? MOVING FROM THE NEIGHBOURHOOD TO THE CITY LEVEL

To conclude this detailed and extensive review, we present a summary of the various categories of built environment variables studied in Table 4.3, with the finer details of the studies and key findings summarized in Table 4.4. Table 4.5 summarizes the survey instruments employed thus far in built environment–health studies for identifying composite quality and design attributes. A scan of these tables reveals a number of consistent findings, but also shows that the magnitude, direction and significance of associations between neighbourhood-level built environment factors and health outcomes are mixed for some dimensions or variables. As well as possibly reflecting unmeasured effects, this may be attributed to the general lack of uniformity in built environment–health studies. Methodological issues arising are summarized below:

- There is no standard set of rules for the selection of built environment and confounding variables in models. Different studies have employed different criteria.
- There is no standard definition of 'neighbourhood' in BE–health studies. Most of the studies have employed census-defined boundaries as a proxy neighbourhood. More accurate definitions, for example defined by a buffer around a subject's home, have been employed. However, operationalization of the idea of functional neighbourhoods is a challenge on account of variability in the concept and data.
- Contextual built environment factors are often unique and local to a particular neighbourhood and city being studied. Thus two cities may have different land use and street configurations and socio-

economic dynamics. Even within the same city, two neighbourhoods may have contrasting dynamics, for example the dynamics of the city centre may be quite different from the dynamics of the peripheral suburbs.

- Most importantly, the compositional and socio-demographic characteristics of the individuals and population being studied may be quite varied. In other words, the association between a particular contextual built environment factor and the health outcome may differ according to the age, gender, socio-demographics and lifestyle factors. This is something that can best be addressed through larger-scale studies.

Other methodological questions pertain to the robustness and reliability of the strength and significance of associations measured. Most of the studies have a cross-sectional design. Longitudinal studies are scarce, primarily on account of the lack of prospective data on health outcomes, as well as on built environment attributes. Consequently, the question about the impacts of sustained exposure to changes in the built environment still remains to be answered with any degree of certainty.

Similarly, designs that reliably indicate causality are scarce for the same reason. Natural and controlled experiments are difficult to design, especially given the large numbers needed to capture weak (but significant) associations. Again, large longitudinal studies are the way forward for drawing stronger causal conclusions.

As well as increasing numbers and adding temporal change data, another approach to overcome these limitations may be to move up to the next spatial hierarchy in the urban health niche model, focusing empirical studies on the city and regional level. There is a need to conduct within-city studies to compare the associations between the built environment and health between clusters of homogeneous neighbourhoods. Studies with a similar design have been previously conducted (Saelens, Sallis, Black et al., 2003; Handy et al., 2006; Cerin, Macfarlane et al., 2007). Within-city between-neighbourhood studies have the potential to identify differences in health outcomes within the city as well as uncover specific cross-level interactions such as different impacts of the built environment on health in neighbourhoods with different SES. Several between-cities regional-level studies have also been reported (Ellaway et al., 2005; Sallis, Bowles et al., 2009). Nonetheless, care should be taken so that the subjects and cities chosen for such studies have a certain degree of homogeneity. Such a design may have the potential to unearth certain regional-level factors at work. Accompanying such models should be more perceptive behavioural theory that generates plausible explanations for the area effects captured at different spatial scales. For example, at a city scale, differences between cities in a regional study may reflect differences in public transport consumption culture that may tend to develop separately in each city. These might, for example, give rise to minor but systematic differences between cities in the cost of time or perceived cost of distance, which without systematically capturing the 'city effect' would confound just about all measures of accessibility used in the models.

Prospective, cohort or longitudinal studies have the potential to identify the city-wide effects of changes in the built environment upon health. A few built environment–health studies have reported longitudinal models of health outcomes (F. Li, Harmer, Cardinal, Bosworth et al., 2009; Wolch et al., 2011). Nonetheless, there is an urgent need to compile retrospective (or indeed prospective) spatial data on the built environment, as this will make possible the identification of impacts of urban regeneration and other forms of retrofitting urban spatial structure of a city. The impact of exposures to differential environments within a city can be further gathered from longitudinal studies of the impact of mobility on health. Several studies have looked into the impact of moving from one neighbourhood to another (Delgard and Tambs, 1997; Wells and Yang, 2008; I.M. Lee et al., 2009). Longitudinal multi-level studies have the potential to further isolate the effects into neighbourhood-level and individual-level factors, in addition, as we have noted, to moving towards explaining causality (Diez Roux, 2004b). Case-controlled studies or retrospective study designs (Schlesselman, 1982) conducted over a period of time have the potential to isolate the beneficial or detrimental effects of specific built environment attributes upon the vulnerable individuals of the population.

Several US studies have tried to assess the impact of urban sprawl with the help of composite sprawl indices and have consistently reported detrimental effects (Ewing, Schmid et al., 2003; R. Lopez, 2004; Garden and Jalaludin, 2009; I.M. Lee et al., 2009). However, such analysis should not be isolated from the question of economies of urban scale in health and health provision. Almost a generation ago, several authors helped formalize a modern theory of *agglomeration* economies within a city system (Segal, 1976; Moomaw, 1981; Henderson, 1986, 1988). Sprawl might be associated with more car-borne travel, but larger cities might be associated with greater innovation and efficiency in health care. At a population level we may wish to ask if there exist optimal city-size thresholds for health, both outcomes and health service supply.

As suggested in Figure 1.1, it is expected that increasing city size magnifies the agglomeration effects manifested in the form of enhanced economies in infrastructure, services and accessibility, until we reach point P3 of the curve. Beyond P3, the benefits of agglomeration are offset by increasing externalities of pollution, congestion, informality and poverty (on the periphery in the typical developing country and in the core in some Western and transitional countries). We can now add to the interpretation of that curve and of that point all of the alleged and evidenced health 'costs' documented in this review. Of course, point P3 of the curve will be unique to each city, and this is indicative of the necessity to conduct future studies focusing on relationships between urban spatial scale, the urban production function (cost of running cities of different sizes, including running their health care systems) and population health, with the objective of identifying the optimum size in terms of both area and population density and imposing policy constraints accordingly.

With individual-level studies, in addition to neighbourhood-level context variables, the impact of the city as a whole should be taken into consideration as envisaged by the urban health niche model. For example, a pertinent question in the public health context is: do spatial network attributes at the levels of household, surrounding neighbourhood, city and overall region have any impact upon an individual's health, and how do we analytically capture them in order to study the nature of potential correlations? Spatial road networks are the arterial and venal systems of the city. They distribute the benefits of urban agglomeration to individuals and share out the costs. This relative apportionment can be measured using network models of accessibility as independent predictors in the kind of well-founded epidemiological models discussed in this chapter. Measuring the detailed topology and geometry of an urban habitat's connectivity system at different spatial scales is likely to increase the power of models that attempt to find associations between attributes of the built environment and health. This is the overriding hypothesis of this book.

To the present knowledge of the authors, the work in the subsequent chapters (and the related work already published) is the only work to model the simultaneous analysis of the effects of multiple network attributes at different spatial scales upon individual health outcomes. We therefore offer the remaining chapters of this book as a unique contribution to the body of knowledge reviewed in this chapter.

Table 4.3 Summary of the neighbourhood-level built environment variables employed in assessing health outcomes

References	Range of neighbourhood built environment variables															Notes and other measures (if any)
	Density	Land use diversity/ mix	Destinations						Street network and transport system			Pedestrian infra-structure	Cycling infra-structure	Crime	Aesthetics	
	(1)	(2)	3a	3b	3c	3d	3e	3f	4a	4b	4c	(5)	(6)	(7)	(8)	
Cervero and Duncan (2003)		✔*							✔							Others: Block density, residentialness index, residents-to-retail/services balance index, residents-to-job balance index. Note: All the variables were assessed within a neighbourhood, both the trip origins and the destinations.
Ewing, Schmid et al. (2003)	✔	✔							✔							Note: Composite sprawl indices* were developed: metropolitan sprawl index (also considered degree of centrality) and county sprawl index (also considered block measures).
Giles-Corti et al. (2003)					✔*		✔*		✔*			✔*	✔			Note: The variables included both objective and perceived self-reported measures.

Saelens, Sallis, Black et al. (2003)	✔*	✔*		✔				✔*	✔	✔	✔	✔*	✔*	Note: These constituted the self-reported Neighbourhood Environment Walkability Scale (NEWS).
Burdette and Whitaker (2004)						✔	✔					✔		Note: No significant results.
Ewing et al. (2004)	✔[a]	✔[b]		✔				✔		✔*	✔			a → Residents + jobs density. b → Job–residence balance, job mix. Others: Accessibility indices.
Frank et al. (2004)	✔	✔*						✔						Others: Time spent in cars*, distance walked*.
R. Lopez (2004)	✔													Urban Sprawl Index* based on population density.
M. Duncan and Mummery (2005)	✔[a]*		✔*		✔*			✔		✔*		✔	✔*	a → Number of active people in 1 km radius. Others: Also included number of registered dogs within buffer. Some of the measures were perceived self-reported.

Table 4.3 (continued)

References	Range of neighbourhood built environment variables															Notes and other measures (if any)
	Density	Land use diversity/ mix	Destinations						Street network and transport system			Pedestrian infra-structure	Cycling infra-structure	Crime	Aesthetics	
	(1)	(2)	3a	3b	3c	3d	3e	3f	4a	4b	4c	(5)	(6)	(7)	(8)	
Ellaway et al. (2005)															✔[a]*	a → Objectively assessed scale based on amount of graffiti, litter and dog mess, as well as the level of vegetation and greenery visible on the dwelling and streets immediately surrounding it.
Hoehner et al. (2005)	✔[a]		✔	✔			✔*			✔	✔*	✔*	✔*	✔	✔*	a → Number of non-residential/specific-purpose destinations. Note: The variables included both objective and perceived self-reported measures.
W.C. King et al. (2005)	✔[a]		✔	✔*		✔*	✔									a → Housing characteristics of participants' neighbourhoods (measured as a percentage of residents living in poverty*, with less than

											a bachelor's degree, non-White and unemployed; median household income; urbanicity; and median year that homes were built*).
van Lenthe et al. (2005)		✔	✔*	✔	✔*				✔*	✔a*	a → Noise pollution. Note: Based on self-reported scores of general attractiveness of neighbourhoods, proximity to neighbourhood facilities and crime.
F. Li, Fisher, Brown-son et al. (2005)	✔a*	✔*	✔	✔*		✔*	✔	✔	✔*		a → Number of households, places of employment. Note: Some of the measures were perceived self-reported.
Rutt and Coleman (2005)	✔a*	✔	✔			✔		✔			a → Population density, density of non-residential buildings. Others: Slope, overall health*, SES*, number and type of morbidities*, television time, fruit and vegetable consumption*, perceived barriers to physical activity*. Note: Some of the measures were perceived self-reported.

Table 4.3 (continued)

Refer-ences	Range of neighbourhood built environment variables															Notes and other measures (if any)
	Density	Land use diversity/ mix	Destinations						Street network and transport system			Pedestrian infra-structure	Cycling infra-structure	Crime	Aesthetics	
	(1)	(2)	3a	3b	3c	3d	3e	3f	4a	4b	4c	(5)	(6)	(7)	(8)	
Gordon-Larsen et al. (2006)			✔[a]	✔[a]		✔[a]	✔[a]									a → Number of physical activity facilities per census blocks*.
Inagami et al. (2006)								✔[a]*								a → Access to grocery stores, disadvantage score difference between grocery store neighbourhood and residential neighbourhood. Others: neighbourhood SES.
C. Lee and Moudon (2006b)	✔[a]*		✔	✔	✔	✔		✔		✔	✔	✔*			✔	a → Net and parcel-level residential density. Others: block size, slope*. Note: Some of the measures were perceived self-reported.
Mobley et al. (2006)		✔*		✔[a]*				✔[a]						✔*		a → Number of fitness facilities, full-sized grocery stores, fast-food establishments, restaurants and minimarts per 1000 residents. Others: Neighbourhood affluence*.

Morland et al. (2006)							✔*		–
Nelson et al. (2006)				✔				✔[a]	a → Three-way and four-way intersection density, α index, γ index and cyclomatic index within buffer. Others: Also included road type. Note: The study compared self-reported physical activity in six neighbourhood clusters.
Norman et al. (2006)	✔[a]	✔	✔*		✔[b]*	✔*		✔*	a → Residential density. b → Retail floor area ratio. Other: Index of neighbourhood walkability.
Berke, Koepsell et al. (2007)	✔[a]*				✔		✔*		a → Dwelling units per acre. Others: block size*, size of closest office complex*, number of educational parcels*. Note: The variables were employed to construct the neighbourhood walkability score.

Table 4.3 (continued)

References	Range of neighbourhood built environment variables															Notes and other measures (if any)
	Density	Land use diversity/ mix	Destinations						Street network and transport system			Pedestrian infra- structure	Cycling infra- structure	Crime	Aesthetics	
	(1)	(2)	3a	3b	3c	3d	3e	3f	4a	4b	4c	(5)	(6)	(7)	(8)	
Boehmer et al. (2007)	✔[a*]						✔			✔	✔	✔*			✔*	a → In terms of presence of non-residential destinations. Note: The variables included both objective and perceived self-reported measures.
Boer et al. (2007)	✔[a]	✔[b*]							✔*							a → Housing density. b → Business diversity score; number of different types of businesses in a neighbourhood. Others: block length, parking pressure.
Cerin, Leslie et al. (2007)	✔[a*]	✔	✔		✔*	✔	✔	✔								a → Objective profile of LUM, based on clustering of neighbourhoods with similar proportion of land uses. Perceived proximity* to non-residential destinations was

															based on the sub-scale of Neighbourhood Environment Walkability Scale.
Cerin, Macfarlane et al. (2007)	✔[a]	✔			✔	✔			✔	✔		✔	✔	✔	a → Residential density. Note: These constituted the self-reported Chinese version of Neighbourhood Environment Walkability Scale (NEWS)*.
Diez Roux et al. (2007)			✔	✔*			✔								–
Jilcott et al. (2007)			✔[a]	✔[a]*			✔[a]								a → Proximity to physical activity resource. Note: The variables included both objective and perceived self-reported measures.
Rundle et al. (2007)	✔[a]*	✔*							✔		✔[b]*				a → Population density. b → Bus stops/km², subway stops/km².
Stafford, Cummins et al. (2007)	✔[a]*			✔		✔	✔*	✔					✔*	✔*	a → Population density. Others: Policing levels, perceived social disorders and participation in physical activity.
Tilt et al. (2007)			✔			✔	✔	✔							Others: NDVI index of greenness, self-reported destinations, natural features, satisfaction

Table 4.3 (continued)

References	Range of neighbourhood built environment variables															Notes and other measures (if any)
	Density	Land use diversity/ mix	Destinations						Street network and transport system			Pedestrian infra-structure	Cycling infra-structure	Crime	Aesthetics	
	(1)	(2)	3a	3b	3c	3d	3e	3f	4a	4b	4c	(5)	(6)	(7)	(8)	
																with greenness, and perceived importance of destinations. Note: Composite measures of objective and subjective accessibility and greenness were significant.
Forsyth et al. (2008)	✔	✔	✔	✔	✔	✔	✔	✔a*	✔*		✔	✔*			✔	a → Density of food store employees. Others: Also included perceived environmental measure.
Leslie and Cerin (2008)	✔	✔*	✔			✔*			✔*	✔*		✔*	✔		✔*	Note: These constituted the Australian version of self-reported Neighbourhood Environment Walkability Scale (NEWS).
F. Li et al. (2008)		✔*	✔*					✔*	✔*		✔*					–

Mujahid, Diez Roux, Shen et al. (2008)					✔					✔	✔	Note: In addition, measures of walking environment, safety and social cohesion were used to construct two self-reported indices of neighbourhood physical environment* and neighbourhood social environment*.
Nagel et al. (2008)			✔	✔*		✔	✔	✔[a]	✔			a → Calculated as number of bus lines. Others: Street volume*.
Smith et al. (2008)	✔[a]					✔*						a → Population density in block group. Others: Housing age*, proportion walking to work*.
Wells and Yang (2008)	✔[a]	✔[b*]				*			✔			a → Population density, employment density, housing density, service job density. b → Service jobs/population ratio, job/resident ratio. Others: Design features of the lot and building.

Table 4.3 (continued)

References	Range of neighbourhood built environment variables															Notes and other measures (if any)
	Density	Land use diversity/ mix	Destinations						Street network and transport system			Pedestrian infra-structure	Cycling infra-structure	Crime	Aesthetics	
	(1)	(2)	3a	3b	3c	3d	3e	3f	4a	4b	4c	(5)	(6)	(7)	(8)	
B.B. Brown et al. (2009)	✔[a]*	✔[b]	✔						✔*		✔*					a → Areas under six land uses. b → Six-, three- and two-category land use mix. Others: Proportion of residents who walk to work, tract housing age*.
Dengel et al. (2009)	✔[a]	✔[b]		✔			✔	✔*	✔							a → Residential density. b → Employment density, percentage land use under residential, parks and recreation, vacant. Others: Distance to schools.
Garden and Jalaludin (2009)	✔[a]															a → Population density-based sprawl index*. Others: 2001 Index of Relative Socio-Economic Disadvantage.
I.M. Lee et al. (2009)	✔[a]															a → Sprawl index* based on population density and block size.

Pan et al. (2009)				✔			✔			✔	✔	✔		Others: Social support. Note: The measures were perceived self-reported. The overall index of facility availability remained a significant predictor of physical activity.
Sallis, Bowles et al. (2009)	✔[a]	✔			✔[b≍]				✔					a → Net residential density. b → Retail FAR. Note: These constituted the census-block-level walkability index.
Santana et al. (2009)			✔	✔		✔[a*]	✔	✔		✔[b]			✔*	a → Including public health services. b → Traffic accidents. Others: Household inadequacy, neighbourhood deprivation.
Black et al. (2010)	✔[a*]			✔*				✔*					✔	a → Percentage of residential and commercial land use. Others: Composite index of neighbourhood amenities* and neighbourhood vulnerability.

Table 4.3 (continued)

References	Range of neighbourhood built environment variables															Notes and other measures (if any)
	Density	Land use diversity/ mix	Destinations						Street network and transport system			Pedestrian infra-structure	Cycling infra-structure	Crime	Aesthetics	
	(1)	(2)	3a	3b	3c	3d	3e	3f	4a	4b	4c	(5)	(6)	(7)	(8)	
Gómez et al. (2010)		✔	✔*				✔*		✔*	✔*	✔	✔				Note: The measures were both objective and perceived self-reported.
Owen et al. (2010)	✔[a]	✔			✔[b]				✔							a → Dwelling density. b → Net retail area ratio. Note: These constituted the composite walkability index*. A Dutch version of the Neighbourhood Environment Walkability Scale instrument was also employed.
Pouliou and Elliott (2010)	✔[a]*	✔*					✔	✔	✔*							a → Residential density. Others: Composite walkability index*.

Troped et al. (2010)	✔[a*]	✔[*]			✔[*]					a → Residential population density and housing unit density. Others: Greenness measured by NDVI*.
Wood et al. (2010)	✔[a]	✔[*]	✔[b*]	✔	✔	✔		✔	✔	a → Net residential density. b → Commercial FAR. Others: Presence of steep hills* and interesting sites*. Note: The variables included both objective and perceived self-reported measures.
Yan et al. (2010)	✔[a]	✔[b]	✔		✔	✔[*]	✔[c]	✔[*]	✔	a → Tract population density, density of housing units, 3D population density. b → Diversity index, HHI, acreage of commercial area. c → Residential and commercial transit. Others: Access to central business district (CBD).

Table 4.3 (continued)

References	Range of neighbourhood built environment variables															Notes and other measures (if any)
	Density	Land use diversity/ mix	Destinations						Street network and transport system			Pedestrian infra-structure	Cycling infra-structure	Crime	Aesthetics	
	(1)	(2)	3a	3b	3c	3d	3e	3f	4a	4b	4c	(5)	(6)	(7)	(8)	
Burgoine et al. (2011)	✔[a]*	✔						✔	✔							a → Residential density.
Saarloos et al. (2011)	✔[a]	✔*			✔[b]*	✔[b]	✔[b]		✔							a → Residential density. b → Presence/absence of retail, community services, business and offices. Others: Composite walkability index.

Notes:
1: Density (residential/population); 2: Land use mix; 3a: Public spaces and open spaces; 3b: Sports and physical activity facilities; 3c: Retail/ commercial establishments; 3d: Services; 3e: Recreational facilities; 3f: Food environments; 4a: Connectivity characteristics of streets; 4b: Traffic safety (speed/volume); 4c: Access to public transit stops and stations; 5: Pedestrian infrastructure; 6: Cycling infrastructure; 7: Crime; 8: Aesthetics.
* → Significant association.

Table 4.4 Summary of research evidence from the studies of the association between the neighbourhood-level built environment variables and health outcomes

Reference	Sample size/ geographical extent	Outcome variables	Neighbourhood definition	Key neighbourhood environmental variables	Key socio-economic and demographic variables	Model type	Significance results
Balfour and Kaplan (2002)	A one-year follow-up study of 883 older adults who participated in the 1994 and 1995 waves of the Alameda County Study in Alameda County, California.	Functional loss (a nine-item score consisting of pushing a large object, lifting a weight of more than 10 pounds, reaching the arms up above the shoulders, writing or handling small objects, stooping or crouching, getting up from a stoop, standing in place for more than 15 minutes, walking a quarter-mile, and walking	Census tract.	Rating the seriousness of six potential neighbourhood problems associated with urban living (crime, lighting at night, traffic, excessive noise, trash and litter, and access to public transportation).	Age, sex, family income, household size, educational level, race/ ethnicity, social connectivity (marital status, membership in social, political and community groups, and degree of social isolation), health (self-rated health, levels of depressive symptoms, count of chronic conditions), smoking, alcohol consumption, body mass	Logistic regression using generalized estimating equations.	In reference to individuals living in no-problem neighbourhoods, those who resided in multiple-problem neighbourhoods reported higher odds of overall functional loss (OR=2.23, 95% CI: 1.08, 4.60) and lower extremity functional loss (OR=3.12, 95% CI: 1.15, 8.51). Neighbourhood problems identified to be associated with the largest increase in risk were excessive noise, inadequate lighting and heavy traffic.

Table 4.4 (continued)

Reference	Sample size/ geographical extent	Outcome variables	Neighbourhood definition	Key neighbourhood environmental variables	Key socio-economic and demographic variables	Model type	Significance results
		up a flight of stairs).	Census tract.		index and scale of physical exercise.		
Takano et al. (2002)	A cohort of 3144 older adults born in 1903, 1908, 1913 or 1918 in two cities of Tokyo metropolitan area and followed up between 1992 and 1997.	Five-year survival of older adults.	–	Residential environment questionnaires with components of: presence of space for taking a stroll near residence, parks, noise from automobiles and factories, levels of crime, hours of sunlight, existence of gardens, whether residence faced a road with a regular bus service, active communication among neighbours, preference to continue to live in the current community.	Age, sex, marital status and living expenses.	Chi square, Kruskal–Wallis test, principal component analysis and logistic regression.	Probability of five-year survival was beneficially associated with presence of space for taking a stroll near residence ($p<0.01$), presence of parks and tree-lined streets ($p<0.05$) and preference to continue to live in the current community ($p<0.01$). Principal component analysis identified two factors. After controlling for individual-level variables, the five-year survival was significantly associated with the factor of walkable green streets and spaces near residence (OR=1.13, 95% CI: 1.03, 1.24).

Weich et al. (2002)	A cross-sectional sample of 1887 individuals in two electoral wards of North London.	Depression measured by the Center for Epidemiologic Studies Depression Scale (CES-D).	Housing areas (areas with homogeneity in housing form).	A 31-item Built Environment Site Survey Checklist (BESSC) with items of predominant form, height and age of housing, number of dwellings and type of access, provision of gardens, use of public space, amount of derelict land, security, and distances to local shops and amenities.	Age, gender, ethnicity, marital status, employment status, educational qualifications, access to cars or vans, and dwelling-level factors (tenure, floor level, presence of structural problems of dampness, leaking roof, rot in wood, infestation, and length of stay in current dwelling).	Logistic regression. Sensitivity analysis through OLS regression.	Prevalence of depression was significantly associated with living in housing areas characterized by properties with predominantly deck access (OR=1.28, 95% CI: 1.03, 1.58) and recent/ post-1969 construction (OR=1.43, 95% CI: 1.06, 1.91).
Cervero and Duncan (2003)	Cross-sectional sample of 7889 randomly selected households in the nine-county San Francisco Bay Area who participated in the Bay Area Travel Survey (BATS).	Non-motorized travel (walking and cycling).	1-mile radii of trip origins and destinations.	Factor analysis identified four factors: pedestrian- and bicycle-friendliness of origins and destination, land use diversity of origins and destination. The following variables were included: average square metres per block within 1 mile of origin/destination, proportion of three-way, four-way, five-way or more	Gender, race/ ethnicity, disability, number of vehicles in household, neighbour-hood income. Constraints to walking/ cycling: trip distance, slope,	Discrete choice logit modelling.	The only built environment factor reported to be significant to walking was land use diversity at the trip origin (β=0.098, p=0.021). In the case of the cycling choice model, the urban design and land use diversity factors were positively associated but not significant at 5% probability level.

Table 4.4 (continued)

Reference	Sample size/ geographical extent	Outcome variables	Neighbourhood definition	Key neighbourhood environmental variables	Key socio-economic and demographic variables	Model type	Significance results
				intersections within 1 mile of origin/destination, dead-end proportions within 1 mile of origin/destination, mixed-used entropy within 1 mile of origin/destination, 'residentialness' at origin/destination, residents-to-retail/services balance index and residents-to-job balance index within 1 mile buffer of origin/destination.	rainfall on day of trip, trips made during nightfall.		
Ewing, Schmid et al. (2003)	Cross-sectional sample of 206 992 adults of 448 US counties and 175 609 adults from 83 US metropolitan areas who participated in the Behavioural Risk Factor Surveillance System (BRFSS) study.	Health behaviour and health status: any physical activity, recommended physical activity, minutes walked, BMI, obesity and morbidity (hypertension, diabetes and coronary heart disease).	County and metropolitan levels.	Metropolitan sprawl index (residential density, land use mix, degree of centring, street accessibility). County sprawl index (gross population density, percentage of population living at densities 1500 persons/square mile, percentage of population living at densities 12 500 persons/square mile, county population/amount of urban land in square mile, average block size, percentage of blocks 1/100 of a square mile or less).	Age, gender, race/ethnicity, education, smoking, diet.	Hierarchical linear and non-linear modelling.	Fully controlled models indicated that the residents of sprawling counties were likely to spend fewer minutes walking ($\beta=0.275$, p=0 .004). Also the residents of sprawling counties were likely to have higher BMI ($\beta=-0.0034$, $p=0.005$), be more obese ($\beta=-0.0021$, $p<0.001$) and have higher risks of hypertension ($\beta=-0.0011$, $p=0.018$). At a metropolitan level, sprawl was reported to be negatively associated with minutes walked as a leisure time activity ($\beta=0.338$, $p=0.040$).

Giles-Corti et al. (2003)	A cross-sectional survey of 1803 healthy sedentary adults, aged 18–59 years, who participated in the Study of Environmental and Individual Determinants (SEID1) in metropolitan Perth, Western Australia.	BMI based on self-reported height and weight.	–	Three objectively measured variables: type of street in which the respondent lived (cul-de-sac, highway or other), presence of sidewalks (none or on one or both sides of the road), spatial access to four or more recreational facilities. Two perception measures: presence of walking or cycle paths within walking distance or a five-minute drive, presence of a shop within walking distance.	Demographic factors (age, sex, education, occupation, SES of area of residence). Lifestyle factors (hours per week spent watching television, recreational physical activity, access to a motor vehicle). Social environmental factors (degree of physical activity).	Logistic regression.	Fully adjusted model reported that overweight was significantly associated with living on a highway (OR=4.24, 95% CI: 1.62, 11.09), streets with no sidewalks or sidewalks on one side only (OR=1.35, 95% CI: 1.03, 1.78) and perceiving no paths within walking distance (OR=1.42, 95% CI: 1.08, 1.86). Obesity was associated with poor access to four or more recreational facilities (OR=1.68, 95% CI: 1.11, 2.55) and sidewalks (OR=1.62, 95% CI: 0.98, 2.68) and perceiving no shop within walking distance (OR=1.84, 95% CI: 1.01, 3.36).
Saelens, Sallis, Black et al. (2003)	Cross-sectional samples of 54 residents from a high-walkability neighbourhood and 53 residents from a low-walkability neighbourhood,	Physical activity (measured by accelerometer), self-reported walking, and leisure time physical activity	–	Neighbourhood Environment Walkability Scale (NEWS): self-reported survey of residential density (frequency of various types of neighbourhood residences); land use mix–diversity (walking proximity from home to	Age, gender, ethnicity, education status.	ANOVA and ANCOVA, logistic regression.	Residents of high-walkability neighbourhoods reported higher residential density, land use mix, street connectivity, aesthetics and safety and had more than 70 more minutes of physical activity and had lower obesity prevalence (adjusted

Table 4.4 (continued)

Reference	Sample size/ geographical extent	Outcome variables	Neighbourhood definition	Key neighbourhood environmental variables	Key socio-economic and demographic variables	Model type	Significance results
	aged 18–65 years, from San Diego, California.	(assessed with the Godin–Shephard Leisure Time Exercise Questionnaire).	–	various types of stores and facilities between 1 and 5 minutes and ≥30 minutes); land use mix–access; street connectivity; walking/ cycling facilities, such as sidewalks and pedestrian/ bike trails; aesthetics; pedestrian/traffic safety; and crime safety (test–retest reliability=0.58–0.80).			for individual demographics) than did residents of low-walkability neighbourhoods. Also, 60% of low-walkability neighbourhood residents being overweight, prevalence estimates only 35% of high-walkability neighbourhood residents being overweight.
de Vries et al. (2003)	Cross-sectional sample of 10197 respondents from 1155 neighbourhoods who participated in the Dutch National Survey of Morbidity and Interventions in General Practice.	Self-reported health indicators (percentage of symptoms experienced in the last 14 days, perceived general health, Dutch version of GHQ score).	Netherlands was divided up into about 10000 neighbourhoods (average 1500 inhabitants). The environment of a neighbourhood was defined as a circle with a radius of 3 km around the centre of the neighbourhood.	Percentage of green space (urban green, agricultural green, forests and nature areas); percentage of 'blue' space (fresh and salt water surface); presence of a garden (from survey); urbanity (based on a five-point score).	Gender, age, number of life events in the past year, level of education, household income, number of rooms in house, type of health insurance.	Linear multiple regression (multi-level).	The percentage of green and blue space as well as the presence of a garden was positively associated with improved health outcomes expressed in terms of percentage of symptoms, perceived general health and GHQ. The relationship of green space and all the three health indicators was stronger for lower-educated people, while with number of self-reported symptoms the relationship tended to be stronger for housewives and the elderly.

Burdette and Whitaker (2004)	Cross-sectional study of 7020 low-income children enrolled in the WIC Program, aged 3–4 years and living in Cincinnati, OH, USA.	Overweight (based on body mass index scores).	–	Playground proximity, fast-food restaurant proximity and neighbourhood safety.	Age, sex, race, child's poverty ratio.	Logistic regression.	No significant association was reported between child overweight and proximity to playgrounds, proximity to fast-food restaurants or level of neighbourhood crime.
Ewing et al. (2004)	Cross-sectional sample of 709 K–12 school trips in Florida, USA for which origin and destination traffic analysis zones.	School mode choice (walkability to schools).	Traffic analysis zone (TAZ).	Overall density, job–residence balance, job mix, commercial floor area ratio. Proportion of street miles with street trees, proportion of street miles with bike lanes or paved shoulders, proportion of street miles with sidewalks, average sidewalk width. Street network density. Accessibility indices.	Annual household income, number of household members, per capita auto ownership, driver's licence owned by student.	Multinomial logit model.	Students with shorter walk or bike times to school proved significantly more likely to walk or bike. The proportion of arterials and collectors with sidewalks along them, as well as sidewalk coverage, proved to have the most significant influence on walking. Built environment did not have a significant effect on biking.
Frank et al. (2004)	Cross-sectional sample of 10878 individual respondents of the Strategies for Metropolitan Atlanta's Regional Transportation and Air Quality (SMARTRAQ) study in the Atlanta, GA region.	Body mass index.	A 1 km network buffer around a household.	Built environment (connectivity, net residential density, land use mix (four categories: residential, commercial, office, institutional)). Physical activity (time spent in cars, distance walked).	Age, education, household income, gender and ethnicity (Black male, Black female, White male, White female).	Logistic regression.	Each quartile increase in land use mix was associated with a 12.2% reduction in the odds of obesity (OR = 0.878, 95% CI: 0.839, 0.919). Each kilometre walked was associated with a 4.8% reduction in the odds of obesity (OR = 0.952, CI: 0.910, 0.997). An additional 60 minutes per day spent in cars translated to additional 6% odds of being obese (OR = 1.001, CI: 1.001, 1.002).

Table 4.4 (continued)

Reference	Sample size/ geographical extent	Outcome variables	Neighbourhood definition	Key neighbourhood environmental variables	Key socio-economic and demographic variables	Model type	Significance results
R. Lopez (2004)	Cross-sectional sample of 104084 US adult participants of the 2000 Behavioural Risk Factor Surveillance System (BRFSS).	Overweight and obesity (based on self-reported measures of height and weight to calculate the BMI).	Census tract.	Urban sprawl index developed by the Boston University School of Public Health (scale of 0–100 based on population density of census tracts).	Age, gender, race/ethnicity, income and education.	Multi-level analysis.	Urban sprawl was significantly associated with the risk of being overweight (PR = 1.002, 95% CI: 1.0006, 1.003) and obese (PR = 1.005, 95% CI: 1.004, 1.006).
M. Duncan and Mummery (2005)	Computer-assisted telephone interview (CATI) survey of 1281 residents, aged 18 years and over, and living in Rockhampton, Queensland, Australia (1215 of respondents' residential locations could be geo-coded).	Physical activity (based on Active Australia Physical Activity Questionnaire).	Radii of 0.5, 0.8, 1.0 and 1.5 km, from each respondent's home.	Objective GIS measures: Euclidean and street network distances to the nearest parkland, shopping centre, pathway network of 300 m, busy street (≥60 km/hr speed limit) and newsagent; number of 'sufficiently active' people, total amount of roadway within 20 m of a streetlight and the number of registered dogs in radii of 0.5, 0.8, 1.0 and 1.5 km, connectivity of parklands. Perceptions of physical environment: assessed on a five-point Likert scale:	Age, gender, income, level of education. Self-efficacy for performing physical activity and social support (both assessed using a five-point Likert scale).	Logistic regression.	Physical activity was reported to be significantly associated with GIS-derived measures of connectivity or route directness to parklands (OR = 1.41, 95% CI: 1.00, 1.98), network distance to parkland (OR = 1.41, 95% CI: 1.01, 1.97), the number of active people in a 1 km radius (OR = 1.64, 95% CI: 1.11, 2.43), as well as self-reported perceptions of neighbourhood cleanliness (OR = 2.67, 95% CI: 1.28, 5.55). Recreation walking was found to be negatively associated with having

				items related to safety, aesthetics, accessibility, proximity to infrastructure, and opportunities for physical activity.			footpath networks beyond 400 m (OR=0.31, 95% CI: 0.18, 0.55 in reference to within a buffer of 400 m). People whose home was classed as being in the middle tertile of registered dog numbers within 0.8 km had a positive association (OR=1.66, CI: 1.13, 2.43). Network distance to newsagents (OR=1.65, 95% CI: 1.05, 2.58), as well as good perceptions of footpath condition (OR=1.38, 95% CI: 1.00, 1.91), was positively associated with recreational walking.
Ellaway et al. (2005)	Cross-sectional sample of 6919 European residents from Angers (France), Bonn (Germany), Bratislava (Slovakia), Budapest (Hungary), Ferreira do Alentejo (Portugal), Forlì (Italy), Geneva (Switzerland)	Physical activity. Overweight and obesity.	Immediate residential environment.	Objectively assessed scale of immediate residential environment based on amount of graffiti, litter and dog mess, as well as the level of vegetation and greenery visible on the dwelling and streets immediately surrounding it.	Age, sex, socio-economic status and city of residence.	Logistic regression.	In residential environment containing high levels of greenery, the likelihood of being more physically active was reported to be more than three times (OR=3.32, 95% CI:2.46, 4.50), and the likelihood of being overweight and obese was about 40% less (OR=0.63, 95% CI: 0.49, 0.82) compared to environments with low greenery. In a residential environment containing high levels of

Table 4.4 (continued)

Reference	Sample size/ geographical extent	Outcome variables	Neighbourhood definition	Key neighbourhood environmental variables	Key socio-economic and demographic variables	Model type	Significance results
	and Vilnius (Lithuania) who participated in the Review of European Housing and Health Status (LARES) study.						incivilities, the likelihood of being more physically active was about 50% less (OR=0.53, 95% CI: 0.43, 0.72), while the likelihood of being overweight or obese was about 50% higher (OR=1.42, 95% CI:1.15, 1.96) than in areas with lower levels of incivilities.
Hoehner et al. (2005)	Cross-sectional sample of 1053 adults from high- and low-income study areas within census tracts of St Louis, MO and Savannah, GA in the US.	Physical activity behaviour, transportation activity and recreational activity (assessed from long version of the International Physical Activity Questionnaire).	A 400 metre buffer around each individual respondent's dwelling or a five-minute walk.	Perceived measures: land use (perception of many destinations within walking distance, perceived counts of specific destinations), recreational facilities (perception of places to exercise, presence of parks, trail, private fitness facility, perceived count of facilities), transport environment (perception of presence of sidewalks and bike lanes, availability of public transit, safety from traffic), aesthetics (pleasantness	Age, gender, race/ethnicity and education.	Logistic regression.	Fully adjusted models reported transportation activity to be negatively associated with objective measures of sidewalk levelness and perceived and objective neighbourhood aesthetics. It was positively associated with perceived and objectively measured number of destinations and public transit, perceived access to bike lanes, and objective counts of active people in the neighbourhood. Recreational activity

of neighbourhood, trees along streets, free of garbage, litter or broken glass, neighbourhood maintenance), social environment (perception of safety from crime, neighbourhood physical activity). Objective measures: land use (number of non-residential destinations, specific-purpose destinations), recreational facilities (number of parks with facilities, presence of at least one park, walking trail or indoor fitness facility, total number of recreational facilities), transport environment (percentage of street segments with sidewalks with no or a little unevenness, presence of bike lanes, number of bus stops, street safety score), aesthetics (segments with attractive features, trees, benches, etc., minimal garbage, litter or broken glass, physical disorder score), social environment (count of crime watch signs, count of people engaging in active behaviours).	was positively associated with perceived access to recreational facilities and objective measures of attractive features.

Table 4.4 (continued)

Reference	Sample size/ geographical extent	Outcome variables	Neighbourhood definition	Key neighbourhood environmental variables	Key socio-economic and demographic variables	Model type	Significance results
W.C. King et al. (2005)	Cross-sectional sample of 158 overweight Caucasian and African American post-menopausal women from the randomized clinical trial Women on the Move through Activity and Nutrition (WOMAN) study in south-western Pennsylvania, USA.	Total physical activity level (pedometer measured).	Census block groups, sub-divisions of US Census tracts.	Housing characteristics of participants' neighbourhoods (percentage of residents living in poverty, with less than a bachelor's degree, non-White and unemployed; median household income; urbanicity; and median year that homes were built). Proximity of businesses and facilities – within 1500 metres along the road networks (including department, discount and hardware stores, libraries, post offices, parks, walking and biking trails, golf courses, shopping centres, and museums and art galleries).	Age, race/ ethnicity, marital status, highest level of educational attainment, nature of employment, smoking status, BMI.	ANOVA, stepwise multiple linear regression.	After controlling for individual-level covariates, measures of low neighbourhood SES, i.e. percentage of residents living in poverty (β=0.3807, p=0.0259), living within walking distance of a golf course (β=8.9218, p=0.0104) and a post office (β=7.0140, p=0.0357), the proxy measure of urban form, i.e. living in a neighbourhood with homes built between 1950 and 1969 (β=7.3638, p=0.0068), were all independently associated with more physical activity.
van Lenthe et al. (2005)	A cross-sectional sample of 8767 respondents of the GLOBE Study from 78	Physical inactivity (walking and cycling to shops or	City neighbour-hoods based on infra-structural	Scores of: general attractiveness of neighbourhoods (general physical design of the neighbourhood, the quality	Age, sex, education, occupational level of the breadwinner,	Multivariate logistic regression.	Among participants aged 20–49 years of age, the odds of almost never walking or cycling to shops or work was lower

neighbourhoods of Eindhoven, Netherlands.	work; walking, cycling and gardening in leisure time, and participation in sports activities).	characteristics with an average of 2200 residents.	of green facilities, amount of noise pollution from traffic); proximity to neighbourhood facilities (availability of food shops, availability of sport and recreational facilities); safety (amount of police attention required in the area).	employment status. Neighbourhood socio-economic environment.		in neighbourhoods with the most noise pollution of traffic (OR=0.80, 95% CI: 0.66, 0.97) and poor physical design (OR=0.83, 95% CI: 0.69, 1.01). Among participants aged 50–70 years, residents in the neighbourhoods with less proximity to food shops reported significantly higher walking or cycling (OR=1.36, 95% CI: 1.09, 1.69). Probability of almost never walking, cycling and gardening in leisure time was significantly higher in the tertile of neighbourhoods with the poorest general physical design (OR=1.40, 95% CI: 1.17, 1.69) and highest level of noise pollution of traffic (OR=1.20, 95% CI: 1.01, 1.44). Probability of almost never participating in sports activities was significantly increased in neighbourhoods with the poorest proximity to sports facilities (OR=1.23, 95% CI: 1.05, 1.45) and in those requiring the most police attention (OR=1.17, 95% CI:1.00, 1.38).

Table 4.4 (continued)

Reference	Sample size/ geographical extent	Outcome variables	Neighbourhood definition	Key neighbourhood environmental variables	Key socio-economic and demographic variables	Model type	Significance results
F. Li, Fisher, Brownson et al. (2005)	Cross-sectional sample of 577 older adults aged 65–94 years from Portland, OR, USA.	Self-reported neighbourhood walking.	City defined neighbourhoods (56 in number) 0.5 mile radius around the resident's household.	Neighbourhood level: number of residential households, number of places of employment (offices and commercial buildings, workplaces, etc.), number of street intersections including those with traffic lights and those without (excluding freeway ramps), and total green and open spaces for recreation. Household level (0.5 mile radius): number of street intersections, total area of green and open spaces for recreation. Self-reported perceived measures of proximity to local recreational facilities, physical activity facilities, safety from traffic, and number of nearby recreational facilities.	Age, sex, marital status, education, household income and health status.	Multi-level modelling.	Density of places of employment in the neighbourhood ($\beta=0.15$), household density ($\beta=0.27$), number of street intersections ($\beta=0.37$), and area of green and open spaces ($\beta=0.23$) were all significantly related to walking activity at the neighbourhood level. Neighbourhood-level factors accounted for 28% of the reported variations in walking activity. At the housing level, number of recreational facilities ($\beta=0.22$) and areas reported by the residents that were safe for walking ($\beta=0.12$) were significantly related to walking activity. In addition, significant interaction was found between the variables of number of street intersections and perceptions of safety from traffic.

Rutt and Coleman (2005)	Cross-sectional sample of 943 adults, primarily Hispanic population, from El Paso, TX (452 samples were geo-coded).	Body mass index.	A 0.25 mile radius was employed for transportation and other variables; a 2.5 mile radius was used to enumerate the number of physical activity facilities around an individual's home.	Population density, land use (percentage of non-residential buildings), distance to physical activity facilities, number of physical activity facilities within a 2.5 mile radius, perceived barriers to exercise, sidewalk availability, slope, intersection number and type.	Age, SES, overall health, number and type of morbidities, acculturation, number of children, television time, fruit and vegetable consumption, and physical activity.	Structural equation modelling.	BMI was positively associated with moderate-intensity physical activity ($p=0.05$), overall health ($p=0.0004$), SES ($p=0.0003$) and living in areas with more mixed land use ($p=0.03$). Increased fruit/vegetable consumption ($p=0.04$) and younger age ($p=0.02$) acted as predictor of moderate physical activity. Time spent in light physical activities was associated with the number of co-morbidities ($p=0.02$). Increased fruit/vegetable consumption ($p=0.04$) was significantly associated with vigorous physical activity. A significant mediating relationship was found between self-reported overall health, perceived barriers to exercise, moderate physical activity and BMI, such that people with worse overall health self-reported more barriers to physical activity, less moderate physical activity and higher BMI.

Table 4.4 (continued)

Reference	Sample size/ geographical extent	Outcome variables	Neighbourhood definition	Key neighbourhood environmental variables	Key socio-economic and demographic variables	Model type	Significance results
Frank et al. (2006)	A cross-sectional sample of 1228 individuals who participated in the Neighbourhood Quality of Life Study (NQLS) in King County, WA, USA. Travel and demographic data were obtained from 5766 King County respondents.	Body mass index. Transportation-related physical activity (based on self-reported International Physical Activity Questionnaire). Vehicle miles travelled. Air pollution.	A 1 km network buffer around a household.	Neighbourhood walkability index based on net residential density, street connectivity, six-category land use mix and retail floor area ratio.	Age, gender, education, ethnicity, annual household income and presence of children below 18.	Ordinary regression.	A 5% increase in neighbourhood walkability was significantly associated with a per capita 32.1% increase in time spent in physically active travel, a 0.23-point reduction in body mass index, 6.5% fewer vehicle miles travelled, 5.6% fewer grams of oxides of nitrogen (NOx) emitted, and 5.5% fewer grams of volatile organic compounds (VOCs) emitted.
Glass, Rasmussen et al. (2006)	Cross-sectional sample of 1140 older adults aged 50–70 years from Baltimore Memory Study cohort of Baltimore, USA.	Obesity (based on BMI scores).	65 contiguous city neighbourhoods created by the Baltimore City Department of Planning.	Townsend Index of Socio-Economic Deprivation. Index of Neighbourhood Affluence. Neighbourhood Psychosocial Hazards Scale.	Age, gender, race/ethnicity, education, household wealth, alcohol consumption, tobacco use, self-reported physical activity, and dietary intake.	Multi-level logistic regression.	Residents of neighbourhoods in the highest quartile of the Neighbourhood Psychosocial Hazards Scale were nearly twice as likely to be obese compared to residents in the least-hazardous neighbourhoods (OR = 1.96, CI: 1.18, 3.28). Residents

							of neighbourhoods in the highest quartile of the Townsend Index of Socio-Economic Deprivation had higher odds of obesity as compared to those in the least deprived neighbourhoods (OR = 1.48, CI: 0.95, 2.31). The most affluent neighbourhoods had lower odds of obesity as compared to the least affluent ones (OR = 0.63, CI: 0.39, 1.02).
Gordon-Larsen et al. (2006)	Cross-sectional sample of 20 745 US adolescents from the National Longitudinal Study of Adolescent Health.	Overweight (calculated from BMI based on self-reported measures of height and weight). Achievement of five bouts per week of moderate to vigorous physical activity.	An 8.05 km (5 mile) buffer was drawn around each respondent's residence.	Number of physical activity facilities per census block (schools, public facilities, youth organizations, park, YMCA, public fee facilities, instruction, outdoor sporting or recreation camp, swimming pool, athletic club and gymnasium, tennis club, basketball club, etc.).	Population density, proportion of population with college degree or higher, and non-White proportion of the population, educational level.	Logistic regression.	Having just 1 physical activity facility per block group was associated with a 5% decrease in the relative odds of overweight relative to having no such facilities (OR = 0.95, 95% CI: 0.90, 0.99). Having just one physical activity facility was associated with increased relative odds of engaging in five or more bouts of moderate to vigorous physical activity (MVPA) per week by 3% relative to having no such facilities (OR: 1.03, 95% CI: 1.01, 1.06). Individuals who lived in census block groups with seven physical activity

Table 4.4 (continued)

Reference	Sample size/ geographical extent	Outcome variables	Neighbourhood definition	Key neighbourhood environmental variables	Key socio-economic and demographic variables	Model type	Significance results
							facilities were 32% less likely to be overweight and 26% more likely to be highly active than those who lived in block groups with no physical activity facilities.
Guite et al. (2006)	A cross-sectional sample of 854 adults derived from a survey of 2696 adults in 1610 households from four areas of Greenwich, London.	SF-36v2 mental health and vitality scores.	–	Internal environment: degree of satisfaction with level of control over heat, light, noise, damp and draughts. Density: overcrowding in home, road, estate or area. Valued escape: satisfaction with facilities for green space; shopping facilities; social and entertainment; community facilities; sports facilities. Design and maintenance: extent to which people liked the look of their neighbourhood, satisfaction with the maintenance of grassy areas and open spaces, flower beds, trees and bushes; play areas; and	Age, sex, ethnicity, duration of residence in the area, the number of dependent children, number of adults in the household, paid employment, type of dwelling and number of storeys, tenure, housing benefit, rent arrears, requesting rehousing,	Logistic regression.	Fully controlled model indicated that neighbour noise (OR=2.71, 95% CI: 1.48, 4.98 for mental health), feeling overcrowded in the home (OR=2.22, 95% CI: 1.42, 3.48 for mental health and OR=1.51, 95% CI: 0.99, 2.30 for vitality), dissatisfaction with green spaces (OR=1.69, 95% CI: 1.05, 2.74 for mental health), feeling unsafe to go out in the day (OR=1.64, 95% CI: 1.02, 2.64 for mental health and OR=1.58, 95% CI: 1.00, 2.49 for vitality) and dissatisfaction with community facilities (OR=1.92, 95% CI: 1.24, 3.00 for vitality) all remained

				entrances to blocks. Crime and fear of crime: safety while walking around in the day and night; sufficient street lighting; existence of blind spots; vandalism; graffiti; rubbish; dog mess; abandoned cars; presence of needles and syringes. Noise: street noise, neighbourhood noise, noise in the home, etc.	density of dwellings and local crime rates.		significant predictors of low SF-36v2 mental health or vitality scores or both.
Inagami et al. (2006)	Cross-sectional sample of 2144 adult respondents of the Los Angeles Family and Neighborhood Study (L.A.FANS).	BMI (based on self-reported height and weight).	Census tract.	Residential neighbourhood disadvantage score (DSR). Disadvantage score of the census tract where the respondents indicated that they shopped for groceries (DSG). DSG−DSR, i.e. the disadvantage score difference between grocery store neighbourhood and residential neighbourhood for each person, averaged for each census tract, access to grocery stores (centroid-to-centroid distance between the residential census tract and the grocery store census tract).	Age, gender, race/ethnicity, marital status, educational status, income, employment status, car ownership, neighbourhood SES.	Multi-level linear regressions.	Individuals reported higher BMI if they resided in disadvantaged areas and if the area where the average person frequented grocery stores was located in more disadvantaged neighbourhoods ($\beta=0.24$, $p \leq 0.01$). Shopping at grocery stores located ≥ 1.76 miles was an independent predictor of increments of BMI by 0.775 unit ($\beta=0.78$, $p \leq 0.05$).
C. Lee and Moudon (2006b)	Cross-sectional sample of 438 adults, aged 18 years or older	Survey based on walking for recreation and transport.	A 1 km/0.6 mile buffer area around the home (for	Perceived environmental variables: neighbourhood perception (neighbourhood type, visual look, social	Demographics: age, gender, race, marital status.	Multinomial logit models.	The study reported that utilitarian destinations were beneficially associated with transportation walking.

Table 4.4 (continued)

Reference	Sample size/ geographical extent	Outcome variables	Neighbourhood definition	Key neighbourhood environmental variables	Key socio-economic and demographic variables	Model type	Significance results
	and participants of the Walkable and Bikeable Communities (WBC) project in the city of Seattle, USA.		calculation of type and intensity of land uses) or 3 km from the home (for proximity calculations).	interaction, traffic problems and pollution), attitude (awareness of physical activity, agreement to walk/bike, awareness of congestion and pollution). Objective environmental variables: distance to the closest grocery store, restaurant, fitness centre, park, trail, number of retail stores within a 1 km buffer, total length of sidewalks within a 1 km buffer, mean traffic volume within a 1 km buffer, total number of street trees, mean block size, total number of bus rides within a 1 km buffer. Net and parcel-level residential density, mean slope within a 1 km buffer. Others: distance to the closest bank, day care, office, church, convenient store, school and post office, parcel density.	Behavioural: transit use, walking in the neighbourhood, vehicle miles travelled per month, frequency of walking for transportation purposes, recreational purpose. Household: car ownership, dog ownership.		However, recreational destinations were not associated with both categories of walking. Residential density was correlated with both categories of walking, and sidewalks with recreational walking only. Hilly terrain, as well as proximity to day care, was positively associated with recreational walking.

J. Maas et al. (2006)	Cross-sectional sample of 250 782 Dutch residents registered to 104 GPs from the second Dutch National Survey of General Practice data set.	Perceived general health (self-rated).	A 1.0 and 3.0 km radius around the respondent's residence.	Total percentage of green space (urban green, agricultural green, forests and nature conservation areas) within a 1 km radius and within a 3 km radius around a respondent's home. Urbanity (based on a five-point score).	Socio-demographic: age, sex, income and education. SES: highest level of completed education, the work situation, type of health insurance and ethnicity.	Multi-level logistic regression.	The percentage of green space inside a 1 km and a 3 km radius had a significant relation to perceived general health. Perceived general health was associated with both agricultural green (1 km: β=0.004, SE=0.000; 3 km: β=0.004, SE=0.001) and natural green (1 km: β=0.004, SE=0.001; 3 km: β=0.006, SE=0.001) in a person's living environment. The relation was generally present at all degrees of urbanity.
Mobley et al. (2006)	Cross-sectional sample of 2692 women enrolled in the WISEWOMAN programme from Connecticut, Nebraska, North Carolina and South Dakota, USA.	Body mass index. Log of ten-year risk for coronary heart disease (CHD).	Zip code level (from the US Census and US Geological Survey data, 222 in all).	Zip code level: land use mix, number of fitness facilities, full-sized grocery stores, fast-food establishments, restaurants and minimarts expressed as per 1000 residents. County level: percentage of workforce commuting outside the county.	Individual: age, race/ethnicity, education level, smoking. Socio-ecologic: index of racial segregation and income factor at the zip code level; number of robbery arrests per 100 000 residents and income inequality at the county level.	Ordinary least squares regression.	The average BMI for women living in an environment of maximum mixed land use was 2.60 kg/m^2 lower ($p<0.05$), and CHD risk was 20% lower ($p<0.05$), than for women living in a single-use environment. An additional fitness facility per 1000 residents was associated with significantly lower BMI and CHD risk, by 1.39 kg/m^2 and 15.1%, respectively ($p<0.05$). Crime was positively associated with BMI and CHD risk, whereas neighbourhood affluence was negatively associated.

Table 4.4 (continued)

Reference	Sample size/ geographical extent	Outcome variables	Neighbourhood definition	Key neighbourhood environmental variables	Key socio-economic and demographic variables	Model type	Significance results
Morland et al. (2006)	Cross-sectional sample of 10 763 respondents participating in the Atherosclerosis Risk in Communities (ARIC) study from Mississippi, North Carolina, Maryland and Minnesota, USA.	Cardio-vascular disease (CVD) risk factors: two categories of body weight (overweight and obesity), diabetes, hypertension and hypercholesterolemia.	Census tracts containing approximately 3000 to 4000 individuals were used as proxies for neighbourhoods (207 in total).	Presence of food stores/ service places (supermarket, grocery store, convenience store, full-service restaurant, franchised fast-food restaurant, limited-service restaurant) per census tract.	Age, gender, education, income, race/ ethnicity and physical activity.	Binomial regression using random effects generalized linear models.	The presence of supermarkets was associated with a lower prevalence of obesity (PR=0.83, 95% CI: 0.75, 0.92) and overweight (PR=0.94, 95% CI: 0.90, 0.98). On the contrary, the presence of convenience stores was associated with a higher prevalence of obesity (PR=1.16, 95% CI: 1.05, 1.27) and overweight (PR=1.06, 95% CI: 1.02, 1.10). Also overweight and obesity were positively associated with the presence of supermarkets and convenient stores (PR=1.11 95% CI: 1.00, 1.23) as well as grocery stores and convenience stores (PR=1.18 and PR=1.60).
Nelson et al. (2006)	Nationally represented cross-sectional sample of 20 745 adolescents of	Self-reported daily physical activity and obesity.	A 3 km Euclidean buffer around each	Number of physical activity facilities. Walkability (three-way and four-way intersection density, α index, γ index, cyclomatic	Age, census block group measures: education (proportion	Cluster analysis. Poisson regression (parameter	Six robust neighbourhood clusters were identified: rural working class; exurban; newer suburban; upper-middle-class, older

	Health in the USA.		respondent's residence.	index). Road type (proportion of A1 and A4 roads and their absolute total length).	of adults with college degree), SES (housing unit's occupancy status, home age, mobility, proportion working in county of residence), poverty (proportion of people with incomes <185% of poverty level), ethnicity (minority, proportion of non-Whites), crime (serious crimes/100 000 persons).	estimates – adjusted risk ratio).	suburban; mixed-race urban; and low-socio-economic-status (SES) inner-city areas. Compared to adolescents living in newer suburbs, those in rural working-class (ARR = 1.38, 95% CI: 1.13, 1.69), exurban (ARR = 1.30, 95% CI: 1.04, 1.64) and mixed-race urban (ARR = 1.31, 95% CI: 1.05, 1.64) neighbourhoods were more likely to be overweight, independent of individual SES, age and race/ethnicity. Adolescents living in older suburban areas were more likely to be physically active than residents of newer suburbs (ARR = 1.11, 95% CI: 1.04, 1.18).
Norman et al. (2006)	Cross-sectional sample of 799 adolescents, ages 11–15, from San Diego County, USA.	Physical activity (accelerometer measured). Body mass index.	A 1 mile buffer around the residence, with distances based on the street network.	Access to recreational facilities. Community design: residential density, intersection density, land use mix, retail floor area ratio, and an index of neighbourhood walkability.	Age, ethnicity, highest adult household education.	Hierarchical multiple linear regression.	Number of nearby recreation facilities ($\beta = 0.11$, $p < 0.05$) and number of nearby parks ($\beta = 0.14$, $p < 0.01$) were positively associated with girls' physical activity, while intersection density ($\beta = -0.14$, $p < 0.01$) was inversely related to girls' physical activity. Retail floor

Table 4.4 (continued)

Reference	Sample size/ geographical extent	Outcome variables	Neighbourhood definition	Key neighbourhood environmental variables	Key socio-economic and demographic variables	Model type	Significance results
							area ratio ($\beta=0.12$, $p<0.05$) was beneficially associated positively with boys' physical activity.
Araya et al. (2007)	A cross-sectional sample of 3870 adults in the Greater Santiago area, Chile.	Psychiatric disorders (assessed with the Revised Clinical Interview Schedule, CIS-R).	Boroughs and small geographical sectors (based on the Chilean Office of National Statistics).	25-item Built Environment Assessment Tool (BEAT) scores measured for geographical sectors. They consisted of four component factors (general quality of the area; facilities, noise and traffic in the area; public green areas; and empty sites).	Age, gender, presence of disease, income, education, marital status, housing type, number of supportive individuals and alcohol use, episodes of violent crime (sector level) and borough variables (education budget per capita, health budget per capita and number of social organizations).	Multi-level regression modelling.	Fully controlled model reported a beneficial association between factor 1 (overall quality of the built environment) and CIS-R-based psychiatric disorder ($\beta=-0.30$, 95% CI: −0.49, −0.11). There was a significant negative association between factor 4 (presence of empty sites) and mental health ($\beta=0.17$, 95% CI: 0.06, 0.28).

Berke, Gottlieb et al. (2007); Berke, Koepsell et al. (2007)	Cross-sectional sample of 740 and 936 respondents from the Walkable and Bikeable Communities Project in King County, WA, USA.	Self-reported walking for exercise, body mass index and Center for Epidemiologic Studies Depression Scale.	A 100, 500 and 1000 metre Euclidean buffer around a respondent's dwelling.	Neighbourhood walkability score, which consisted of components of: shorter distance to closest grocery store; more dwelling units per acre; more grocery store, restaurant or retail density; fewer educational parcels; fewer grocery stores or markets within a 1 km buffer; smaller size of closest office complex; longer distance to closest office/mixed-use complex and smaller size of block where residence is located.	Age, ethnicity, income, education, chronic disease burden score, smoking.	Logistic regression.	Living in highly walkable neighbourhoods was significantly associated with more walking for exercise (OR = 5.86, 95% CI: 1.01, 34.17 to OR = 9.14, 95% CI: 1.23, 68.11 for men and OR = 1.63, 95% CI: 0.94, 2.83 to OR = 1.77, 95% CI: 1.03, 3.04 for women). Living in highly walkable neighbourhoods was also associated with lower odds of depression only among men (OR = 0.31, 95% CI: 0.12, 0.81 to OR = 0.33, CI: 0.14, 0.82).
Bernstein et al. (2007)	Cross-sectional sample of 1355 residents of New York City, USA.	Alcohol use in the past 30 days.	59 community districts of New York City.	External built environment: percentage of buildings in a dilapidated condition, deteriorating condition, with external wall problems, window problems, interior or exterior stairway problems, and number of structural fires. Internal built environment: percentage of housing units with toilet breakdowns, non-functional kitchen facilities, experiencing more than three heating breakdowns in winter, with internal water leakage, with large area of peeling paint or plaster.	Age, race/ethnicity, sex, educational attainment and income.	Multi-level logistic regression.	Those living in a neighbourhood characterized by units with large areas of peeling paint or plaster (OR = 1.33, 95% CI: 1.08, 1.65) and internal water leakage (OR = 1.30, 95% CI: 1.01, 1.66) had greater odds of drinking in the last 30 days. Heavy alcohol use was significantly associated with the percentage of buildings with window problems (OR = 2.05, 95% CI: 1.03, 4.09) or stairway problems (OR = 2.34, 95% CI: 1.13, 4.86), and the percentage

Table 4.4 (continued)

Reference	Sample size/ geographical extent	Outcome variables	Neighbourhood definition	Key neighbourhood environmental variables	Key socio-economic and demographic variables	Model type	Significance results
							of units with more than three heating breakdowns in winter (OR = 2.42, 95%, CI: 1.33, 4.43), needing additional heat in winter (OR = 2.18, 95% CI: 1.21, 3.93), with large areas of peeling paint or plaster (OR = 2.02, 95% CI: 1.18, 3.46) or with internal leakage (OR = 2.55, 95% CI: 1.61, 4.05).
Boehmer et al. (2007)	Cross-sectional sample of 1032 randomly selected urban residents of the two US cities of Savannah, GA and St Louis, MO.	Obesity (obese vs normal weight, obese/ inactive vs normal weight/active) measured from self-reported body mass index.	A 400 metre (equivalent to five minutes' walk) radius surrounding each respondent's residence.	Perceived and objective environmental indicators: recreational facilities (number and access to recreational facilities, presence of equipment for physical activity); land use (non-residential destinations); transportation (sidewalks, access to transit stops, traffic safety); aesthetics (pleasantness of the community, presence of interesting locations;	Age, gender, education.	Logistic regression.	Being obese was significantly associated with perceived indicators of no nearby non-residential destinations (OR = 2.2, 95% CI: 1.3, 3.5), absence of sidewalks (OR = 2.2, 95% CI: 1.1, 4.3), unpleasant community (OR = 3.1, 95% CI: 1.5, 6.5) and lack of interesting sites (OR = 4.8, 95% CI: 2.4, 9.8) as well as observed indicators of poor sidewalk quality (OR = 2.1, 95% CI: 1.3, 3.6), physical disorder

				presence of garbage, litter, broken glass; maintenance).			(OR=4.0, 95% CI: 2.3, 7.0) and presence of garbage (OR=3.7, 95% CI: 2.1, 6.6).
Boer et al. (2007)	Cross-sectional sample of 29 724 respondents from ten largest consolidated metropolitan statistical areas of Boston, Chicago, Dallas, Detroit, Houston, Los Angeles, New York, Philadelphia, San Francisco and Washington, USA who participated in the National Personal Transportation Survey (NPTS).	Walking trips.	A 0.25 mile radius of the centroid of the block group of the household.	Housing density, fraction of four-way intersection, block length, land use mix (business diversity score; number of different types of businesses in a neighbourhood), parking pressure (number of residents per foot of parkable street length).	Age, gender, household size, Hispanic ethnicity, race, consolidated metropolitan statistical area (CMSA), individual education, job status and household life cycle.	Logistic regression.	Higher levels of business diversity and higher percentage of four-way intersections were beneficially associated with walking. Moving from two different business types in the neighbourhood to three types (OR=1.15, 95% CI: 1.001, 1.320) as well as four different business types (OR=1.24, 95% CI: 1.11, 1.39) significantly improved the probability of walking. Neighbourhoods with 50–74% four-way intersections had higher odds of walking (OR=1.4, 95% CI: 1.09, 1.78) relative to those with 25–49% four-way intersections.
Cerin, Leslie et al. (2007)	Cross-sectional sample of 2650 residents from 32 urban neighbourhoods aged 20–65 from the Physical Activity in Localities and	Weekly minutes of walking for transport (based on the long version of the International Physical Activity	Census collection districts (CCDs), 154 in total.	Objective index of land use mix (LU entropy). Objective profile of LUM (based on clustering of CCD with similar average proportion of land uses). Perceived LUM (number of reported destinations within 5, 6–10 and 11–20 minutes).	Age, gender, educational attainment, marital status, annual household income before taxes, employment	Generalized linear modelling.	No significant associations between objective index of LUM. Weekly minutes of walking for transport. Objective profile of LUM was positively correlated with walking for transport. Residents of commercial or industrial areas reported

Table 4.4 (continued)

Reference	Sample size/ geographical extent	Outcome variables	Neighbourhood definition	Key neighbourhood environmental variables	Key socio-economic and demographic variables	Model type	Significance results
	Community Environments (PLACE) study in Adelaide, Australia.	Questionnaire, IPAQ), monthly frequency of walking to specific destinations.		Perceived proximity of access to non-residential destinations (commercial, home/car commercial destinations, schools, workplace, bus/train stop, recreational, beach/river destinations), based on sub-scale of the Neighbourhood Environment Walkability Scale (NEWS). Neighbourhood selection (Likert-type scale of perceived importance of neighbourhood in terms of closeness to open space, jobs or school, public transport, shops and services, recreational facilities).	status, ethnicity, number of children under 18, children's age, household size.		39.6 more weekly walking minutes (95% CI: 0.4, 78.9) than the residents of recreational CCDs. Positive association was reported between different types of destinations within 5 minutes from home and weekly minutes of walking (β=3.8, 95% CI: 1.2, 6.3). Positive association was reported between perceived proximity of commercial and workplace destinations and weekly minutes of walking (β=15.1, 95% CI: 3.3, 26.8). Significant association existed between proximity of types of destinations and monthly frequency with and without controlling for neighbourhood selection, with the exception of train/ bus stops.

Cerin, Macfarlane et al. (2007)	124 participants aged 20–65 years from four objectively identified neighbourhoods (with extreme values of walkability and SES representing high walkable–high SES, high walkable–low SES, low walkable–high SES, low walkable–low SES) of Hong Kong.	Reliability and concurrent validity study of Chinese version of Neighbourhood Environment Walkability Scale for measuring the objective and perceived attributes of the neighbourhood environment for walking.	A 400 metre crow-fly buffer surrounding the specific street block.	Chinese version of Neighbourhood Environment Walkability Scale (NEWS-A), consisting of: multi-item scales of residential density, land use mix diversity, access to services, street connectivity, infrastructure and safety for walking, aesthetics, traffic safety and safety from crime; single-item scales of access to parking, hilly streets, physical/natural obstacles, and presence of cul-de-sacs. Neighbourhood SES.	–	Intra-class correlation coefficient to examine the variance in Chinese NEWS-A sub-scale owing to between-neighbourhood differences. Spearman's correlation to test the reliability of single items.	Residents from highly walkable neighbourhoods provided ratings indicative of higher residential density, land use mix diversity, access to services, street connectivity, infrastructure and safety for walking and fewer cul-de-sacs and hills, less traffic, lower levels of environmental aesthetics.
Diez Roux et al. (2007)	Cross-sectional sample of 2723 adult residents, aged 45–84 years from the Multi-Ethnic Study of Atherosclerosis (MESA) and living in New York City, Baltimore, MD and Forsyth County, NC, USA.	Physical activity (based on semi-quantitative questionnaire adapted from Cross-Cultural Activity Participation Study).	A 0.5 (0.8 km), 1, 2 and 5 mile buffer of each participant's residence.	Total number of parks. Population adjusted density of recreational resources (team sports, dual sports, running areas, water activities, tai-chi, Pilates, yoga, martial arts, aerobics, cardiovascular equipment weight training, gymnastics, dancing, skating, skiing, golf and others), total number and acreage of parks within the buffer.	Age, gender, race/ethnicity, income, and perceived neighbourhood violence.	Binomial regression.	Density of resources was positively associated with physical activity for neighbourhoods ranging from 1 mile to 5 miles (PR = 1.15, 95% CI: 1.04, 1.27 for 1 mile; PR = 1.15, 95% CI: 1.04, 1.27 for 2 miles; and PR = 1.06, 95% CI: 0.96, 1.18 for 5 miles). These associations were slightly stronger among minority and low-income residents.

Table 4.4 (continued)

Reference	Sample size/ geographical extent	Outcome variables	Neighbourhood definition	Key neighbourhood environmental variables	Key socio-economic and demographic variables	Model type	Significance results
Jilcott et al. (2007)	Cross-sectional sample of 199 women enrolled in the randomized trial conducted by the WISEWOMAN programme from three counties in south-eastern North Carolina, USA.	Moderate to vigorous physical activity (MVPA), accelerometer measured.	A 1 and 2 mile Euclidean or crow-fly buffer of the respondent's dwelling.	Perceived proximity to resources: perceived distance to nearest school, gym or recreation centre and park; presence of school, gym or recreation centre and park within a ten-minute drive from home. Objectively measured proximity: road network distance of the participant's home to the closest physical activity resource and number of each type of physical activity resource in the 1 and 2 mile buffer.	Age, race, BMI, education, baseline self-reported annual household income, smoking status, and urbanicity.	Multiple linear regression.	Greater perceived distance to gyms ($\beta=-0.19$, $p=0.05$) and objective number of schools ($\beta=-0.17$, $p=0.03$) were negatively associated with fewer minutes of MVPA. No significant relationships were found between physical activity and perceived or objectively measured proximity to parks.
Kligerman et al. (2007)	Cross-sectional sample of 98 White or Mexican American adolescents, aged 14.6–17.6 years from San Diego County, CA, USA.	Physical activity (accelerometer measured).	0.25, 0.5 and 1 mile, with distances based on street networks.	Walkability index (based on land use mix, net residential density, intersection density and retail FAR). Shortest distance to the nearest public or private recreation facility. Total number of recreation facilities within the buffered areas.	Age, gender, ethnicity, BMI, parent-reported marital status, employment status, parent education, household income, number in household, and parentage.	Linear regression.	None of the recreation facility variables was related to moderate to vigorous physical activity (MVPA). Walkability index at 0.5 mile buffer was beneficially associated with MVPA ($\beta=0.278$, 95% CI: 0.285, 1.864) and explained approximately 4% of the variance.

Rundle et al. (2007)	Cross-sectional sample of 13 102 adult respondents of the New York Cancer Project from the 1989 census tracts in five boroughs of New York.	Body mass index.	Census tract.	LU mix, access to public transport, population density, intersection density.	Age, gender, race/ethnicity, education, pre-tax income, census tract-level poverty, and interactions between gender and race/ethnicity.	Multi-level model.	Fully adjusted model reported significant inverse associations between BMI and mixed land use ($\beta=-0.46$, 95% CI: −0.88, −0.04), subway stops ($\beta=-0.04$, 95% CI: −0.08, −0.004) and population density ($\beta=-0.24$, 95% CI: −0.31, −0.17).
Stafford, Cummins et al. (2007)	Cross-sectional sample of 6848 adult respondents of the Health Survey of England and Scottish Health Survey.	Body mass index, waist-to-hip ratio.	Local authority (LA) as well as postcode sector (PCS).	Number of high street services (pharmacies, optical and dental practices, libraries, banks, building societies, bingo halls in PCS), leisure centres (number of swimming pools and expenditure of leisure and recreation in LA), population density in PCS, food environment (number of fast-food outlets and supermarkets), crime (violent crime/1000 residents in LA), policing (number of special constables, police in LA), physical dereliction (number of missed waste collections/100 000, vacant and derelict land area in LA). Perceived social disorder in PCS. Physical	Age, gender, social class.	Structural equation model.	BMI model: neighbourhood social disorder was positively associated with number of police officers and presence of vacant/derelict land and negatively associated with number of special constables. BMI was negatively associated with average sports participation rate (standardized path coefficient (spc)=−0.038), high street facilities (spc=−0.033) and proximity to a post office (spc=−0.019), all at $p<0.05$. Waist-to-hip ratio model: waist-to-hip ratio was positively associated with neighbourhood disorder (spc=0.053) and negatively associated with population density (spc=−0.041).

Table 4.4 (continued)

Reference	Sample size/ geographical extent	Outcome variables	Neighbourhood definition	Key neighbourhood environmental variables	Key socio-economic and demographic variables	Model type	Significance results
				activity (average proportion of people participating in sports club in PCS).			
H. Thomas et al. (2007)	A cross-sectional sample of 1058 respondents who participated in the Housing and Neighbourhood and Health (HANAH) study in the Neath Port Talbot borough of South Wales, UK.	Mental disorders measured by the 12-item General Health Questionnaire.	UK census-defined postcodes.	28-item score of the Residential Environment Assessment Tool (REAT), consisting of components of physical incivilities, territorial functioning, defensible space, natural environment and miscellaneous. Composite geographical accessibility score.	Gender, age, working status, financial status, number of unaffordable lifestyle items, household-level proportion of income from benefits, household crowding, level of social support and postcode-level socio-economic deprivation.	Multi-level modelling.	There was no significant association of residential environment quality and accessibility with mental disorders. Only 2% of the unexplained variations in psychological distress were attributed to the neighbourhood (postcode) level, while 37% existed at the household level.
Tilt et al. (2007)	Cross-sectional sample of 529 residents of Seattle, WA, USA.	Walking trips per month. Body mass index.	0.4 mile of walking distance of residential parcels.	Objective accessibility: number of destinations (churches, community centres, libraries, neighbourhood communal garden spaces, parks, playgrounds, post offices,	Age, gender, education, income.	Multiple regression.	Walking trips per month were beneficially associated with objective accessibility ($\beta=2.269$, $p<0.0001$), subjective greenness ($\beta=2.047$, $p<0.0001$). There was no significant

				schools, swimming pools, theatres, banks, bars, grocery stores and restaurants) that are within the defined neighbourhood. Measure of greenness: Normalized Difference Vegetation Index (NDVI) of walkable neighbourhood for each parcel. Self-reported destinations. Self-reported natural features. Self-reported satisfaction with greenness. Perceived importance of destinations.			relationship with objective measures of actual greenness and satisfaction with greenness. An interaction effect between objective accessibility and objective greenness with respect to BMI. High NDVI areas reported a negative relationship between BMI and objective accessibility, while low NDVI areas reported a slight positive relationship.
Forsyth et al. (2008)	Cross-sectional sample of 715 participants in 36 environmentally diverse areas in Twin Cities metropolitan area, Minnesota.	Self-reported walking (transport and leisure), physical activity behaviour (seven-day travel/walking diary and the long form of the International Physical Activity Questionnaire, IPAQ), and total physical activity	Straight-line and network buffers around the participant's residence at 200, 400, 800 and 1600 metres.	Street pattern (road length per unit area; number of access points; intersections per unit area; four-way intersections/all intersections; three-way intersection/all intersections; connected node ratio). Pedestrian-oriented design (sidewalk per unit area; sidewalk length/road length; street light and street trees per length of street; percentage of street segments with marked pedestrian crossings; litter, graffiti or dumpsters; traffic calming; proximity to transit stops;	Age, gender, race, marital status, education, tenure, home ownership, car ownership, household size, and overall health.	Correlation analysis, logistic regression.	Land use mix was reported to be negatively correlated with physical activity outcomes. Significant but weak associations were observed between walk outcomes and intersections per unit area, sidewalk length, and the density of food service employment.

Table 4.4 (continued)

Reference	Sample size/ geographical extent	Outcome variables	Neighbourhood definition	Key neighbourhood environmental variables	Key socio-economic and demographic variables	Model type	Significance results
		(objectively measured by accelerometer).		transit stop density). Destinations (percentage of total parcel area in commercial, industrial, office, parks and recreation, residential, tax-exempt, vacant; percentage of land area in night-time use, social uses, retail, industrial and auto-oriented uses; dissimilarity index, entropy index, Herfindahl–Hirschman Index, employment per unit land area, retail employment per unit area; employee density in general merchandise, food stores, eating and drinking, miscellaneous retail; proximity measures). Perceived measures (street pattern, pedestrian-oriented design and destination elements).			

Leslie and Cerin (2008)	Cross-sectional sample of 2194 respondents from the Physical Activity in Localities and Community Environments (PLACE) study in Australia.	Neighbourhood satisfaction (domains consisting of safety and walkability, access to destinations, social network, travel network, and traffic and noise) and mental health assessed by self-reported SF-12 questionnaire.	Census collection districts (CCDs).	Perceived environmental characteristics were measured using the Australian version of the Neighbourhood Environment Walkability Scale. It consisted of components of perceived neighbourhood density, land use mix, access to services, street connectivity, infrastructure for walking and cycling, aesthetics and greenery, traffic load, traffic safety, crime, hilliness, physical barriers to walking, presence of cul-de-sacs and parking difficulty.	Age, gender, educational attainment, annual household income, and CCD-level median household size and median weekly income.	Generalized linear models.	Perceived environmental characteristics of aesthetics and greenery, land use mix diversity, street connectivity, traffic safety, infrastructure for walking, access to services and barriers to walking were found to be positively associated with neighbourhood satisfaction domains, while traffic load and crime were negatively associated. Three domains of neighbourhood satisfaction – safety and walkability ($\beta=1.53$, CI: 0.77, 2.29), social network ($\beta=1.74$, CI: 1.31, 2.17) and traffic and noise ($\beta=0.80$, CI: 0.36, 1.24) – were significantly associated with mental health.
F. Li et al. (2008)	Cross-sectional sample of 1221 residents aged 50–75 years from 120 neighbourhoods in Portland, OR.	BMI. Physical activity (measured in terms of neighbourhood walking, walking for transportation, walking for household errands and meeting the	798 census block groups within the urban growth boundary of Portland metro-politan area.	Land use mix, density of fast-food outlets, density of street connectivity, density of public transit stations, acreage of green and open spaces.	Age, gender, race/ethnicity, marital status, employment status, education, household income, living situation, home ownership, alcohol use, tobacco use,	Multi-level Poisson regression.	Land use mix was significantly associated with reduced odds of obesity (PR=0.749, 95% CI: 0.624, 0.899). But density of fast-food outlets was associated with increased odds of obesity (PR=1.069, 95% CI: 1.031, 1.108). Furthermore, higher mixed-use land was positively associated with all three types of

Table 4.4 (continued)

Reference	Sample size/ geographical extent	Outcome variables	Neighbourhood definition	Key neighbourhood environmental variables	Key socio-economic and demographic variables	Model type	Significance results
		physical activity recommendation).			general health status, BMI, fruit and vegetable intake, and fried food consumption.		walking activities and the meeting of physical activity recommendations. Higher street connectivity, density of public transit stations, and green and open spaces were also related in varying degrees to walking and the meeting of physical activity recommendations.
Mujahid, Diez Roux, Shen et al. (2008)	Cross-sectional sample of 2865 participants of the Multi-Ethnic Study of Atherosclerosis (MESA), aged 45–84 years and residing in Maryland, New York and North Carolina.	Body mass index.	Census tracts as proxy neighbourhoods. Survey measured BE within a 1 mile (1.6 km) buffer surrounding the participant's home.	Self-reported survey identified two factors. Neighbourhood physical environment factor consisting of measures of the walking environment (seven items) and the availability of healthy foods (three items). Neighbourhood social environment factor consisting of measures of aesthetic quality (five items), safety (three items), violent crime (four items) and social cohesion (four items).	Age, gender, race/ethnicity, education, income, time lived in the neighbourhood, diet, energy intake, physical activity.	Factor analysis, marginal maximum likelihood estimation methods.	Fully adjusted models reported that individuals residing in better physical environments had a lower mean body mass index (estimate=−0.69, 95% CI: −1.67, 0.29 for women and estimate=−0.44, 95% CI: −1.09, 0.22 for men) than those residing in worse environments. Men who resided in better social environments had a higher mean body mass index than those residing in worse environments (estimate=0.53, 95%

							CI: 0.03, 1.02). A significant attenuation of the associations after adjustment for diet and physical activity was reported, indicating a mediating role for behavioural factors.
Nagel et al. (2008)	Cross-sectional sample of 546 community-dwelling older adults in Portland, OR from the Senior Health and Physical Exercise (SHAPE) study.	Total weekly walking time (calculated by summing the brisk walking and leisure walking items from the Yale Physical Activity Scale Activities Checklist).	A 0.25 and 0.5 mile buffer around the respondent's dwelling.	Number of commercial establishments, select establishments, percentage of high-, medium- and low-volume streets, percentage of sidewalks, numbers of intersections, number of bus lines, and distance to parks.	Age, gender, race, educational level, household income, self-reported health status, walking self-efficacy, poverty, neighbourhood problems and safety.	Multi-level regression analysis.	Within a quarter-mile radius, a higher number of commercial establishments ($\beta=0.23$, $p<0.001$) and select establishments ($\beta=0.60$, $p=0.024$), and a greater percentage of high-volume streets ($\beta=1.00$, $p=0.048$) were all beneficially associated with increased total walking time, while a higher percentage of low-volume streets ($\beta=-1.16$, $p=0.004$) was associated with fewer minutes walked per week. At the half-mile buffer, similar associations were observed between total walking time and number of commercial establishments ($\beta=0.06$, $p=0.002$) and select establishments ($\beta=0.31$, $p=0.002$), and percentage of high-volume ($\beta=1.50$, $p=0.015$) and low-volume ($\beta=-1.69$, $p<0.001$) streets.

Table 4.4 (continued)

Reference	Sample size/ geographical extent	Outcome variables	Neighbourhood definition	Key neighbourhood environmental variables	Key socio-economic and demographic variables	Model type	Significance results
Smith et al. (2008)	Cross-sectional sample of 453927 residents from 564 block groups of Salt Lake County, UT, aged 25–64 years.	BMI, overweight, obesity.	Neighbourhood definitions varied between census tract, block group, 0.25 mile of resident's home.	Density (population per square mile in block group), number of intersections within 0.25 mile of the resident's home, proportion of workers walking to work in block group), housing age (census tract level).	Age, gender. Block group level: ethnic composition, median family income, and the median age of individuals.	Linear and logistic regression.	Higher intersection density was related to lower risk of being overweight (OR=0.991, 95% CI: 0.985, 0.997) and obese (OR=0.988, 95% CI: 0.980, 0.996) for men and the lower the risk of overweight for women (OR=0.993, 95% CI: 0.985, 1.000). Increases in the proportion of residents in the neighbourhood who walk to work were associated with a lower risk of overweight and obesity for both men (OR=0.958, 95% CI: 0.950, 0.965 and OR=0.911, 95% CI: 0.900, 0.922) and women (OR=0.936, 95% CI: 0.926, 0.946 and OR=0.903, 95% CI: 0.891, 0.915). Furthermore, increases in the age of the housing in the neighbourhood was associated with lower odds of overweight and obesity.

Wells and Yang (2008)	Cross-sectional sample of 70 low-income primarily African American women in the South-Eastern USA for between-group comparison of the difference in post-move walking among those living in neo-traditional and suburban neighbourhoods. Longitudinal sample of 32 women to assess the walking levels prior to and after relocation to new neighbourhoods.	Walking using pedometers.	Area within 0.25 mile of the residence along the street network (network buffer zone, NBZ).	Density (population density, employment density, housing density, service job density); land use mix (service jobs/population ratio, job/resident ratio); street network characteristics (total linear length of street, number of street intersections, number of cul-de-sacs in the NBZ). Design features (mean lot size, setback distance, presence of sidewalks, front porches, public open space).	Age, race/ethnicity, marital status, household size, number of adults in the household, number of children in the household, BMI, ethnicity.	General linear modelling for cross-sectional analysis, mixed modelling for the longitudinal study.	Cross-sectional analysis: levels of walking in neo-traditional neighbourhoods were slightly higher (62 207 steps/week) than in the suburban neighbourhoods (58 617 steps/week). Fully adjusted models indicated that African American women walked 20 184 fewer steps per week (50 320 steps/ week) than non-African American women (70 504 steps/week). Furthermore, women walked approximately 5600 more steps per week for each additional household member. Longitudinal analysis: pre-move to post-move in areas with higher land use mix, i.e. increases in the service-jobs-to-residents ratio from pre- to post-move were negatively associated with walking (31 820 fewer steps per week). Moving to an area with fewer cul-de-sacs predicted more walking (5303 more steps per week).

Table 4.4 (continued)

Reference	Sample size/ geographical extent	Outcome variables	Neighbourhood definition	Key neighbourhood environmental variables	Key socio-economic and demographic variables	Model type	Significance results
B.B. Brown et al. (2009)	Cross-sectional sample of 5000 randomly chosen residents of Salt Lake County, UT, aged 25–64 years.	Body mass index, overweight, obesity.	A 1 km street network buffer around each residence.	Land use mix (six-, three- and two-category); proxy-based measure (proportion of residents who walk to work, tract housing age); area of land uses in the mix scores (multi- and single-family residences, retail, office, education, entertainment); destination-based variables (kilometres to rail, bus stop, park in buffer); and intersection density.	Age, median family income in the census block group (BG), BG racial/ethnic composition, median age of residents in the BG, population density of the BG.	Correlation analysis, generalized estimating equations.	Older neighbourhoods with higher six-category LU mix and nearer to rail stops had better health outcomes. Male: BMI was beneficially associated with more multi-family residences ($\beta = -2.27$, $p = 0.03$) and tract housing age ($\beta = -0.02$, $p < 0.001$), and non-beneficially with intersection density ($\beta = 0.02$, $p = 0.01$). Lower rate of overweight related to more office space ($\beta = -2.35$, $p < 0.01$) and more educational space ($\beta = -3.38$, $p = 0.05$). Female: lower BMI positively associated with higher tract housing age ($\beta = -0.03$, $p < 0.001$), more office space ($\beta = -3.48$, $p = 0.02$), more entertainment space ($\beta = -7.24$, $p = 0.02$), closer to rail stops ($\beta = 0.12$, $p = 0.00$). Higher risks of obesity related to more educational

							space (β=4.16, p=0.04), less entertainment (β=−12.1, p=0.04), more distant to rail stops (β=0.06, p=0.00).
Dengel et al. (2009)	Cross-sectional sample of 188 adolescents from Minnesota, USA who enrolled in the Trans-disciplinary Research on Energetics and Cancer – Identifying Determinants of Eating and Activity (TREC-IDEA) study.	Metabolic syndrome (METS) based on METS cluster score. This was calculated as the sum of the z-scores of percentage body fat, fasting glucose, HDL-C (negative), triglycerides, and systolic blood pressure	A 1.6 km street network buffer around a respondent's dwelling.	Residential density, land use mix (expressed as employment density, percentage land use under residential, parks and recreation, vacant), street pattern (expressed as intersection density, median block size, number of access points), density and distance to fast-food and non-fast-food restaurants, density and distance to grocery stores, convenience/gas, distance to parks, distance to physical activity facilities (gym, recreation centre, walking/biking trail, school).	Age, sex, pubertal status.	Spearman correlation and multivariate regression.	Spearman correlation reported significant relationships between the built environment variables and the components of METS. A significant association was reported between an increased distance to convenience stores and the METS (β=−0.0002, p=0.04).
Garden and Jalaludin (2009)	Cross-sectional sample of 7290 residents of the NSW Population Health Survey of 2002 and 2003, aged 16 and above and living in New South Wales, Australia.	Overweight, obese (both based on self-reported BMI scores), inadequate physical activity, and minutes walked in last week.	Local governing areas (LGAs).	Sprawl (measured by population density). Area variable (2001 Index of Relative Socio-Economic Disadvantage).	Age, gender, household income, highest level of education completed, current smoking status, adequate diet, number of years lived in	Multi-level logistic regression.	The fully controlled model reported that each inter-quartile increase in sprawl was associated with higher odds of being overweight (OR=1.26, 95% CI: 1.10, 1.44), higher odds of being obese (OR=1.47, 95% CI: 1.24, 1.75) and higher odds of inadequate physical activity (OR=1.38, 95%

Table 4.4 (continued)

Reference	Sample size/ geographical extent	Outcome variables	Neighbourhood definition	Key neighbourhood environmental variables	Key socio-economic and demographic variables	Model type	Significance results
					the neighbourhood, and perceived safety.		CI: 1.21, 1.57). The odds of not spending any time walking during the past week were OR = 1.58 (95% CI: 1.28, 1.93) for an inter-quartile increase in sprawl.
I.M. Lee et al. (2009)	Harvard Alumni Health Study, US: Cross-sectional sample of 4997 men in the 1993 study and 4918 men in the 1988 study, as well as a longitudinal sample of 3448 men for longitudinal associations between changes in exposure to urban sprawl for movers and physical activity over the period 1988–93.	Physical activity (self-reported), physician-diagnosed hypertension, high cholesterol, and diabetes.	County.	Sprawl index based on gross population density, percentage living at low and at high densities, county population per square mile of urban land, average block size, and percentage of blocks 500 feet or smaller on a side.	Age, smoking habits, overweight, diet (1988 only).	Logistic regression for cross-sectional analysis. Linear regression for the longitudinal study.	Cross-sectional analysis reported that, in reference to individuals living in high-sprawl areas, those in low-sprawl areas were beneficially associated with more walking for meeting physical activity recommendations (OR = 1.38, 95% CI: 1.09, 1.76 in 1993 and OR = 1.53, 95% CI: 1.19, 1.96 in 1988), lower prevalence of overweight (OR = 0.79, 95% CI: 0.64, 0.98 in 1993 and OR = 0.81, 95% CI: 0.66, 1.00 in 1988), and hypertension (OR = 0.76, 95% CI: 0.61, 0.95 in 1993 and OR = 0.76, 95% CI: 0.60, 0.95 in 1988). Longitudinal analysis results were insignificant.

F. Li, Harmer, Cardinal and Vongjatu-rapat (2009)	Longitudinal study based on one-year follow-up of 1145 older adults from Portland, OR who participated in the Portland Neighbourhood Environment and Health Study.	Systolic and diastolic blood pressure.	Census block group.	Walkability index (consisting of components of land use mix, street connectivity, number of public transit stations, amount of green and open spaces). Density of fast-food restaurants. Eating-out behaviour. Fruit and vegetable intake.	Age, gender, education, household income, race/ethnicity, alcohol use, smoking, use of blood pressure medication, residence density, median household income, percentage of non-Hispanic Black and Hispanic residents.	Multi-level regression.	Significant reduction in systolic and diastolic pressure (−4.46 and −3.63 respectively at $p<0.001$) were reported among respondents living in high-walkable neighbourhoods. For the low-walkable neighbourhoods, density of fast-food restaurants was significantly associated with increases in systolic ($\beta=8.65$, CI: 5.1, 12.2) and diastolic ($\beta=4.07$, CI: 1.05, 7.1) blood pressure. Furthermore, weekly visits to fast-food restaurants were associated with increases in systolic ($\beta=3.11$, CI: 0.19, 6.0) and diastolic ($\beta=1.94$, CI: 0.17, 3.70) blood pressure.
Pan et al. (2009)	5167 Canadian adult respondents of the Physical Activity Monitor, aged 15–79 years.	Physical activity based on the short-form version of the International Physical Activity Questionnaire (IPAQ).	–	Self-reported physical environment variables (number of places to safely walk, number of places to safely ride a bike, number of publicly owned multi-purpose recreation trails, number of facilities, places and programmes designed for physical activity and sports, number of other places that could be used for physical activity). Social	Age, gender, education level, marital status, employment status, number of children, household income, self-rated health, intention, perceived health benefits, self-efficacy.	Multiple logistic regression.	Self-efficacy and intention exhibited strongest positive correlations with physical activity. Family income, self-rated health and perceived barriers were also consistently associated with physical activity. The effects of the perceived health benefits, education and family income were more salient to older people, whereas the influence

Table 4.4 (continued)

Reference	Sample size/ geographical extent	Outcome variables	Neighbourhood definition	Key neighbourhood environmental variables	Key socio-economic and demographic variables	Model type	Significance results
				environmental variables (information for physical activity, health and well-being; help in planning daily schedule; professional help for choosing best types of activities; convenient public transportation; affordable facilities, services and programmes; affordable support services; affordable services to link with other people).			of education was more important to women and the influence of perceived barriers was more salient to women and younger people. Facility availability was more strongly associated with physical activity among people with a university degree than among people with a lower education level.
Sallis, Bowles et al. (2009)	Cross-sectional sample of 11 541 adults aged 18–65 years and residents of 11 countries (Belgium, Brazil, Canada, China–Hong Kong, Colombia, Japan, Lithuania, New Zealand, Norway, Sweden and the US) who	Physical activity (International Physical Activity Questionnaire measured the frequency and duration of walking, and moderate-intensity and vigorous physical activity,	Area within a 10- to 15-minute walk from home.	Physical Activity Neighbourhood Environment Survey (PANES): housing type, shops within the neighbourhood, transit stop within the neighbourhood, sidewalks on streets, facilities to bicycle, access to low-cost recreation facilities, crime rate.	Age, gender, educational attainment.	Logistic regression.	Physical activity prevalence was beneficially associated with the presence of shops (OR = 1.29, 95% CI: 1.15, 1.44), access to transit stops (OR = 1.32, 95% CI: 1.16, 1.54), presence of sidewalks (OR = 1.47, 95% CI: 1.32, 1.65), bicycle facilities (OR = 1.21, 95% CI: 1.10, 1.33) and access to low-cost recreation facilities (OR = 1.16, 95% CI: 1.05, 1.27).

	participated in the International Physical Activity Prevalence Study (IPS).	for leisure, transportation and occupational purposes, and of inactivity).					
Sallis, Saelens et al. (2009)	A cross-sectional sample of 2199 adult respondents of the Neighbourhood Quality of Life Study (NQLS) from 32 neighbourhoods of Seattle–King County and Baltimore–Washington, DC.	Daily minutes of moderate to vigorous physical activity (MVPA), body mass index, mental and physical quality of life (QoL) based on SF-12.	Census block group.	Neighbourhood walkability index based on net residential density, street connectivity, six-category land use mix and retail floor area ratio. Neighbourhood income.	Age, gender, education, ethnicity, number of motor vehicles/adults in household, marital status, number of people in household, and years at current address.	Mixed effect regression modelling.	In the case of percentage overweight/obese, the walkability main effect was significant ($p=0.007$). With respect to the high-walkable neighbourhoods, those living in low-walkable neighbourhoods reported higher odds (OR=1.35, 95% CI: 1.09, 1.69). In the case of percentage obese, the income main effect was significant ($p=0.007$). With respect to the high-income neighbourhoods, those living in low-income neighbourhoods reported higher odds (OR=1.53, 95% CI: 1.12, 2.07). Physical QoL was higher in high-income neighbourhoods, but unassociated with walkability ($p=0.006$). Total MVPA was 5.8 minutes/day higher in high-walkability neighbourhoods than the low-walkable neighbourhoods ($p=0.0002$).

Table 4.4 (continued)

Reference	Sample size/ geographical extent	Outcome variables	Neighbourhood definition	Key neighbourhood environmental variables	Key socio-economic and demographic variables	Model type	Significance results
Santana et al. (2009)	Cross-sectional sample of 7669 individuals aged 18 and over from 143 neighbourhoods of Lisbon metropolitan area, Portugal.	Overweight and obesity (based on self-reported body mass index), healthy diet, moderate and vigorous physical activity.	Administrative boundaries of the wards.	Environmental opportunity (number of groceries, supermarkets, green parks, sports facilities, swimming pools, post offices). Social capital (number of clubs for recreational or sports activities, local newspaper, local newspaper circulation per inhabitant). Diverse local resources (number of dental practices, banks, ATMs, shopping centres, opticians, sports shops, book shops). Public health services (number of nursery staff, public health doctors in primary care services per 1000 inhabitants, GPs and family doctors per 1000 inhabitants). Unsafe environment (crimes, traffic accidents/1000 inhabitants).	Age, gender, marital status, educational level, economic activity, occupational class, self-rated health, income, smoking. Housing inadequacy. Deprivation.	Multi-level logistic model.	Higher crimes against property were associated with higher BMI (OR=1.02, 95% CI: 1.01, 1.03), less healthy diet (OR=0.98, 95% CI: 0.98, 0.99) and moderate physical activity (OR=0.98, 95% CI: 0.97, 0.99). Density of public health services was beneficially associated both with weight outcomes (OR=0.84, 95% CI: 0.74, 0.95) and with moderate physical activity (OR=1.38, 95% CI: 1.14, 1.66). Social cohesion was beneficially associated with both moderate (OR=1.28, 95% CI: 1.09, 1.52) and vigorous (OR=1.24, 95% CI: 1.01, 1.52) physical activity.

Black et al. (2010)	Cross-sectional sample of 9916 non-institutionalized adult respondents of New York City Community Health Survey (CHS).	Obesity calculated from self-reported body mass index ($BMI \geq 30kg/m^2$).	Based on United Hospital Fund geographic units used in 2005 Community Health Survey (34 neighbourhoods in total).	Population adjusted (per 100 000) availability of supermarkets, restaurants, emergency food providers, small grocers, fast-food outlets, beverage and snack stores, physical activity facilities. Percentage of residential and commercial land use. Violent crime. Factor analysis-based measures of neighbourhood amenities and neighbourhood vulnerability.	Age, gender, racial/ethnic identity, marital status, nativity, highest educational attainment, employment status, annual household income, and smoking status.	Multi-level Poisson regression.	Availability of large supermarkets (PR for z-score=0.88, 95% CI: 0.84, 0.93), restaurants (PR for z-score=0.87, 95% CI: 0.81, 0.93), fast-food outlets (PR for z-score=0.89, 95% CI: 0.84, 0.95), beverage and snack stores (PR for z-score=0.88, 95% CI: 0.82, 0.93) and fitness facilities (PR for z-score=0.87, 95% CI: 0.81, 0.93), and commercial land use (PR for z-score=0.89, 95% CI: 0.83, 0.94) were associated with reduced risks of obesity. Increased neighbourhood-level income (PR for z-score=0.89, 95% CI: 0.84, 0.95) was also associated with reduced risks of obesity. Higher residential land use was associated with enhanced obesity (PR=1.00; PR for z-score=1.07, 95% CI: 1.01, 1.14). Neighbourhood amenities score was a significant predictor of obesity (PR for z-score=0.85, 95% CI: 0.80, 0.91).

Table 4.4 (continued)

Reference	Sample size/ geographical extent	Outcome variables	Neighbourhood definition	Key neighbourhood environmental variables	Key socio-economic and demographic variables	Model type	Significance results
Gómez et al. (2010)	A cross-sectional sample of 1886 older adults from 50 neighbourhoods of Bogotá, Colombia.	Physical activity (adapted version of International Physical Activity Questionnaire – Short Form.	Bogotá neighbourhood as defined by Mayor's Office. Built environment was measured within a 500 metre buffer around the centroid of each neighbourhood.	GIS-based objective measures: number of TransMilenio stations, presence/absence of *Ciclovía corridor* (a recreational strategy), public park density, street connectivity index, land use mix. Perception of built environment: safety from traffic, satisfaction with quality and maintenance of sidewalks.	Age, gender, education level, years of residence in the neighbourhood, limitation to engaging in physical activity, slope, and neighbourhood SES.	Multi-level modelling.	People residing in neighbourhoods with middle tertile of park density (4.53%–7.98% of land) were more likely to walk for at least 60 minutes during a usual week (prevalence OR [POR]=1.42, 95% CI: 1.02, 1.98). Residents of areas with the highest connectivity index were less likely to report walking for at least 60 minutes (POR=0.64, 95% CI: 0.44, 0.93). Participants who reported feeling safe or very safe from traffic were more likely to report walking for at least 60 minutes (POR=1.50, 95% CI: 1.11, 2.03). The presence of *Ciclovía* was marginally associated with having walked at least 150 minutes in a usual week (POR=1.29, 95% CI: 0.97, 1.73).

Huang et al. (2010)	Cross-sectional sample of 523 primary school children, aged 11–12 years, of ten primary schools in urban and rural areas of Taipei City, Taiwan.	Physical activity assessed by: modified Chinese version of Child/ Adolescent Activity Log (CAAL). Questionnaire adapted from the short form of the International Physical Activity Questionnaire (IPAQ).	–	Modified Neighbourhood Environment Walkability Scale (NEWS): 11 component items measuring the aspects of aesthetics (four items), convenience (four items) and safety (three items).	Gender, grade in school, monthly household income, educational level of head of school.	ANOVA, multiple regression.	No significant difference in walkability was found between the urban and rural areas. There was a significant difference in accessibility of places for physical activity between the urban and rural areas, with urban children reporting better accessibility. Total hours of physical activity were beneficially associated with accessibility ($\beta=6.21$, $p=0.03$). The urban children reported more physical activity after school, on holidays and weekends, and also in total amount compared with the rural children.
Owen et al. (2010)	Cross-sectional study involving a total of 2159 (aged 20–65 years) nested within 32 communities of Adelaide and 382 (18–65 years) residents from Ghent, respectively.	Bicycle use for transport – measured by International Physical Activity Questionnaire – Long Form.	A 10- to 15-minute walk around the resident's home.	Adelaide study: walkability index based on dwelling density, street connectivity, land use mix, and net retail area ratio. Ghent study: 40-item questionnaire, which was a modified Dutch version of the Neighbourhood Environment Walkability Scale instrument.	Age, gender, educational attainment, and working status, as well as area-level SES (for Adelaide study).	Logistic regression, multi-level logistic modelling.	Higher neighbourhood walkability was associated with a higher likelihood of bicycle use for transport in Adelaide (OR$=1.82$, 95% CI: 1.24, 2.66, $p<0.01$). Also, less bicycling with increasing age. In Ghent, those living in the higher- and highest-walkability neighbourhoods had approximately a 2.5 times higher likelihood of using a bicycle for transport

Table 4.4 (continued)

Reference	Sample size/ geographical extent	Outcome variables	Neighbourhood definition	Key neighbourhood environmental variables	Key socio-economic and demographic variables	Model type	Significance results
							(OR = 2.42–2.62, p = 0.004). Also, those who were working reported less bicycle use, compared to the non-working populations. Statistically significant associations for gender in both samples, with women having a lower likelihood of bicycle use compared to men.
Parra et al. (2010)	Cross-sectional sample of 1863 older adults from 50 residential neighbourhoods of Bogotá, Colombia.	Health-related quality of life (HRQoL) employing the Short Form 8 (SF-8) instrument for self-rated health.	City neighbourhoods. All built environment (BE) variables were measured within a 0.5 km crow-fly buffer around the centroid of each neighbourhood.	Objective BE measures: public park density, number of TransMilenio stations and presence/ absence of *Ciclovía corridor* (a recreational strategy). Perceived BE measures: safety of parks, green spaces and public recreational spaces, safety from traffic, street noise levels. Walking levels based on International Physical Activity Questionnaire.	Age, gender, neighbourhood SES, education level, time of residence in the neighbourhood, living alone and proximity to family members.	Hierarchical linear regression.	The physical dimension of HRQoL was negatively associated with perception of noise level ($\beta = -1.75$, $p < 0.001$), while positively associated with perception of safety from traffic ($\beta = 3.02$, $p < 0.001$), as well as walking levels ($\beta = 9.50$, $p < 0.001$ for 150 or more minutes/week). The mental health dimension of HRQoL was negatively associated with perception of noise level ($\beta = -3.51$, $p = 0.003$), while positively associated

							with perception of safety from traffic (β=2.09, p=0.002), park safety (β=1.72, p=0.001) and walking levels (β=5.58, p<0.001 for 150 or more minutes/week). Self-rated health was beneficially associated with park safety (OR=1.40, 95% CI: 1.13, 1.73), safety from traffic (OR=1.54, 95% CI: 1.25, 1.89) and areas with more than 8% park coverage (OR=1.31, 95% CI: 1.01, 1.70).
Pouliou and Elliott (2010)	Cross-sectional sample of 5418218 respondents aged 20 years and older from the Canadian Community Health Survey (CCHS) and living in metropolitan areas of Toronto and Vancouver, Canada.	Overweight and obesity (based on BMI).	1 km buffers, with distances based on the street network.	Built environment variables: land use mix, street connectivity, residential density, density of fast-food restaurants, density of convenience stores, density of grocery stores and supermarkets and density of recreational activity facilities. Walkability index (consisting of residential density, street network connectivity and land use mix variables).	Demographic variables: age, gender, marital status, period of arrival in Canada, race/ethnicity. Socio-economic variables: income adequacy, employment status, home ownership, education level. Health status: chronic disease status, such as	Stepwise multivariate linear regression.	BMI was significantly associated with age, sex, race, participants diagnosed with chronic conditions, education. Self-reported smoking status was found to be inversely associated with BMI. Residential density was also negatively associated with BMI for both Toronto (β=−0.0534, p<0.01) and Vancouver (β=−0.2997, p<0.05). Individuals living in areas with mixed land uses (β=−1.107, p=0.001) and higher street connectivity (β=−0.00494, p=0.001)

Table 4.4 (continued)

Reference	Sample size/ geographical extent	Outcome variables	Neighbourhood definition	Key neighbourhood environmental variables	Key socio-economic and demographic variables	Model type	Significance results
					cardiovascular diseases, rheumatoid arthritis and anxiety mood disorders. Lifestyle: smoking status, drinking, physical activity, fruit and vegetable consumption.		have lower BMIs only for Vancouver, but the results were insignificant for Toronto. Individuals living in more walkable areas had lower BMI on average (0.04kg/m^2 for Toronto and 0.06kg/m^2 for Vancouver) than those living in the least walkable areas.
Troped et al. (2010)	Cross-sectional sample of 148 adults aged 19–78 years from Massachusetts, USA.	Moderate to vigorous physical activity (MVPA), calculated as total, home and office MVPA within 50 m and 1 km home and work buffers. Respondents wore	A 1 km street network buffer around the home and work locations.	Intersection density (connectivity), land use mix, residential population density, housing unit density, greenness (based on NDVI index within buffer using Landsat ETM+ satellite image).	Age, gender, race/ethnicity, education.	Multiple linear regression.	The study reported a non-significant association between built environment variables and total MVPA. Significant positive associations were reported for intersection density (β=0.4337, p=0.0004), land use mix (β=3.0128, p=0.0001), residential population density (β=0.0001, p=0.0004) and housing unit density (β=0.0001, p=0.0001)

		accelerometer and GPS unit.					within a 1 km home buffer and MVPA in buffer; vegetation index was inversely associated with home MVPA ($\beta=-5.3704$, $p<0.0001$). Significant positive associations were reported for population density ($\beta=0.00001$, $p=0.0004$) and housing unit density ($\beta=0.00001$, $p=0.0006$) within a 1 km work buffer and MVPA in buffer.
Van Dyck et al. (2010)	Cross-sectional sample of 1166 adult respondents of the Belgian Environmental Physical Activity Study (BEPAS) conducted in Ghent, Belgium.	Self-reported physical activity was collected using the long Dutch International Physical Activity Questionnaire, objectively assessed accelerometer-measured physical activity.	Census statistical sector.	Neighbourhood walkability index based on residential density, intersection density, and five-category land use mix. Neighbourhood SES based on annual household income data.	Age, gender, education, living situation, working situation, working status and BMI.	Multi-level modelling.	Living in a high-walkable neighbourhood was beneficially associated with significantly more walking for transport ($\beta=0.746$, $p<0.001$), more cycling for transport ($\beta=0.447$, $p<0.001$), more recreational walking ($\beta=0.334$, $p<0.01$) and more accelerometer-based moderate to vigorous physical activity ($\beta=0.095$, $p<0.001$), but less motorized transport ($\beta=-0.125$, $p<0.05$). Living in a high-SES neighbourhood was associated with significantly less walking for transport ($\beta=-0.360$, $p<0.05$) and more motorized transport ($\beta=0.215$, $p<0.001$).

Table 4.4 (continued)

Reference	Sample size/ geographical extent	Outcome variables	Neighbourhood definition	Key neighbourhood environmental variables	Key socio-economic and demographic variables	Model type	Significance results
Wood et al. (2010)	Cross-sectional sample of 609 participants drawn from the Strategies for Metropolitan Atlanta's Regional Transportation and Air Quality (SMARTRAQ) study in 13 county metropolitan areas of Atlanta region.	Six-item composite measure of sense of community (SofC).	A 1 km road network buffer around each participant's household.	Objective measures of built environment (land use mix, connectivity, commercial FAR, net residential density). Perception of neighbourhood (see neighbours when walking, walkable shops and services, interesting sites, good sidewalks, safe street crossings, adequate street lighting, safety from traffic when walking, safety from crime when walking, no steep hills).	Age, gender, race, number of dependent children, educational level, household income, percentage renting or owning home, length of residence, median income in the neighbourhood, percentage home ownership in the neighbourhood, and self-reported physical activity.	General linear model.	SofC was positively associated with leisure walking (days/week) ($\beta=0.329$, $p=0.000$), home ownership ($\beta=2.564$, $p=0.000$), seeing neighbours when walking ($\beta=0.682$, $p=0.000$) and the presence of interesting sites ($\beta=0.617$, $p=0.001$). SofC was also beneficially associated with higher commercial floor space to land area ratios (FAR) ($\beta=2.315$–2.607, $p=0.018$–0.046). The presence of more mixed use ($v=3.260$, $p=0.002$ in reference to high land use mix) and perceptions of steep hills ($\beta=-0.365$, $p=0.010$) were inversely associated with SofC.

Yan et al. (2010)	Cross-sectional sample of 350 high school students from the Baltimore Active Living Teens Study (BALTS) in Baltimore, MD.	Physical activity-related environmental perceptions based on the Neighbourhood Environment Walkability Scale (NEWS).	Census tracts.	Neighbourhood form: land use mix (diversity index, Herfindahl–Hirschman index, acreage of commercial land use). Density (tract population density, 3D population density, housing unit). Street pattern and circulation system (internal connectivity, external connectivity, intersection density, distance to CBD, road density). Accessibility measures (commercial distance, commercial gravity, residential transit, commercial transit). Environmental perception: access, traffic safety, neighbourhood safety.	Age, gender, race/ethnicity, grade in school.	Factor analysis and cluster analysis for classification of neighbourhood types, multinomial logistic regression.	Four neighbourhood types: arterial development, inner-city area, suburban residential and central business district were identified. Girls who lived in suburban residential areas were less likely than their central business district counterparts to perceive the facilitating effects of crosswalks (OR=0.44, 95% CI: 0.20, 0.94) and pedestrian traffic signals (OR=0.37, 95% CI: 0.18, 0.78). Girls living in inner-city neighbourhoods were more likely to perceive traffic as slow compared to central business district counterparts (OR=2.75, 95% CI: 1.04, 7.27). Boys' perceptions of their neighbourhoods did not vary by neighbourhood types.
Burgoine et al. (2011)	Cross-sectional sample of 893 individual participants of the Health Survey for England (HSE) data set from North-East England.	Body mass index and fruit and vegetable intake.	Lower super output area (LSOA).	Availability of food that is generally consumed outside the home (pizza delivery and takeaway, takeaway and restaurant), availability of food that is generally consumed within the home (supermarkets, greengrocers and convenience stores), residential density, street connectivity and land use mix.	Age, sex, ethnicity, social class, urban/rural, index of multiple deprivation, perceived vandalism and access to shops.	Correlation, ANOVA and chi square, and logistic regression.	A higher residential density was associated with increased odds of being overweight (OR=2.704, 95% CI: 1.062, 6.885 for the highest quintile). None of the other walkability and food availability variables were significantly associated with BMI and fruit and vegetable intake.

Table 4.4 (continued)

Reference	Sample size/ geographical extent	Outcome variables	Neighbourhood definition	Key neighbourhood environmental variables	Key socio-economic and demographic variables	Model type	Significance results
Saarloos et al. (2011)	Cross-sectional sample of 5218 older adults drawn from the Health in Men Study (HIMS) from Perth metropolitan area, Australia.	Prevalence of depression assessed by the self-rated 15-item Geriatric Depression Scale.	Census collection districts (CCDs).	GIS-based measures of street connectivity, residential density, land use mix, neighbourhood walkability (standardized from the preceding three variables) and land use availability expressed in terms of presence or absence of retail, other retail, business/offices, community services and recreation facilities.	Age, education, migrant status, smoking, Charlson comorbidity, living alone, housing type, index of relative socio-economic disadvantage, Duke Social Support Index (DSSI), family and friends adaptation, partnership, growth, affection, resolve (APGAR) scale, sense of community.	Multivariate logistic regression.	A higher land use mix was independently associated with higher odds of depression (OR = 1.54, 95% CI: 1.10, 2.16, and OR = 1.52, 95% CI: 1.08, 2.14 for the second and third tertiles respectively). Also retail availability was associated with a 40% increase in the odds of depression (95% CI: 1.04, 1.90).

Wolch et al. (2011)	Longitudinal (eight years) study of 3173 children aged 9–10 years from 12 communities of Southern California.	Body mass index.	A 0.5 km Euclidean buffer.	Park space in acres within a 0.5 km buffer and number of recreation programmes within a 10 km buffer. Adjustments in the models were made for traffic density within a 150 metre buffer, distance to nearest highway, population density, average urban imperviousness, average tree canopy within a 0.5 km buffer, agricultural land use, number of 'X' intersections, NDVI.	Age, ethnicity, town, gender, percentage poverty in census block of home, forcible rape rate.	Multi-level growth curve model.	Access to both parklands ($\beta = -0.1389$, 95% CI: −0.032, −0.246) and recreational programmes ($\beta = -1.4429$, 95% CI: −0.671, −2.215) was beneficially associated with BMI attained at the age of 18. Gender differences were notable, but significant only for access to recreation.
Ball et al. (2012)	Cross-sectional sample of 1062 respondents who participated in the Greater Glasgow Health Board (GGHB) Health and Well-Being Survey from 198 neighbourhoods of Glasgow, UK.	Body mass index.	Census-defined data zones (DZs).	Index of street connectivity based on measures of direction density, intersection density (for three or more directions of travel), density of cul-de-sacs, street density, length density, beta index and eta index.	Age group, gender, socio-economic position and Scottish Index of Multiple Deprivation.	Linear multi-level modelling.	No evidence of significant association between street connectivity and BMI or BMI category.

Table 4.5 Audit tools developed to study the built environmental correlates of physical activity and mental health

Audit tool	Reference	Objective	No. of items covered	Component variables	Reliability
Observational measure for urban neighbourhoods	Caughy et al. (2001)	Assessment of the neighbourhood characteristics relevant to the studies of health and well-being of families and children.	17	Physical incivilities (presence of graffiti, poorly maintained resident buildings and resident grounds, moderate or significant litter, presence of vacant/burned residences and commercial establishments, poorly maintained public space). Territoriality (presence of Crimewatch/security/'No trespassing' signs, residents react to presence of raters, a third or more of homes with borders/hedges, security bars, decorations, visible sign denoting neighbourhood name). Availability of play resources (a third or more of homes with gardens, public playground in good condition, children visible playing, street not a busy thoroughfare).	A total of 1135 hundred blocks for the 57 neighbourhoods in Baltimore City, USA were rated. The neighbourhood-level reliability for the scales of physical incivilities, territoriality, and play resources was 0.96, 0.93 and 0.94 respectively. At the street level, the reliability of the physical incivilities was 0.74; however, the street-level reliability of the territoriality and play resources scales was low at 0.33 and 0.42 respectively.
Built Environment Site Survey Checklist (BESSC)	Weich et al. (2001)	Evaluation of the psychometric properties of a set of objective measures of the built environment.	27	Housing form, number of storeys of buildings, type of access to dwellings, number of dwellings per entrance, number of dwellings in a housing area, age of housing, number of trees in public domain, nature of spaces outside dwellings, proportion of private gardens, proportion of balconies, shared	Kappa coefficients were 0.5 for 15 categorical items, and intra-class correlation coefficients exceeded 0.6 for a further three continuous measures.

				recreational space, number of vehicular entrances, number of pedestrian entrances, entrances visible from roads, footpaths, parking arrangements, number of children's play areas, footpaths overlooked, open spaces overlooked, disused buildings, derelict land, evidence of vandalism, evidence of graffiti, territorial functioning, Neighbourhood Watch signs.	
Systematic Pedestrian and Cycling Environmental Scan (SPACES)	Pikora et al. (2002)	Measurement of the physical environmental factors that may influence walking and cycling in local neighbour hoods.	35	Functional factors associated with: walking/cycling surface – path type, surface type, path maintenance, path continuity, route directness, path width, gradient; street – street width, vehicle parking, kerb type; traffic – volume, speed, traffic control devices; permeability: street design, intersection distance and design, other access points. Safety factors associated with: personal safety – lighting, surveillance, path obstruction; traffic safety – crossing, crossing aids, verge width, driveway crossovers, lane marked, path/lane continuity. Aesthetic factors associated with: streetscape – trees, garden maintenance, maintenance, pollution, cleanliness, parks; views – sights, architecture. Destination factors associated with: facilities – parks, shops, services, local facilities, vehicle parking, public transport, bike parking. Subjective assessment based on: attractiveness and difficulty for walking and cycling.	Sixteen observers assessed a total of 12925 street segments in metropolitan Perth, Western Australia. Of the 67 variables, 48 had excellent–fair inter-rater reliability (kappa ≥ 0.4), while 64 out of the 71 variables had excellent–fair intra-rater reliability (kappa ≥ 0.4).

Table 4.5 (continued)

Audit tool	Reference	Objective	No. of items covered	Component variables	Reliability
Walking Suitability Assessment Form, Bicycling Suitability Assessment Form	Emery et al. (2003)	Assessment of the suitability of sidewalks for walking and roads for bicycling.	15 (walking), 27 (bicycling)	Walking Suitability Assessment Form, consisting of: continuous items (annual average daily traffic, posted speed, number of through lanes, sidewalk presence, sidewalk condition, sidewalk width, sidewalk material, buffer width, kerb ramps, adequate lighting, isolated problem spots); and categorical items (if any busy intersections need arrow-marked cross-walks, traffic signal lights, pedestrian walk signals; if any wide intersections need refuge island for safer crossing). Bicycling Suitability Assessment Form, consisting of: general road factors (annual average daily traffic, number of through lanes, speed, outside lane width, bike lane width); pavement factors (pavement condition, presence of kerb and gutter, rough railway crossing, storm drain grate); and location factors (angle parking, parallel parking, right-only turn lanes, centre (both) turn lane, physical median, paved shoulder, marked bike lane, severe grades, moderate grades, frequent curves, restricted sight distance, numerous	Intra-class reliability correlations for the walking and bicycling assessment instruments were r=0 .79 and 0.90, respectively. Inter-coder reliability of the experts' Likert response system was r=0.73 for the walking form and r=0.77 for the bicycling form.

				driveways, numerous intersections, difficult intersections, commercial land use, industrial land use, sidewalk only one side, sidewalks don't exist).	
Neighbourhood Environment Walkability Scale (NEWS)	Saelens, Sallis, Black et al. (2003)	Assessment of neighbourhood environment characteristics hypothesized to be related to physical activity.	8	Residential density; proximity to, and ease of access to, non-residential land uses, such as restaurants and retail stores (land use mix–diversity and land use mix–access); street connectivity; walking/cycling facilities, such as sidewalks and pedestrian/bike trails; aesthetics; traffic safety; crime safety.	Intra-class correlations for the test–retest reliability of the NEWS sub-scales were all ≥0.58, and the majority of test–retest values were ≥0.75.
Walkable Places Survey (WPS)	Shriver et al. (2003)	Enables common people to assimilate site-specific physical and perceptual data evaluations for collaborative community-based neighbourhood planning.	30	30 streetscape characteristics all scored on a three-point Likert scale: traffic and parking: traffic speeds, noise/fumes, driver behaviour, parking; buildings and land use: signs, visual interest, building setback, sidewalk building links, occupancy, convenience; sidewalks: gaps/rips, width, kerb, utilities; trees and greens: buffers, bushes/grounds, trees; amenities and comforts: seating, transit shelter, lighting, information/maps, public art; intersections: crosswalks, kerb ramps, road width, kerb radius; perceptual: eyes on the street, enclosure, well-being.	Evaluation was conducted along a ten-block length of Baltimore Avenue in West Philadelphia, PA. WPS was primarily designed to be implemented by laypeople with a view to fostering community-based neighbourhood planning.
Self-reported questionnaire instrument	Echeverria et al. (2004)	Assessment of self-reported measures of the neighbourhood environment of	6 scales of 36 items and 4 indices	Six scales: aesthetic quality scale (7 items); walking/exercise environment scale (11 items); access to healthy foods scale (6 items); social cohesion scale (5 items); safety from crime scale (3 items); and	The study consisted of a face-to-face and telephone interview administered twice to 48 of a largely Latino and African

Table 4.5 (continued)

Audit tool	Reference	Objective	No. of items covered	Component variables	Reliability
		possible relevance to cardiovascular disease.		violence scale (4 items). Four indices: presence and quality of recreational facilities (2 recreational facilities indices); participation in neighbourhood activities (neighbourhood participation index); potentially stressful neighbourhood problems (neighbourhood problems index).	American study sample recruited from a public hospital setting in New York City. Cronbach's α ranged from 0.77 to 0.94 for the scales corresponding to these domains, with test–retest correlations ranging from 0.78 to 0.91. Test–retest reliability measures for neighbourhood indices of presence of recreational facilities, quality of recreational facilities, neighbourhood participation and neighbourhood problems ranged from 0.73 to 0.91.
Senior Walking Environmental Assessment Tool (SWEAT)	Cunning ham et al. (2005)	Assessment of the effects of the physical environment on walking among seniors.	188	Functionality: structural aspects of the environment, including types of buildings (32 items), sidewalks (48 items) and buffer zone/street life (54 items). Aesthetics: quality and visual appeal of the surroundings (12 items). Destination: availability of services, transportation and	Thirty-six neighbourhood segments in the city of Portland, OR were randomly selected and analysed for inter-rater reliability. The raters had acceptable agreement for

				parking in the neighbourhood (12 items). Safety: personal safety (24 items), traffic safety (6 items).	67% of the items. Almost 80% of the sidewalk and street life items were reliable, while items assessing buildings and destinations were also less reliable than other categories (44% and 42% of items reliable, respectively).
Residential Environment Assessment Tool (REAT)	Dunstan et al. (2005)	Assessment of the physical conditions of neighbourhood and residential environment.	28	A 28-item index with five sub-indices, consisting of: physical incivilities (broken/boarded-up windows, vandalism to public and private property, abandoned cars, stray roaming dogs, illegal parking, burned-out properties, dog litter in the street, littered pathway/street; territorial functioning (low external beautification, poor garden and property maintenance, absence of Neighbourhood Watch signs); defensible space (low defensible space, property density); natural environment (few trees in front garden, predominant outlook green, no trees in public space, no planted vegetation, no green space); and miscellaneous (absence of recreational space, poor path condition, vacant properties, presence of derelict land, undesirable parking, poorly maintained shared areas, industrial outlook, commercial outlook).	The REAT score ranged from 0 to 68. Four raters worked in pairs to survey the 51 postcode units of Neath Port Talbot, South Wales, UK. Inter-rater reliability was assessed for individual items and also for the total REAT score and indicated a lowest kappa of 0.58 for the condition of the paths, while the maintenance of shared space had a kappa of 0.67. Kappa values for the density of housing and maintenance of houses were between 0.7 and 0.8. Intra-class correlations were all greater than 0.9.

Table 4.5 (continued)

Audit tool	Reference	Objective	No. of items covered	Component variables	Reliability
Neighbourhood Active Living Potential (NALP)	Gauvin et al. (2005)	Neighbourhood-level measurement of active living potential.	18	Activity friendliness (expressed in terms of limits of pedestrian system to pedestrian, efforts to walk around, limits of bicycle system to cyclist's needs, efforts to cycle around, if the pedestrian system addresses the pedestrian's and cyclist's needs). Safety (degree of threat from traffic to pedestrians and cyclists, if feeling threatened with the potential for crime, if feeling comfortable with the potential for crime). Density of destinations (exclusiveness and inclusiveness of people, number of people-oriented destinations, environmental stimuli, socially dynamic/static, visual interest, variety of destinations, overwhelming).	Eight observers performed ratings of 112 neighbourhoods of Montreal, Canada. The average reliability indices across neighbourhoods were 0.78, 0.76 and 0.83, for activity friendliness, safety, and density of destinations, respectively.
Irvine–Minnesota Inventory	Day et al. (2006)	Measure the wide range of built environment features that are potentially linked to active living, especially walking.	162	Items were associated with the four domains of: accessibility (62 items); pleasurability (56 items); perceived safety from traffic (31 items); and perceived safety from crime (15 items). Some items pertain to more than one domain.	University of California–Irvine study: 76.8% of the variables had >80% agreement among the three raters. University of Minnesota study: 99.2% of the variables had >80% agreement among the two raters.

RESIDential Environment project (RESIDE)	Giles-Corti et al. (2006)	Design of Neighbourhood Physical Activity Questionnaire (NPAQ) to differentiate and measure recreational- and transport-related walking undertaken within and outside the neighbourhood and to provide an overall index of physical activity behaviour.	–	A list of behaviour-specific destinations was provided. Transport-related walking destinations included work, public transport, shops and cafés. Recreation-related walking destinations included parks, the beach, walking trails/paths, cafés and sidewalks. Participants ticked the main destinations used for walking and recorded the frequency and duration (total minutes on each occasion) of walks to each destination.	The study comprised over 82 participants, aged 20–71 years, in Western Australia. NPAQ was reported to be reliable for studies examining environmental correlates of walking within the neighbourhood (reliability of recall of whether participants had walked within the neighbourhood was kappa = 0.84, and outside the neighbourhood was kappa = 0.73).
Pedestrian Environmental Data Scan (PEDS)	Clifton et al. (2007)	Assessment of a range of micro-scale elements of the built and natural environment that predicts pedestrian movement.	40 questions, 83 measures	Segment type (low volume/high volume/ bike–pedestrian path). Environment (land uses in the segment, slope, cul-de-sacs/ dead ends in the segment). Pedestrian facility (type, path material, path obstructions, buffers between road and path, sidewalk continuity/completeness, sidewalk connectivity, sidewalk condition and maintenance). Road attributes (condition, number of lanes, posted speed limit, on-street parking, off-street parking lot spaces, whether walk through the parking lots to most buildings, driveways, traffic control devices, kerb cuts in the	A total of 71.5 miles of street and pedestrian pathways, equal to 995 segments, in the city of College Park, MD, USA were surveyed. The rater reliability testing showed that only a small number of items in the audit consistently garnered kappa scores below 0.40. These were mainly the questions involving more subjective assessment or more abstract

Table 4.5 (continued)

Audit tool	Reference	Objective	No. of items covered	Component variables	Reliability
				segment, presence of crossing aids). Walking/cycling environment (lighting, amenities, way-finding aids, number of trees shading walk areas, degree of enclosure, power lines along the segment, cleanliness, articulation in building design, building setbacks from streets, bicycle lane, transit facilities).	concepts, like amount of street lighting, articulation of building designs and degree of enclosure. On the other hand, many items (such as land uses, traffic control features, and presence of sidewalk) in the audit received very high kappa scores (0.75 or above).
Scottish Walkability Assessment Tool (SWAT) (builds upon SPACES tool to suit Northern European conditions)	Millington et al. (2009)	Objective record of the aspects of the physical environment that promote walkability in urban Scotland.	112	37 destination items: parks (2); parking (10); services (18); public transport (7). 25 safety items: personal safety (8); road safety (17). 30 aesthetics items: streetscape (20); architecture (3); views (7). 20 functional items: walking surface (16); permeability (4).	Eighteen items showed good inter- and intra-rater reliability, showing adequate variability ($0.4 \leq kappa < 0.7$), namely 5 destination items (3 parking and 2 services), 2 safety items (both traffic safety items), 7 aesthetics items (4 streetscape, 2 architecture and 1 views items) and 4 functional items (3 walking surface and 1 permeability items). Twenty-five items

					proved unreliable, and 69 items lacked adequate environmental variability.
Montreal Neighbourhood Assessment Tool (MoNAT)	Paquet et al. (2010)	Assessment of the structural and contextual environmental characteristics of urban neighbourhoods related to urban form, negative attributes, especially social disorder and negative physical attributes, and positive physical attributes.	44	Physical characteristics/condition of streets and throughways (14 items). Negative physical characteristics/condition of public spaces (9 items). Positive physical characteristics/condition of public spaces (8 items). Physical characteristics/condition of dwelling units (13 items).	Two trained evaluators rated the condition of the streets, public spaces and dwelling units and the presence or absence of specific characteristics of 250 street blocks within 30 socio-economically diverse census tracts of the Montreal metropolitan census area in 2003. Inter- and intra-rater reliability was excellent (kappa > 0.80) for items pertaining to urban form, and substantial (kappa > 0.60) for domains pertaining to positive and negative characteristics. Internal consistency was acceptable (Cronbach's alpha > 0.70) for urban form and negative characteristics, but not for positive characteristics.

5. Spatial Design Network Analysis for Urban Health (sDNA-UH)

5.1 URBAN CONFIGURATION, ACCESSIBILITY AND HEALTH BEHAVIOUR

The relationship between the structure of configured urban space in a city and human behaviour has long been established in architecture and urban design scholarship. In his seminal work on environmental cognition Lynch articulated the idea that the cognitive maps with which people perceive and navigate through urban space depend on the legibility of the city structure (K. Lynch, 1960). He proposed that cognitive maps of urban settings consist of a set of five basic types: paths, path intersections (nodes), landmarks, districts and boundaries (edges). Paths form the predominant element in urban morphology and may include channels along which individuals move, which may be in the form of roads, walkways, transit lines, canals and railways. Districts act as distinct internally homogeneous subsections or neighbourhoods, which an individual is 'inside of'. Edges constitute boundaries between two phases, representing breaks in continuity, for example shores, railway cuts, a boundary between two districts, and so on. Paths connect within and between districts, while nodes are strategic points acting as destinations, and landmarks act as meta-level points of reference. Norberg-Schulz (1971) proposed a similar topological schema. The relationship between human functioning and perception psychology within an urban space was conceptualized to evolve as a result of the three intrinsic sensations of centres or place (proximity), directions or paths (continuity) and areas or domains (enclosure). Another study reported an association between route angularity and spatial orientation of pedestrians, with oblique routes producing more disorienting effects than linear ones (Montello, 1991). Hillier proposed a formal mathematical relationship between urban spatial configuration and social processes (Hillier and Hanson, 1984; Hillier et al., 1993; Hillier, 1996). He reasoned that urban space evolves intelligibly with an inherent social logic; continuous urban space (buildings and street networks) is configured into a set of discrete interconnected units (subspaces). According to him, these subspaces may be classified into three types: linear space in the form of street segments through which people move; convex space comprising squares and public spaces in which people interact; and the ever changing visual field through which they perceive the surroundings. In Hillier's theory, it is primarily the boundaries, physical connectivity and accessibility between these sub-spaces that govern the individual's mental and behavioural responses and social interactions within them. Thus, the environmental psychology of a place is defined by the physical structure of configured urban space, which in turn governs how people perceive it and are likely to move about within it. How they move about, in turn, has a fundamental impact on an urban economy, on urban society – and on urban health.

Thus, one of the primary emergent paradigms in the study of contextual health variations has been the influence of *accessibility to health-promoting community resources* upon an individual's health. Accessibility in an urban activity space may be defined as the relative ease with which goods, services, activities and, generally, 'destinations' or 'opportunities' can be reached from a given origin, essentially the dwelling location of an individual (Litman, 2003). Handy and Niemeier (1997) define accessibility to be a function of the spatial distribution of potential destinations, the ease of reaching each destination, and the magnitude, quality and character of the activities found there, and it is quantified in terms of travel costs, travel choice and destination choice. Koenig (1980) describes two major components of accessibility: a transportation element and an activity element. The transportation element is the resistance or impedance, that is, the role played by the characteristic topology of the urban route network in facilitating or inhibiting travel between two points in space, measured in terms of travel distance, time or cost. The activity element indicates the spatial distribution of activities in the given urban space, in other words reflecting the existing land use pattern. It is often termed the 'attractiveness' of a particular location or as a trip destination. The importance of accessibility in health research stems from the spatial logic that the impedance of distance shapes mobility and individual spatial behaviour in and through urban space. Both the distance to health-promoting community resources and the spatial distribution of these offer lifestyle choices and influence individual activity behaviours (Knox, 1982). As the studies reviewed in Chapter 4 show, it is now well established that the configuration of urban space, namely land use and street network configuration, shapes physical accessibility and seems thereby to have a purchase on health.

Several studies have highlighted the associations between health and access to health-promoting community resources, including: green spaces and recreational facilities (Norman et al., 2006; Diez Roux et al., 2007; Nielsen and Hansen, 2007; Björk et al., 2008; Wolch et al., 2011); transit stops (Bassett et al., 2008; B.B. Brown and Werner, 2008; R.D. Edwards,

2008); supermarkets (Inagami et al., 2006; Morland et al., 2006; Black et al., 2010); sports facilities (Giles-Corti et al., 2003; Rutt and Coleman, 2005); community services (Field et al., 2004; J. Pearce et al., 2006); and health care facilities (Lovett et al., 2002; Luo and Wang, 2003).

Sarkar et al. (2013a, 2013b), Sarkar (2013) and Ball et al. (2012) considered the health effects of land use and street network configurations in an urban space. Some studies have also highlighted the inhibitory health effects of specific land uses, such as the density of alcohol outlets (Fone et al., 2012). Fone et al. (2012) place this within a network accessibility model. As well as affecting access to specific health-promoting or -detracting destinations, street network configuration, it is hypothesized, has intrinsic qualities that affect individual health through making walking more or less attractive. This relates both to environmental psychology theory such as that already discussed and to urban economic theory. C. Webster (2010) discusses the distinction between specific and general accessibility in the creation and intra-city distribution of urban agglomeration benefits.

Building upon these notions of accessibility in urban space, this chapter describes a novel methodology for testing and monitoring accessibility–health associations. It is a GIS model of high-resolution urban morphological metrics (morphometrics) constructed through a series of spatial network analysis techniques. We refer to it for convenience as *spatial Design Network Analysis for Urban Health* (sDNA-UH). sDNA-UH has been operationalized for the Caerphilly assembly constituency, South Wales, UK, with the objective of constructing detailed data for built environment–health epidemiological models for the population cohort of a long-standing and internationally prominent panel cohort study of adult men: the Caerphilly Prospective Study (CaPS). The use of a GIS framework enables the linking of data from diverse sources, as well as the performing of extensive spatial analyses and queries with respect to the specific attributes of the built environment. More than 100 broad categories of objectively measured morphometrics were created. Spatial analysis, data integration and compilation were performed in ArcGIS 10.0.

5.2 METHODS

5.2.1 Health Data Source

The Caerphilly Prospective Study, initiated in 1979–83 with the objective of studying the aetiology of heart disease in adult men, provided the source of health data for this research (Elwood, 1984; SS&CM,

2007). Over the past 34 years, this population-based male cohort has subsequently been used as an epidemiological laboratory for studying the various parameters of health in older adults with the progression of age. Briefly, the initial wave of the study comprised a cohort of 2512 men aged 45–59 years. Their health was followed up in four subsequent waves: phase II, 1984–88; phase III, 1989–93; phase IV, 1993–97; and phase V, 2002–04. The present research employed living members of CaPS who had participated in the third, fourth and fifth examinations and resided within the study area. The geographical extent of the study covered the assembly constituency of Caerphilly, South Wales, spreading across 114.54 square kilometres (see Figure 7.1, p. 287). The third examination was employed as a baseline in our study, while the latest follow-up comprised 1225 surviving men aged 65–84 years. The maximum follow-up period was 13.9 years, with an average of 11.7±1.0 (standard deviation) years. In each phase, the respondents answered a series of self-completion questionnaires on health, lifestyle and socio-demographic variables. Furthermore, the individual respondents attended a clinic, where they completed another set of questionnaires that included a psychiatric health section to measure mental health indices based on the General Health Questionnaire (GHQ-30) and Hospital Anxiety and Depression Scale (HADS), as well as a section on cognition and memory. Physiological data were collected through an extensive clinical examination, including anthropometry, blood pressure assessment and an electrocardiogram, and donation of a fasting blood sample. The respondents gave written consent at the time of recruitment, and the research protocol for phase III was approved by Cardiff Local Research Ethics Committee, with the protocols for phases IV and V being approved by the Gwent Research Ethics Committee.

5.2.2 Built Environment Data Source

The UK Ordnance Survey MasterMap (OSM) data layers – the Topography Layer, Integrated Transport Network (ITN) Layer and Address Layer 2 of Caerphilly – formed the basis for the construction of the morphometrics. The OSM Topography Layer contains information on detailed surface features of the landscape categorized under nine themes (buildings, roads, tracks and paths, rail, water, terrain and height, heritage and antiques, structures and administrative boundaries). The OSM Address Layer 2 provides the geo-referenced grid coordinates and the land use classifications for each and every Royal Mail address point, surveyed with a spatial accuracy of less than 1 metre. The OSM Topography Layer and Address Layer 2 were cleaned and the buildings and dwellings tables extracted. These tables enabled us to calculate the number of dwellings per building, the Royal Mail address and the OSM land use classes contained within each building unit. Data on transit stops (bus stops) were obtained from the Caerphilly Borough Council. A land use GIS of Caerphilly was extracted containing detail of each and every building in the Topography Layer. We used the same land use classification as used by the Ordnance Survey (Ordnance Survey UK, 2011). The OSM ITN Layer provides a topologically structured representation of the road network with respect to geometry of road links, road type (expressed in terms of motorway, A road, alleyway, etc.), junctions, grade separation, road names and numbers and information about the nature of road the link represents (for example single carriageway, dual carriageway or slip road). Geometric information consists of the length of the link as well as references to the node features at the ends of it. As a first step, the three layers of the OSM were linked together using a unique id known as the *topo id* (see Figure 5.1). The OSM ITN Layer was subjected to network analysis techniques to evaluate the topological accessibility indices of the street network.

5.3 BUILT ENVIRONMENT MORPHOMETRICS OF SDNA-UH

The built environment was measured within a predefined street network buffer around an individual respondent's dwelling unit. Four buffer distances of 0.5 mile, 0.8 mile (i.e. 1 kilometre), 1 mile and 1.5 miles were employed in the study for testing the effect of various health outcomes. A series of four sets of built environment morphometrics were constructed and were integrated within a GIS on the basis of the typological framework proposed by Lynch. Thus, each variable fell within one of the typologies of paths, nodes, edges and districts, while landmarks were excluded from the study, as the focus was solely on objective measurements of built environment rather than on the individual's perceptual information. The detailed architecture of sDNA-UH is shown in Figure 5.2.

5.3.1 Land Use Morphometrics

Land use mix

Land use mix reflects the degree of heterogeneity of land uses within the defined buffers. It is usually measured with an indicator that ranges from 0 to 1, with 0 representing a homogeneous, single land use environment and 1 representing a perfectly heterogeneous neighbourhood comprising all possible permutations and combinations of land use categories. Heterogeneity (entropy) is usually synonymous with smaller trip lengths,

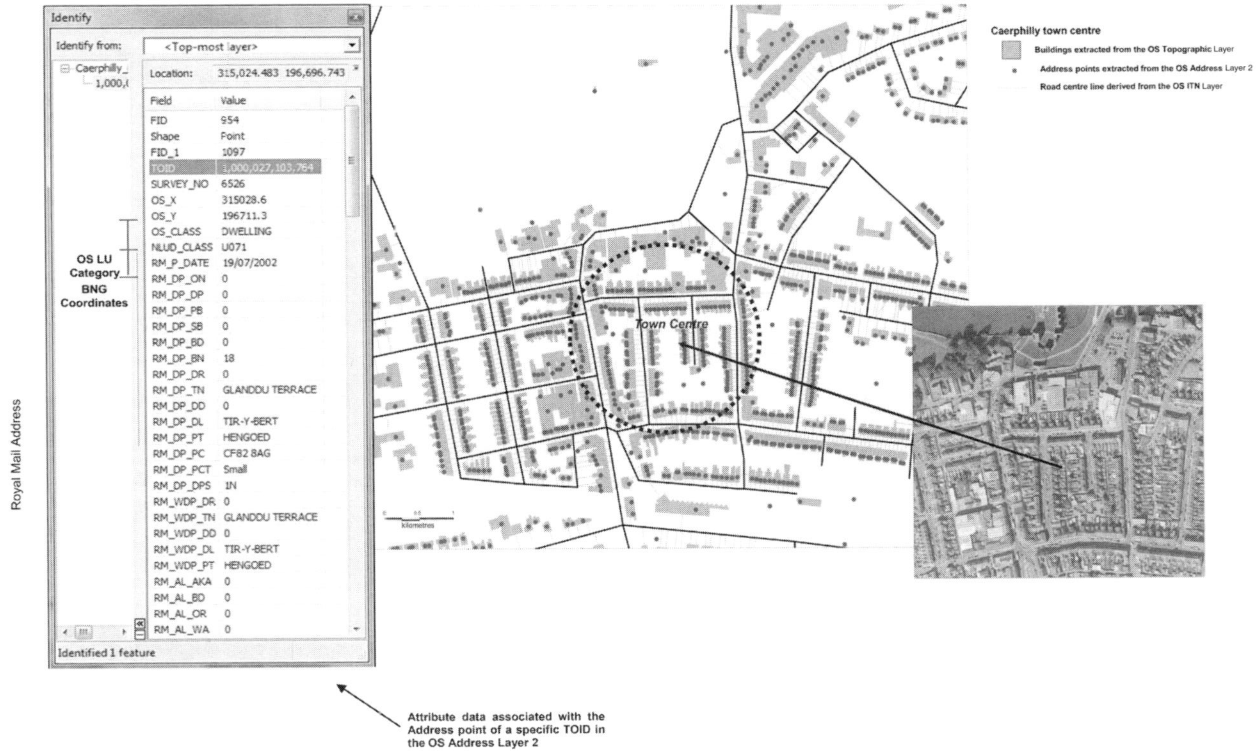

Source: Derived from UK Ordnance Survey Mastermap data of Caerphilly. © Crown copyright Ordnance Survey. All rights reserved.

Figure 5.1 Linking of the three layers of UK Ordnance Survey data

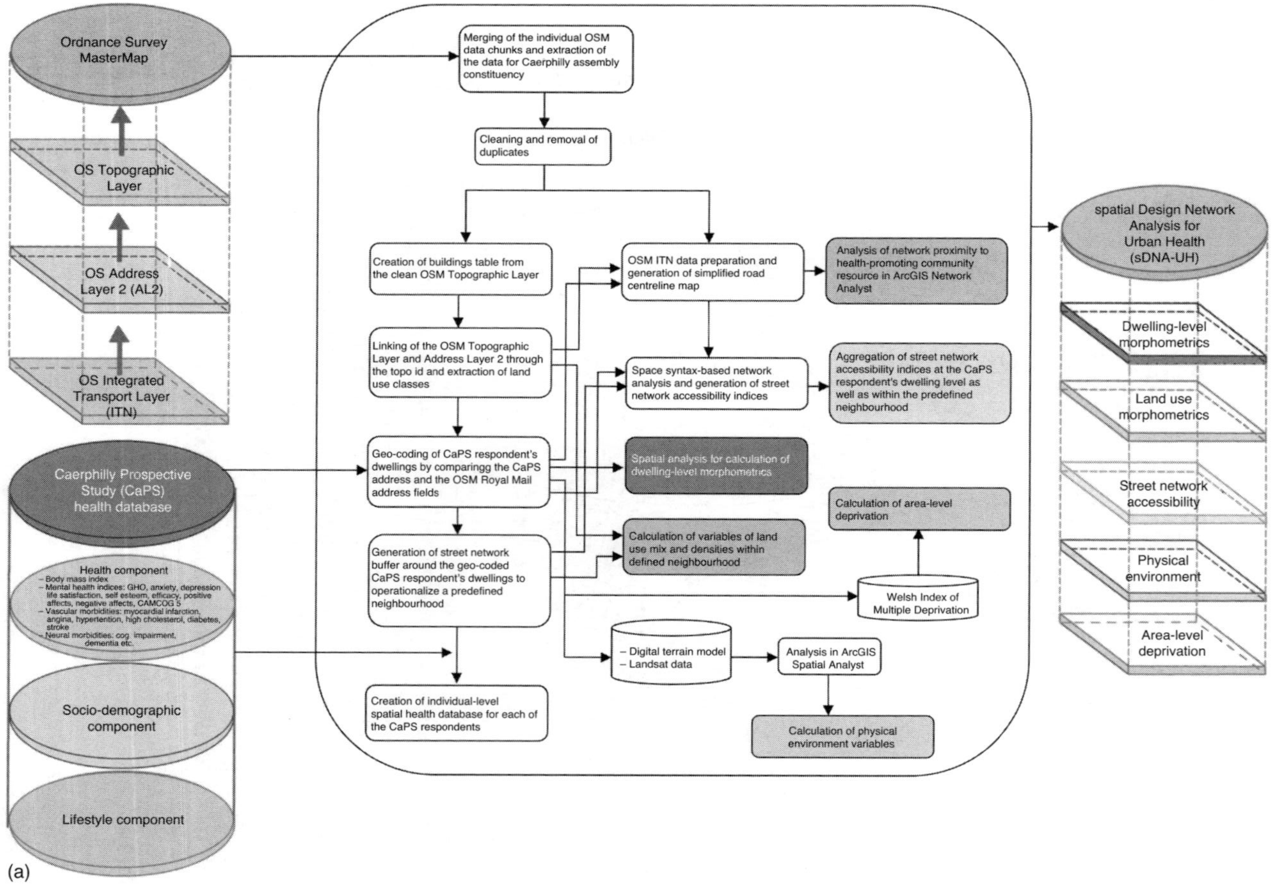

Figure 5.2a *Flow diagram illustrating the architecture of spatial Design Network Analysis for Urban Health (sDNA-UH)*

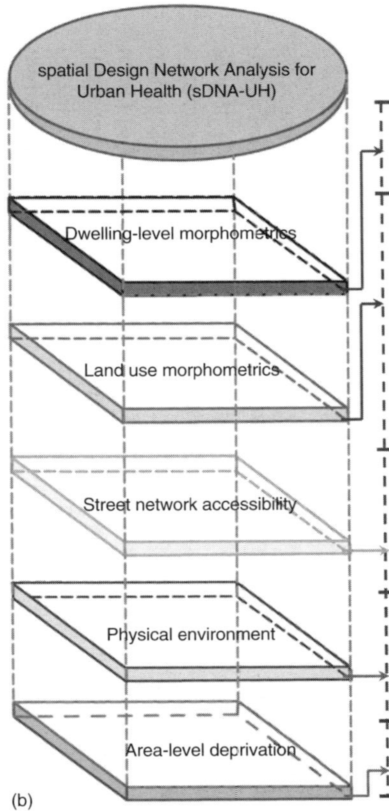

Built environment morphometrics	Description/data source/Lynch typology
Dwelling-level morphometrics (dwelling-level data extracted from OS Topographic Layer and Address Layer 2) – Node	
Dwelling-centred density	Immediate density surrounding the dwelling unit (30m kernel)
Dwelling type	Categorized as detached, semi-detached, terraced and flat
Plot exposure	Number of building fronts/exposed to street segments (Edge)
Dwellings per street segment	Number of dwelling units per segment (Edge)
Land use morphometrics (building-level land use data were extracted from OS Topographic Layer and Address Layer 2) – District	
Land use mix	Land use mix was measured within 11 km street network buffer of an individual respondent's dwelling unit
Density of retail Density of churches Density of community services Density of recreation and leisure facilities Density of business and offices Density of bus stops	Density was measured as area occupied per unit area of predefined street network buffers around an individual respondent's dwelling unit within a GIS
Destination accessibility (spatial location of destinations was extracted from OS Topographic Layer and Address Layer 2) – Node	
Accessibility to nearest green space, sports facility, health care facility, supermarket, takeaway and allotment	Measured as street network distance in metres from an individual respondent's dwelling unit in ArcGIS Network Analyst
Topological accessibilitty of streets (street network was extracted from OS Integrated Transport Network Layer, transformed and subjected to network analysis – Path	
Link connectivity Closeness Betweenness Junction connectivity	Measured for each street segment/link at varying radii to capture the effect multiple urban scales: city scale (N, 5000, 3000 m), and local/walking distance scale (1200, 800, 400 m). Thereafter, accessibility indices were aggregated at the neighbourhood (level of 1 km street network buffer of a respondent's dwelling unit), as well as at dwelling level
Network hull area	Network buffer of an individual's dwelling unit (District)
Physical environment – District	
Topography (slope raster was processed from the Blue Sky 5 metre resolution DTM)	
Neighbourhood slope variability	Measured the standard deviation of slope in degrees within 1 km street network buffer around an individual respondent's dwelling unit
Greenness (30 metre resolution Landsat data)	
NDVI	Expressed as mean Normalized Difference Vegetation Index (NDVI) within a 500 m airline buffer of a dwelling
Area-level deprivation (Welsh Index of Multiple Deprivation 2004) District	
WIMD 2005	Expressed as seven component WIMD 2005 for each census-defined lower super output area (LSOA)

Figure 5.2b *Morphological metrics (morphometrics) of spatial Design Network Analysis for Urban Health (sDNA-UH)*

fewer car trips and hence more walking, while homogeneity is assumed to be associated with more travel, especially car-borne travel, and is a feature of a health-inhibiting environment (as illustrated in Figure 5.3).

In the present study, a five-category land use mix score comprising residential dwellings, retail, community services, business and offices, and recreation and leisure was operationalized using a method proposed by Frank et al. (2004, 2006) using the following formula:

$$\text{LUM} = \left[\frac{-\sum_{k=1}^{n} (p_k . \ln p_k)}{\ln N} \right]$$

where p is the proportion of land area occupied by a specific land use category k, and N is the number of land uses.

Land use density

In section 4.3.1 of Chapter 4, we summarized studies that have found a relationship between land use density and health. A building-level GIS table was generated from the OSM Topography Layer, and each building unit within the study area was classified into one of the OS land use classes from Address Layer 2. Overall, the following categories of land uses were used in the study: single-family dwellings, multi-family dwellings, residential dwellings, non-residential dwellings, retail, community services, business and offices, and recreation and leisure. The densities of walkable community service destinations – bus stops, retail, churches, community services, and recreation and leisure amenities as well as business and offices – were also measured within each grade of buffer distance from a respondent's dwelling unit.

5.3.2 Health Specific Destination Accessibility

In section 4.3.3 of Chapter 4, we summarized the impact of specific health-enhancing facilities. Walkable destinations having the propensity to influence health in a specific way were parameterized in the study area in the form of network distance from a respondent's dwelling to the nearest green space, facility for physical activity, health care facility, supermarket, takeaway and allotment garden. Network proximity was used as opposed to the conventional Euclidean/airline distance, as it provides a more accurate behavioural measurement of accessibility. Street network distance (in metres) was calculated using 'closest facility analysis' in Network Analyst, ArcGIS 10.0. For larger destinations occupying a significant area, such as

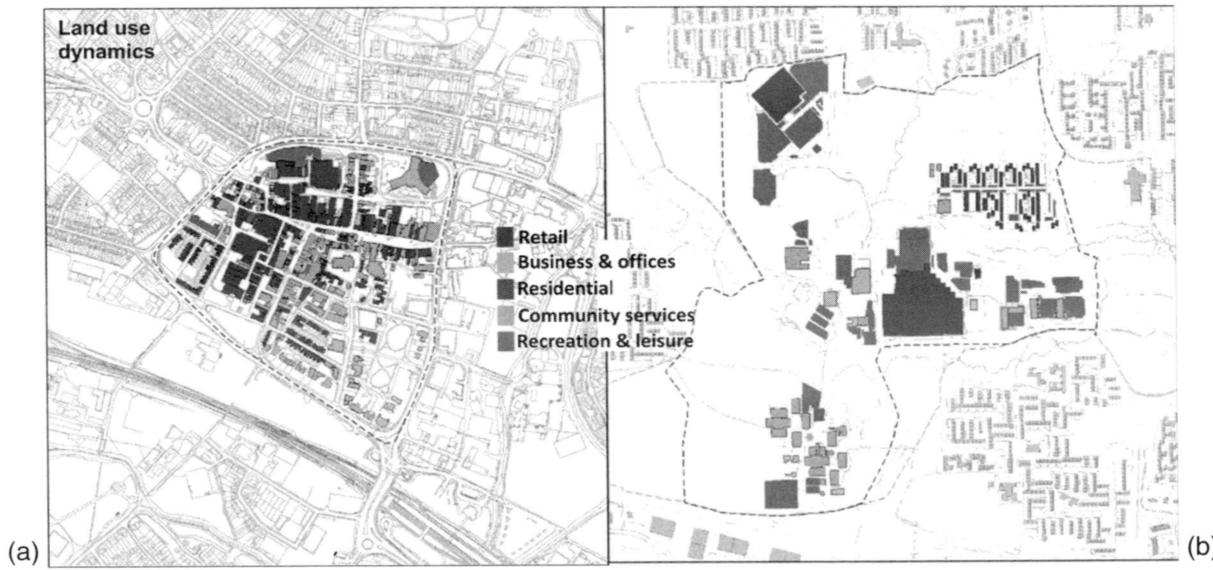

Figure 5.3 *Concept of land use mix*

a) Higher mixed land use is characterized by the presence of heterogeneous destinations and tends to minimize trip length, thereby promoting a walkable community

b) Reduced land use mix represents a zoned community with longer trip lengths and hence more car dependency

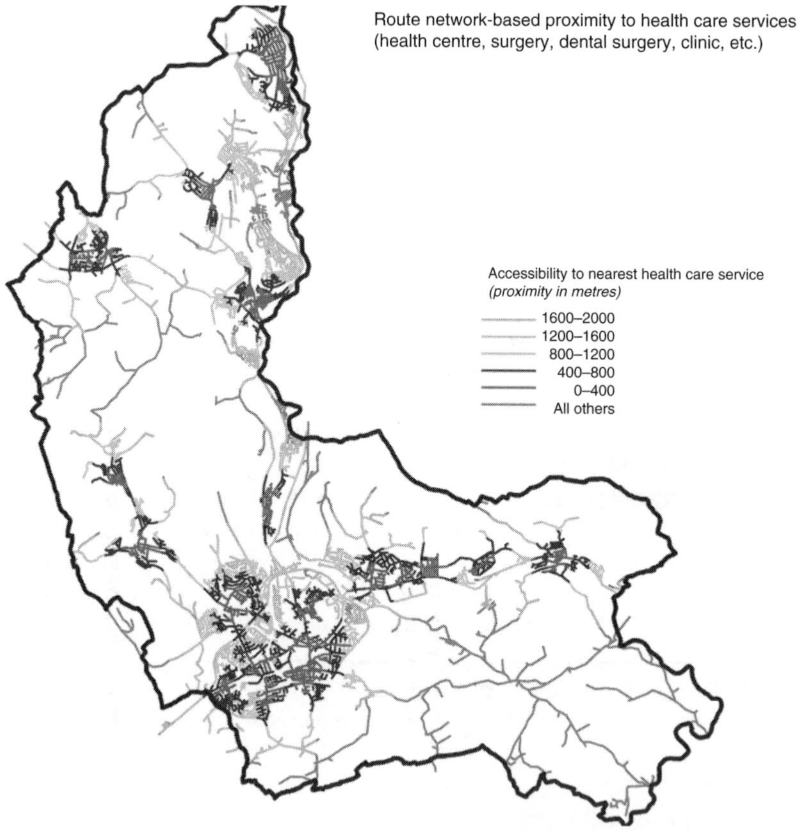

Source: Modelled from UK Ordnance Survey ITN Layer. © Crown copyright Ordnance Survey. All rights reserved.

Figure 5.4 Analysis of network proximity to nearest health care service

green space, allotments and sports facilities, the intersection of the street network with the outer boundary was considered as the point of access, while, for building destinations, a single point was employed as the location of the facility. The network analysis conducted for calculating proximity to the nearest health care facility is shown in Figure 5.4.

5.3.3 Street Network Accessibility

A city's route network defines the evolved and evolving urban form. It shapes the anthropogenic processes affecting an individual's activity patterns, and its attributes are therefore likely to capture something important about the impacts of multi-scale urbanization upon individual health, which collectively builds up to public health. The human movement patterns are not merely random; rather, they are planned, consisting of multiple steps based on individuals' spatial cognition. In an urban space, the individual's cognition may be governed by two components:

a. the location of destinations from a given origin, generally an individual's residence;
b. the configuration of the intervening spaces that must be traversed to move to and fro from the origin to the destinations.

Consequently, in addition to land use accessibility expressed in terms of density, mix, and physical distance to destinations, street network accessibility was included as the second component of accessibility on account of its significant potential in influencing activity behaviours and health. This allows us to test the independent association between health and, respectively, special and general accessibility (access to specifically demanded destinations and access to all other destinations).

Most studies looking at street network effects as part of a model of health have been vague, often parameterizing network characteristics in terms of the number of three- and four-way street intersections within a defined buffer or per unit length of street. Although they capture some measure of route directness by doing this, they nonetheless fail to capture more sophisticated and potentially more important behavioural information about connectivity and the interaction effects of land uses (destinations) adjoining the street network. Furthermore, in any systematic study of the effects of such network attributes, the spatial scale of the effects needs to be examined. This has hardly been covered at all in the spatial-epidemiology literature.

In this respect, the pertinent questions in the public health context are: (a) Do spatial network attributes at the levels of household, surrounding community, city, and the region as a whole have any impact upon an individual's health? (b) How do we analytically capture them in order to study the nature of potential correlations?

As a methodological innovation, the series of models presented in the subsequent chapters of this book conduct a simultaneous analysis of the effects of land use and street network-based systemic multi-scale accessibility and movement potential on individual health outcomes.

Network analysis of urban streets has a long tradition in the fields of transport geography and land use planning. In recent years several terms such as 'proximity', 'connectivity', 'integration', 'choice', 'cost', 'effort' and so on have emerged, with a view to highlighting the basic tenet that some urban spaces are more important than others on account of their being more *accessible*. Most network analysis techniques are driven by simple and tested, yet computationally demanding, mathematical algorithms which owe their origins to *graph theory* (Freeman, 1977; Hillier, 1999; Crucitti et al., 2006b; Porta et al., 2006). The associations between urban morphology and the social phenomena dependent on it are essentially captured by indices of relationality in the graphs. The notion of accessibility captured by these measures acts to formally elucidate how network morphology influences individual activity behaviours and drives various socio-economic processes.

In this book, we initially employed the network analysis concept known as *space syntax* to assess street network accessibility. The epistemological framework of space syntax originated from the seminal works of Bill Hillier and Julienne Hanson of University College, London, with an aim to delve deeper into the intricacies of the urban space utilization and dynamics of cities like London. It eventually evolved into a well-developed and widely adopted set of analytical techniques to represent, quantify and analyse the spatial configuration of cityscapes and building space. The principal driving objective behind space syntax research has been to explain the nature of spatial configuration of urban spaces that evolve as a result of two simultaneous and interactive processes: (a) transformation of the physical urban form consisting of the network of routes and adjoining land uses; and (b) the anthropogenic social interactions that give rise to and are supported by the urban form. There is a specific theory about these interacting evolutionary processes that gave rise to the initial space syntax model that puts emphasis on the perception of space and, particularly, the unhindered lines of visual sight (Hillier et al., 1983; Hillier and Hanson, 1984; Hillier, 1996). The model can be abstracted from the specific theory, however, and is consistent with a variety of urban economic behavioural propositions variously based on effort minimization (C. Webster, 2010). It is also consistent, as we have noted already, with key ideas from environmental psychology. The essential idea is that the topology as well as the geometry of a system of interconnected urban spaces determines movement patterns and thus land use (and land value), and that the patterns created by the interrelationships between spaces are predictive of the kind of use made of different parts of a city. At the same time, those patterns are themselves determined by individuals interacting within the constraints of pre-existing morphological configurations. Global (in the sense of urban-systemic) space-organizing processes tend to shape the micro level of patterns of movement within spaces and vice versa.

In recent years, space syntax-based measures of syntactic accessibility and movement potential of street segments have been shown to correlate well with many social phenomena. They have been employed in studies of pedestrian behaviour (Hillier et al., 1993; Raford and Ragland, 2004), walkability and physical activity in neighbourhoods (Baran et al., 2008; Cutumisu and Spence, 2009), cyclist route choice (Radford et al., 2007; McCahill and Garrick, 2008), geographies of crime (Hillier, 2004), social segregation (L. Vaughan, 2007), real estate value (Matthews and Turnbull, 2007; Chiaradia et al., 2009), city planning and urban design (Hillier and Hanson, 1984; Hillier, 1996; Peponis et al., 1997; Karimi et al., 2007; Volchenkov and Blanchard, 2008; Önder and Gigi, 2010; Chiaradia, Hillier et al., 2012; Karimi, 2012), and land grading, land pricing and rent evaluations (H. Zhao et al., 2007; Enström and Netzell, 2008). At an architectural scale (from where the method originated), the same measures have been employed to generate housing genotypes (Hillier et al., 1987; Bandyopadhyay and Merchant, 2006), and to devise innovative designs of buildings based on perception psychology of way-finding and movement tracing (Ortega-Andeane et al., 2005; R. Li and Klippel, 2010).

In this book, two space syntax modelling techniques described below are employed in the assessment of the impact of street network configurations on individual health outcomes.

Space syntax modelling technique: angular segment analysis (ASA)

As with other network analysis models, space syntax is operationalized through a set of basic indices from graph theory applied to spatial relationality. In order to replicate the linear pattern in which we tend to move, the entire urban space is broken up into a series of components, namely convex spaces (such as public spaces or green spaces) and longest axial lines corresponding to streets, boulevards, avenues, alleys and so on. In space syntax methodology, a so-called *axial map* of the urban space is extracted: the axial map comprising the fewest and longest set of lines representing uninterrupted movement and/or visibility.

In the conventional space syntax analysis paradigm, the model of street segments represented by the axial map is first transcribed into an access graph comprising a set of nodes representing the street segments and edges representing their intersections. The access graph captures the essential topological properties of the built environment. The access graph is then transformed into a justified graph, wherein a node of the access graph is identified as the *root* for the analysis and the rest of the nodes in the graph are ordered into a tree, relative to the root (in the example indicated in Figure 5.5, the root is segment A). In a way, the justified graph drawn from a particular root pulls the configuration close to it if the segment is highly integrated. On the contrary, segregated spaces tend to push the configuration away from the root.

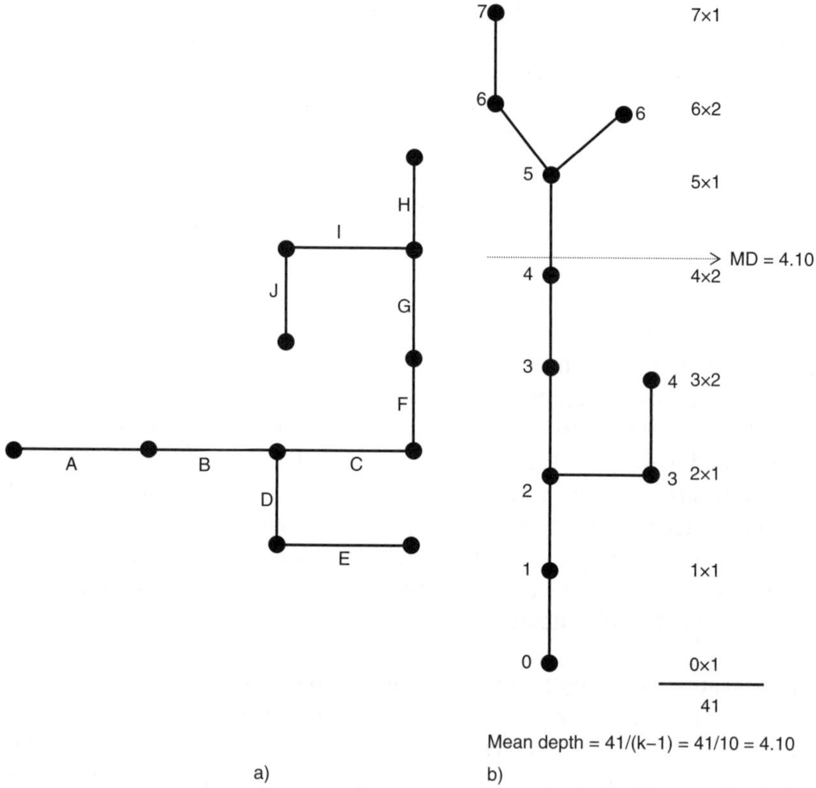

Figure 5.5
a) Configuration of street segments represented by an access graph
b) Justified graph derived from the configuration, with depths and mean depth indicated (the root of the graph is the origin of segment A)

The hierarchical levels in the constructed tree indicate the number of steps or the depth to pass from the location of a specific node to the root. The indices derived from this version of the space syntax model were based on the notion of metric distance and revolved around the calculation of mean depth from a justified graph of the configuration, calculated within a predefined catchment area (expressed in number of steps away from the root of the graph). The total number of spaces at each level of depth is multiplied by the value of the level and added up to arrive at the total depth. Thus,

$$\text{Mean metric depth} = \frac{\text{Total depth}}{(k-1)}$$

where *k* is the total number of nodes in the graph including the root. The root is considered to be at level 0. This is illustrated in Figure 5.5.

As will be described in the following pages, the theory of space syntax evolved over time from the notion of metric distance to that of angular distance between nodes with the development of the more refined angular segment analysis, which accesses configurational properties between the nodes in the graph based on aggregate turning angles between them.

Hillier and Iida (2005) argued that distance costs between two points in a network may be measured in three ways:

- Least length (pertaining to least Euclidean distance): The distance cost may be measured as the sum of segment lengths (in terms of a space syntax model: equivalent to the Euclidean distance between the mid-points of two adjacent segments).
- Fewest turns (pertaining to least topological distance): The distance cost may be measured in terms of the total number of changes of direction that have taken place along a route.
- Least angle change (pertaining to least geometric distance): The distance cost may be measured as the sum of angular changes that are made along a route. A weight can be assigned to each intersection, proportional to the angle of incidence of the two line segments at the intersection.

This is a subset of a wider set of friction-of-separation measures, which include: the time taken to traverse a route; the money cost of doing so; discounted time costs of route traversal (weighting angular turns encountered earlier in the journey more highly than those met later); and, the most commonly used in health–built environment studies (and other spatial analysis of behaviour), crow-flight distance.

Research evidence suggests that, although Euclidean network distance is an intuitively important measure of accessibility, it is nonetheless dependent upon the psychology of navigation choices of individual movers. Hillier and Iida (2005) termed the geometrical and topological properties of the network as *network effects* and through their empirical studies on London concluded that accessibility measures based on geometrical (angular) analysis within a metric distance-defined measurement window (catchment area or radius) are the most powerful approach to capturing the mixed effects of these different kinds of impedance factors. The different impedances are illustrated in Figure 5.6. In Figure 5.6a, although route AB represents the shortest metric path, it is also the one associated with higher geometric and topological costs. On the contrary, in Figure 5.6b, route AB is associated with comparatively lower angular

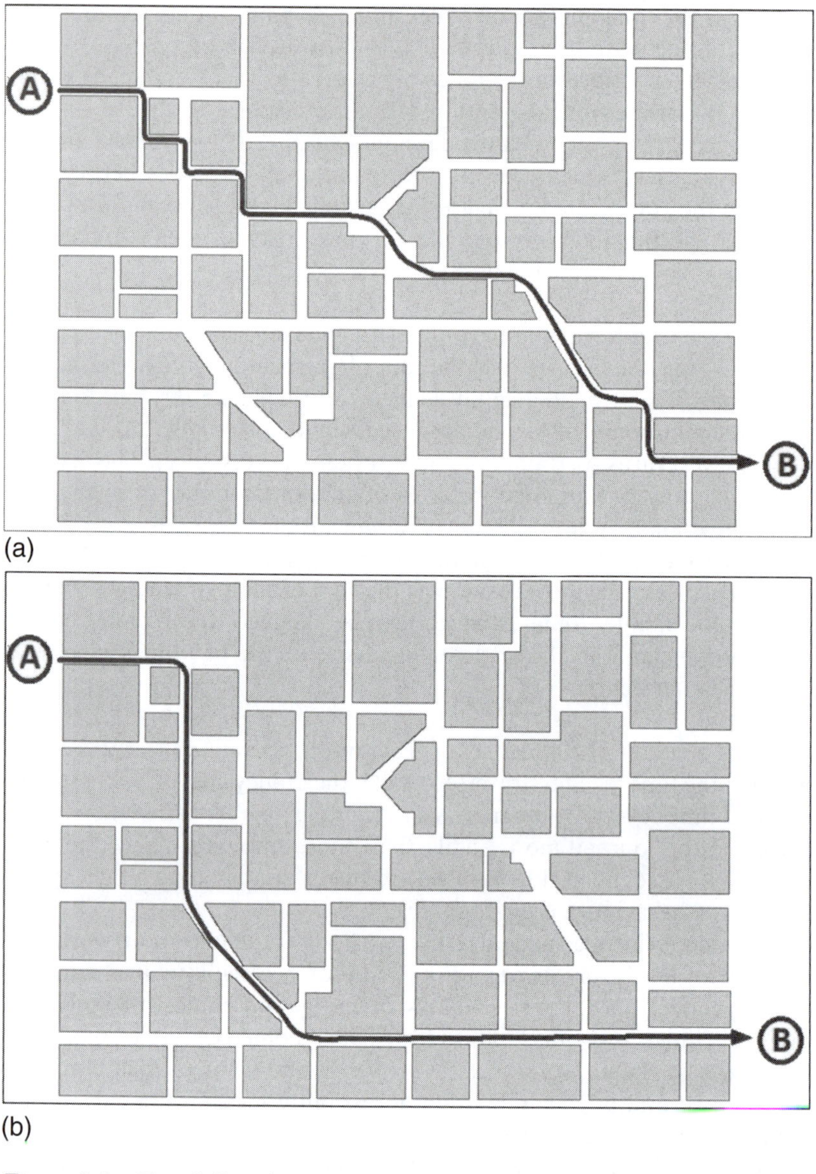

Figure 5.6 *Two different street network configurations*

a) *Route section AB associated with least metric costs and higher geometric and topological costs*

b) *Route section AB associated with least angular costs*

costs and hence is more likely to be taken. The approach therefore measures geometric and topological impedances within a Euclidean-defined radius (to subordinate them to metric distance as a dominant behavioural influence).

Turner (2000) published the space syntax modelling technique termed angular segment analysis wherein he substituted the notion of least metric length (expressed in terms of Euclidean distance between the two centroids of a pair of adjacent line segments or nodes) for the angular depth between them. In simple terms, the angular depth between a set of origin–destination nodes in the graph is simply a function of the aggregate turning angle in radians between the origin and destination nodes. In angular segment analysis, the axial lines in an axial map are first broken into segments; thereafter the corresponding segment map is transcribed into an access graph as described previously. The sum of the angles turned from the origin (starting) node to any other destination node within the system is recorded. This angular sum represents the 'cost' of a putative journey through the graph. The algorithm thus evaluates shortest angular distance (a measure of least cost) from one node to another in the system.

Behaviourally, these graphical accessibility indices are based on two trip-choice criteria that an individual has to make while traversing through urban space:

a. Selecting a destination: This is based on how easy it is to get to a destination, also termed as *to-movement* component. The driving hypothesis is that more accessible destinations are more likely to be selected as locations for higher-activity uses, such as shops, because they are easy to get to.
b. Selecting a route to get to the destination: This determines the places that an individual has to pass through to get to a destination, also termed the *through-movement* component.

Thus, in graphical terms, the total angular depth $D_{\Theta}(x,y)$ is the total angular turn from one graphical node to another following the shortest angular route, where x is the origin node and y is the destination node in the graph. If we consider Figure 5.7, the angular depth from A to segment B will be 0.5, associated with a turn of 45°, while from B to C it is 0.833, corresponding to another turn of 60°. The total depth from A to C is thus 1.333. Similarly, the cost for moving from A to D is 1.333, corresponding to an angular turn of 135°. Directionality is an important criterion in graph analysis, as it is generally assumed that passage through an urban network involves leaving a segment in the same direction as arrival.

The final illustration in Figure 5.7 is called the justified graph, that is, the

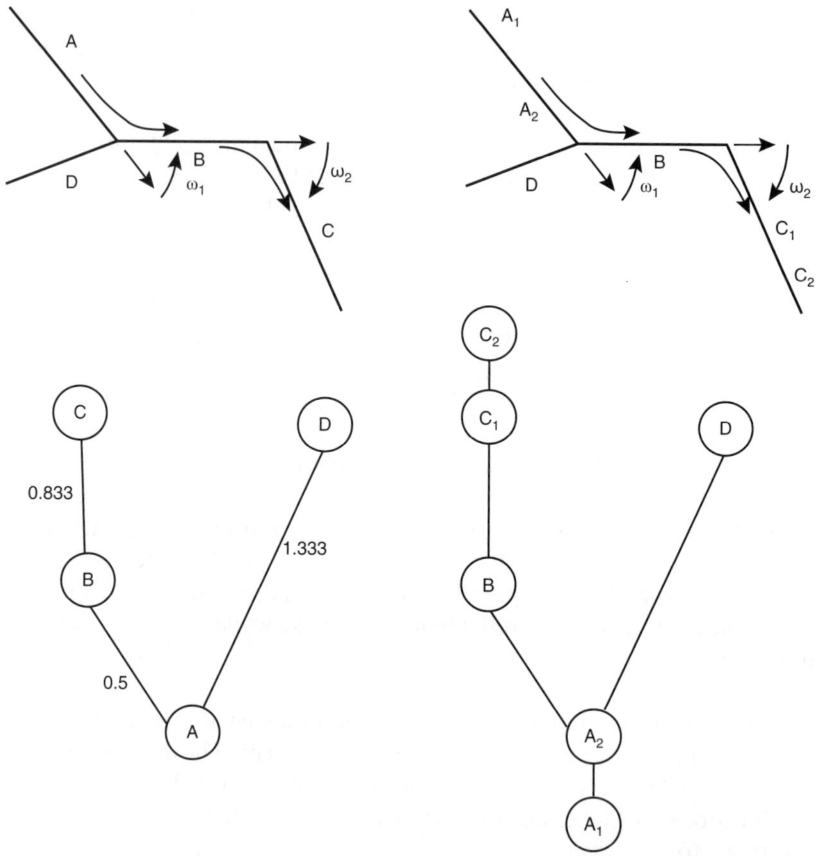

Source: Adapted from Turner (2007, p. 542). Reprinted by permission of the publisher.

Figure 5.7 Paths through a network and their associated justified graph

graph as seen from a particular location (origin), A in this case. The mean depth associated with any node x within a graph of n nodes is calculated as the average length of all the shortest angular paths within the network. It may be expressed as:

$$\overline{D_\theta}(x) = \frac{1}{n}\sum_{i=1}^{n} D_\theta(x, i)$$

Thus in the example in Figure 5.7, the mean depth from A may be calculated as:

$$\overline{D_\theta}(A) = \frac{[D_\theta(A, B) + D_\theta(A, C) + D_\theta(A, D)]}{3} = \frac{(0.500 + 1.333 + 1.333)}{3} = 1.06$$

However, if A and C are further segmented into A_1A_2 and C_1C_2 respectively, the mean depth from A will change accordingly:

$$\overline{D_\theta}(A) = \frac{[D_\theta(A_1, A_2) + D_\theta(A_1, B) + D_\theta(A_1, C_1) + D_\theta(A_1, C_2) + D_\theta(A, D)]}{5}$$

It is generally expected that nodes with longer segment lengths will contain more origins and destinations of journeys than those with shorter segment lengths; hence, some analysts have standardized the depth measure by weighting them with segment length, intuitively overcoming the bias of treating all graphical nodes of different segment lengths as equally important in terms of destination opportunities and so on. Thus, if $l(i)$ represents the segment length of a node i, then the weighted mean depth $\overline{D_\theta^l}(x)$ of any node x in a graph of n segments may be defined as:

$$\overline{D_\theta^l}(x) = \frac{\sum_{i=1}^{n} D(x,i)\, l(i)}{\sum_{i=1}^{l} l(i)}$$

In graph-theoretic terminology, the to-movement potential is termed *closeness* (also called *integration* in space syntax) and measures the ease with which a destination may be accessed within a network. As the mean depth of the central node in an urban network is the minimum, angular closeness has been defined simply as the reciprocal of mean depth as follows:

$$C_\theta(x) = \frac{n}{\sum_{i=1}^{n} D_\theta(x,i)}$$

while segment length weighted closeness is:

$$C_\theta^l(x) = \frac{\sum_{i=1}^{l} l(i)}{\sum_{i=1}^{n} D_\theta(x,i)\, l(i)}$$

The second component of street-level accessibility, the through-movement potential, is captured by the graphical measure of betweenness (Freeman,

1977). It is also termed *route choice* (or just *choice*) in the space syntax literature and measures the degree of potential for movement through a node in the network. In contrast to closeness, which measures the relative ease of reaching potential destinations, the betweenness index indicates how often people are likely to pass through a particular route (hence also called a *path overlap* index). Betweenness can act as an intuitively powerful model of physical movement, especially in studies related to an individual's activity behaviour and walkability. When weighted with land uses, it is a manifestation of the *pull effects* (both attractive and repulsive) of the land uses that are adjacent to a street segment. The superior explanatory power of the betweenness index has been highlighted in several previous studies (Crucitti et al., 2006a; Turner, 2007).

Computing the betweenness measurement involves two steps:

- Generation of journeys with lowest angular costs for each and every potential origin–destination pair of nodes within the graphical network system.
- Giving a value of 1 to a node if it is part of the shortest path from any origin to any destination. The number of journeys made through each node are summed up and then divided by the total number of possible journeys.

In other words, betweenness gives a value to a node proportional to the estimated (simulated) count of movements passing through that node from and to all other parts of the network, assuming that journeys in the network follow the shortest angular path between all origin–destination pairs. Thus, as illustrated in Figure 5.8, segment AB has the highest path overlap and through-movement potential compared to the others.

The betweenness $B_\theta(x)$ of any node x in a graph of n nodes may be defined mathematically as:

$$B_\theta(x) = \frac{\sum_{i=1}^{n} \sum_{j=1}^{n} \sigma(i, x, j)}{\frac{(n-1)(n-2)}{2}}$$

such that $i \neq x \neq j$ where

$\sigma(i, x, j) = 1$, if the shortest path from i to j traverses through x, and
$\sigma(i, x, j) = 0$ otherwise.

Again, given that nodes with longer segment lengths have more origins and destinations along them and thereby support more journeys, it is often customary to use a segment length weighted betweenness:

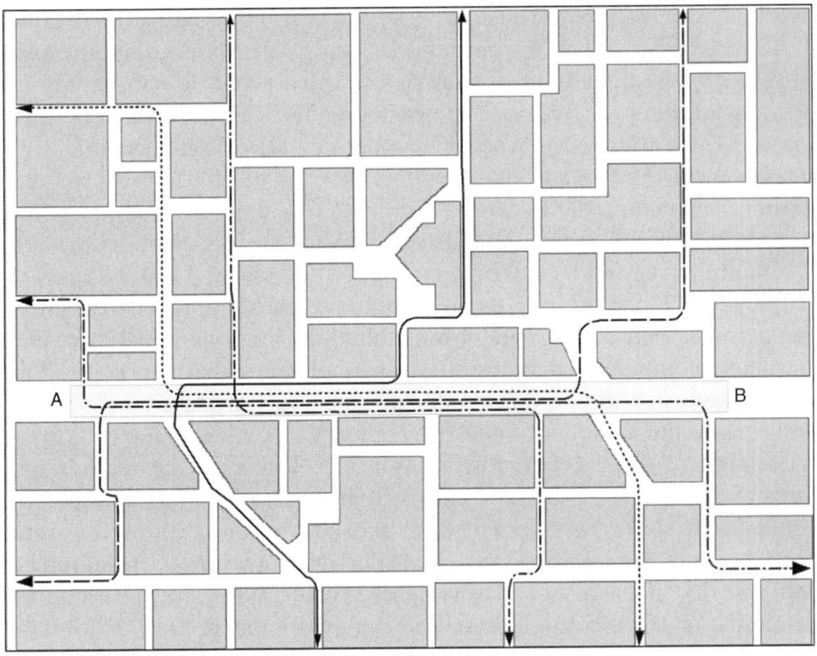

Figure 5.8 The concept of route betweenness: route section AB is associated with high path overlap and high through-movement potential

$$B_\theta^l(x) = \sum_{i=1}^{n}\sum_{j=1}^{n}\sigma^l(i,x,j),$$

such that $i \neq j$ where

$$\sigma^l(i,x,j) = l(i)\,l(j), \text{ if the shortest path from } i \text{ to } j \text{ traverses through } x,$$

$$\sigma^l(i,x,j) = \frac{l(x)l(j)}{2}, \text{ if } x \text{ coincides with the origin } i,$$

$$\sigma^l(i,x,j) = \frac{l(i)l(x)}{2}, \text{ if } x \text{ coincides with the destination } j,$$

$$\sigma^l(i,x,j) = 0, \text{ if } x \text{ is not in the shortest path between } i \text{ and } j.$$

$l(i), l(j), l(x)$ are the segment lengths of nodes i, j and x respectively.

All these graphical street network indices are usually calculated within a user-defined catchment area (termed the *radius*) expressed in metric distance.

Working with road centreline data

It has been argued that, in conventional space syntax modelling, the axial lines generated for graphical analysis are often prone to subjectivity on account of the preferences of the cartographer who drew them. With a view to devising a system to enable analysis of topological networks with *minimum interference and subjectivity*, Turner (2005, 2007) proposed that angular segment analysis can be automated to function using standard geographic road network data sets of street networks (such as the UK Ordnance Survey road centreline map and US national TIGER/Lines) by employing the standardized segment length weighted approach to calculating network metrics. Changing from a hand-drawn axial model representing lines of unhindered visual site to a road centreline map is justified, as such industry-standard network data sets can provide a more realistic insight into the underlying behavioural theory of vehicular and pedestrian movement (Turner, 2007). Furthermore, it overcomes the tedious and somewhat subjective process of cartographic generation of axial line maps. Since 2005, space syntax analysis in the UK has been employed using the Ordnance Survey Integrated Transport Network Layer, including for example one of the most extensive space syntax studies – of the economic potential of urban configuration and design options in the London boroughs, under the i-VALUL project, a part of the UrbanBuzz programme (CABE, 2007; Chiaradia, Hillier et al., 2012).

In Chapters 6 and 7 of the book, angular segment analysis has been performed on the Ordnance Survey ITN Layer of Caerphilly. The ITN Layer was first subjected to a sequence of editing and simplifications before being subjected to angular segment analysis:

1. In order to derive the simplest set of lines from the ITN map, complicated junctions, dual carriageways and other potentially ambiguous parts of the ITN model were first identified and simplified.
2. In an automated routine, all segments in the ITN with an angular threshold less than 5° were joined together to create polylines. Subsequently, another routine performs the operations of thinning, node snapping, and so on to further simplify the geometry. Segmentation of the resulting map produces a segment map, which was then amenable to ASA.

The indices of connectivity, closeness and betweenness were calculated for each road segment (node in the graphical context) at variable metric catchment radius R and subsequently aggregated both at the dwelling level and within a 1 kilometre street network buffer of each CaPS respondent's dwelling unit. This has been illustrated in Figure 5.9.

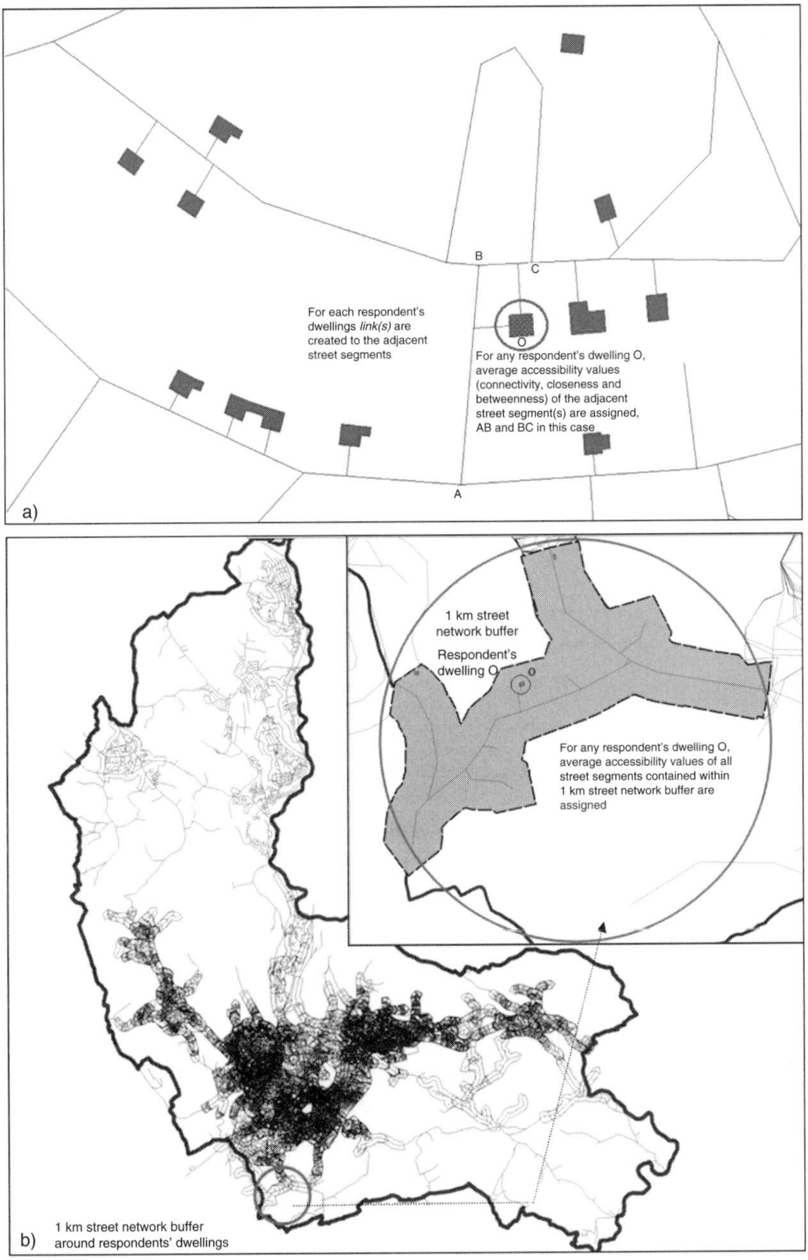

Figure 5.9 Aggregation of network accessibility indices for individual respondents at a) the dwelling level and b) the neighbourhood level

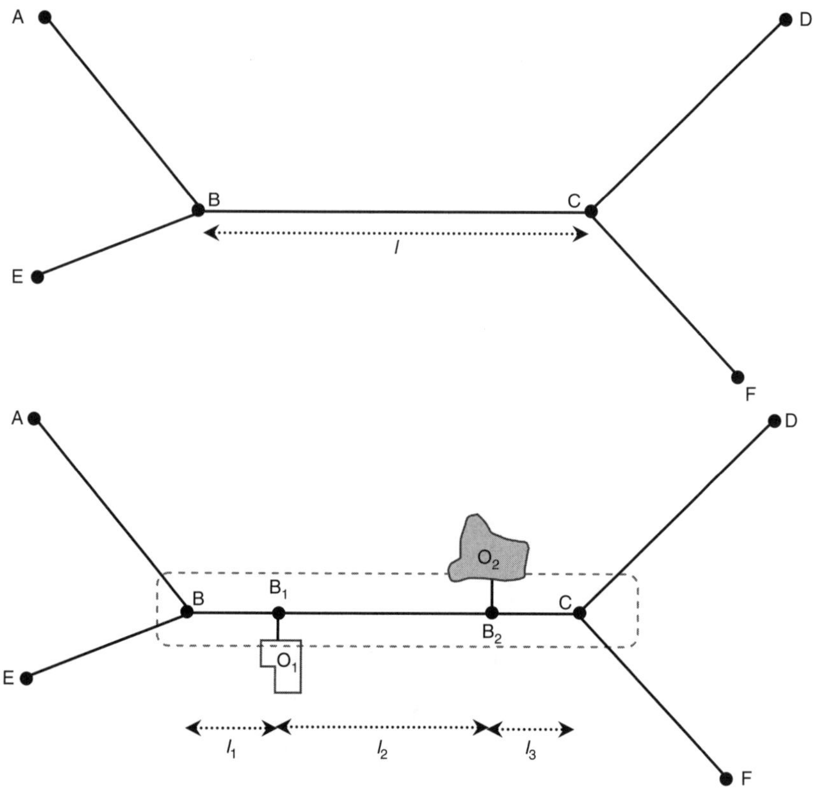

Figure 5.10 *a)* *Normal segment length weighted betweenness*
b) *Betweenness weighted by segment length as well as health-promoting community resources (O_1, O_2) within a 25 metre buffer adjacent to the street*

As has been highlighted previously, in addition to the topological properties of the segment, the pull effects of the land uses adjacent to it are a very important consideration. In order to incorporate this, we have employed a betweenness measure that has been weighted by both the segment length and the presence of a health-promoting service destination adjacent to it in our network models generated for Caerphilly. This is illustrated in Figure 5.10. Figure 5.10a depicts the measurement of normal segment length weighted betweenness, while in Figure 5.10b the presence of walkable destinations (health-promoting community services present within a 25 metre street buffer, O_1 and O_2 in this case) increases the movement potential so that the betweenness of segments BB_1B_2C in Figure 5.10b will be higher than that of the segment BC in Figure 5.10a. Therefore, the weighting scheme involved identification of walkable destinations within 25 metres of a street segment, creating connecting links to the specific segment and thereby dividing the *single* segment into a set of *multiple* segments depending on the density of walkable destinations per street segment. The single segment connecting B and C in Figure 5.10a has been now converted to multiple segments, BB_1, B_1O_1, B_1B_2, B_2O_2 and B_2C in Figure 5.10b, on account of the presence of the adjacent destinations O_1 and O_2.

Network models of closeness and betweenness for Caerphilly are shown in Figures 5.11 and 5.12 respectively.

Spatial Design Network Analysis (sDNA)

Spatial Design Network Analysis (sDNA) is another *state-of-the-art* technique of urban network analysis based on the concept of space syntax. It uses a technically improved network algorithm and has been developed by Cardiff University's School of Planning and Geography (http://www.cardiff.ac.uk/sdna). Representational problems associated with manually prepared axial line models of street networks have been previously highlighted (Ratti, 2004; Porta et al., 2006). As a result, sDNA employs the road centreline data as an input model upon which graphical analyses are performed. Nonetheless, some of the criticisms often made of angular segment analysis pertain to the tedious process of editing and cleaning the road centreline data before processing, as well as the reliability of the model and reproducibility of the results; minor differences in representation of a geographic feature (different segmentation of the same network) can lead to differences in the graphical representations, and hence variations in results. This may be thought of as the *modifiable link problem*. To overcome these limitations, sDNA can function with off-the-shelf street centreline data such as Ordnance Survey ITN data, with minimum preparation. The sDNA Prepare tool automates all the initial processes of removal of traffic islands as well as repairing of split links. sDNA standardizes the *network link* as the fundamental unit of computation. By using such industry-standard link representation, sDNA overcomes the modifiable link unit problem, as well as provides a better physical interpretation of road centreline data. In an urban space, several socio-economic processes such as density of residences, jobs, traffic flows, pedestrian movements and so on have been known to be correlated with the density of street network links. Thus sDNA offers the analyst a diverse choice of refined graphical indices of accessibility, thereby enabling analyses of network centrality (in terms of closeness and betweenness centrality), network detour (in terms of sum of crow flight, mean diversion ratio and diversion ratio), network

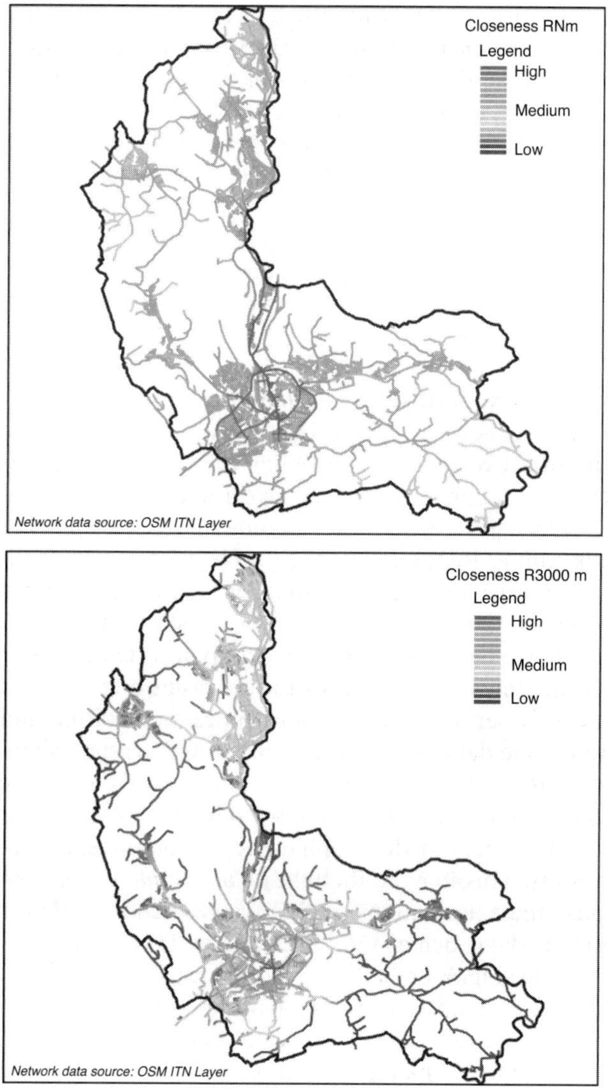

Note: Radius RNm represents the longest distance between two street segments in the spatial model, hence encompasses the entire network. Street accessibility indices modelled over the entire network act as indicators of global accessibility.

Source: Modelled from UK Ordnance Survey ITN Layer. © Crown copyright Ordnance Survey. All rights reserved.

Figure 5.11 Analysis of closeness of street segments at various scales for the study area

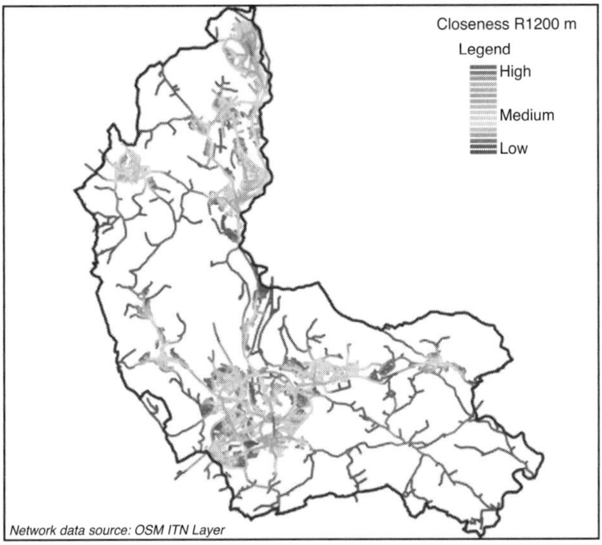

Figure 5.11 (continued)

shape and efficiency (in terms of convex hull area, perimeter and bearing, and network shape index), link characteristics (in terms of length, angular curvature and connectivity) and radius-based indices (in terms of number of links, total network length, total angular distance, total and mean geodesic length and number of junctions within a defined catchment radius). A detailed description of these indices can be found in Chiaradia, Webster et al. (2012). Further, sDNA provides the option of enumerating the centrality indices based on the notion of Euclidean or angular distance, with the choice of several weighting functions such as link weighting, link length weighting or other user-customized weighted indices. As in angular segment analysis, sDNA enumerates all the graphical accessibility indices within a specific user-defined catchment radius; nonetheless, sDNA provides the user with the option of *discrete or continuous space analysis*. In discrete space analysis, each link is considered as a discrete (whole) entity and, if a part of a link falls inside a given radius, the entire link is counted as being within the radius. On the other hand, in continuous space analysis, each link is treated as a continuous entity and only the fractional part of a link falling inside a given radius is counted, leading to fractional (proportional) link counts. The former is computationally faster, while the latter produces more accurate results. Overall, sDNA has been tested and has successfully reproduced results equivalent to or better than those of predecessor space syntax methods. sDNA is also innovative in its

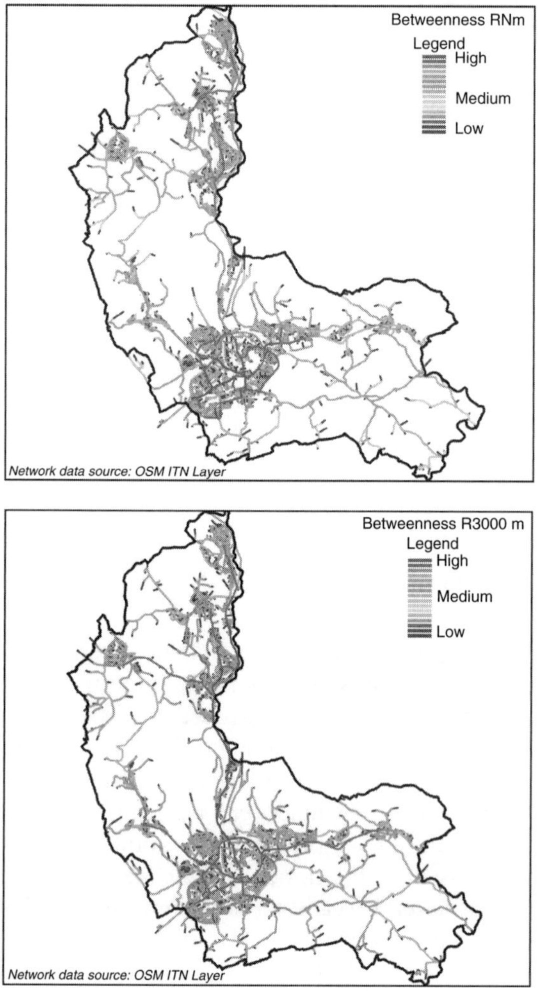

Notes:
Betweenness weighted by segment length and land use destinations was modelled over the Ordnance Survey ITN Layer.
Radius RNm represents the longest distance between two street segments in the spatial model, hence encompasses the entire network. Street accessibility indices modelled over the entire network act as indicators of global accessibility.

Source: Modelled from UK Ordnance Survey ITN Layer. © Crown copyright Ordnance Survey. All rights reserved.

Figure 5.12 Analysis of street movement potential at various scales for the study area

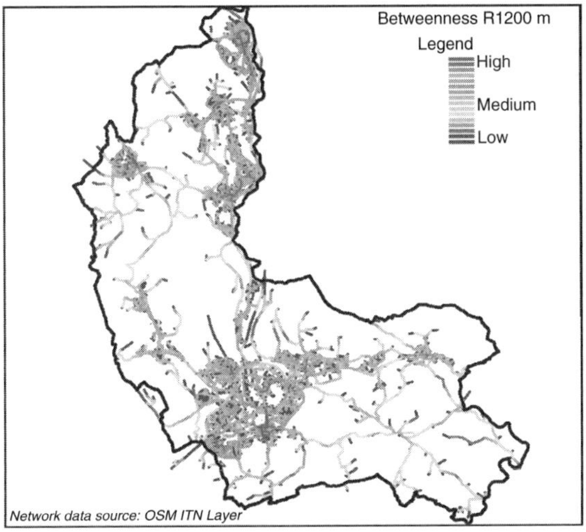

Figure 5.12 (continued)

class in providing a workflow that is fully automated. The UK Ordnance Survey (OS) Topography Layer, Address Layer 2 and Integrated Transport Network Layer linkages are cross-referenced through unique identifiers; the OS supports Digital National Framework identifiers, which facilitate integration and sharing of spatial information from diverse sources.

All the sDNA measured indices of accessibility were calculated for all the street links within the boundaries of the study area (Caerphilly assembly constituency). The indices of connectivity, closeness and betweenness of each link as well as junction connectivity and network hull were considered for inclusion in the models described in Chapter 8. All the sDNA network metrics were measured at spatial radii of 0.5, 1.0 and 1.5 miles and have been subsequently aggregated at the dwelling level, that is, with respect to the dwelling of each CaPS respondent, as has been illustrated in Figure 5.9a. Link connectivity, also termed *degree centrality*, measures the number of connections to other links and is synonymous with the connectivity of a specific link. The network hull area is the convex area containing all the origins and destinations within a defined radius (see Figure 5.13). It is an indicator of the network footprint or the spatial spread of the street network in the urban space. The junction connectivity measures the number of junctions (street intersections) within a defined radius (see Figure 5.14).

We have employed sDNA to arrive at a set of street network accessibility measures in Chapter 8. We include both space syntax and sDNA analysis in the book to demonstrate that this is an area that is rapidly gathering

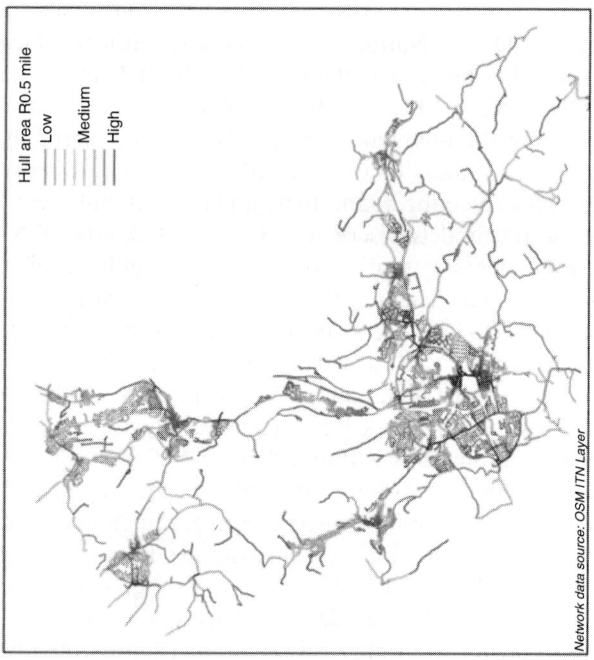
Hull area R0.5 mile
Low
Medium
High
Network data source: OSM ITN Layer

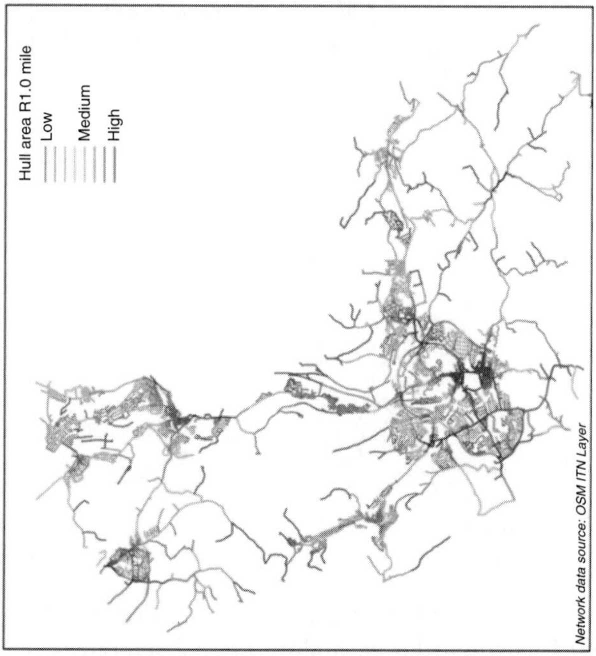
Hull area R1.0 mile
Low
Medium
High
Network data source: OSM ITN Layer

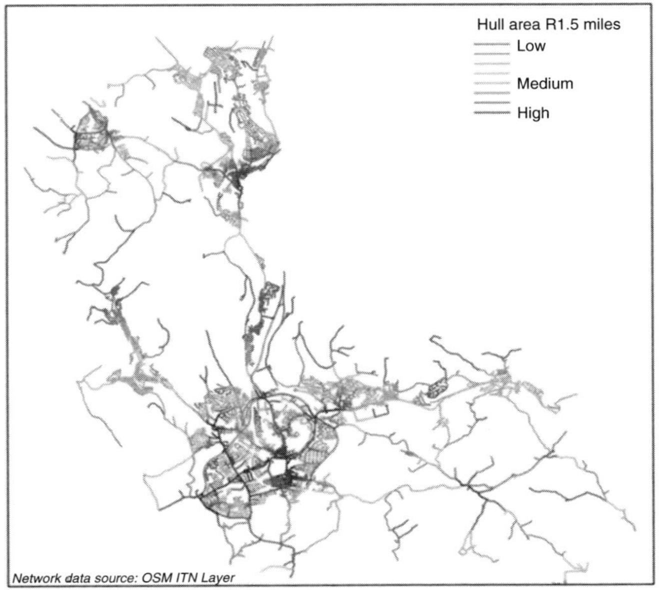

Source: Modelled from UK Ordnance Survey ITN Layer.

Figure 5.13 Analysis of the hull area of the street network links at various scales for the study area

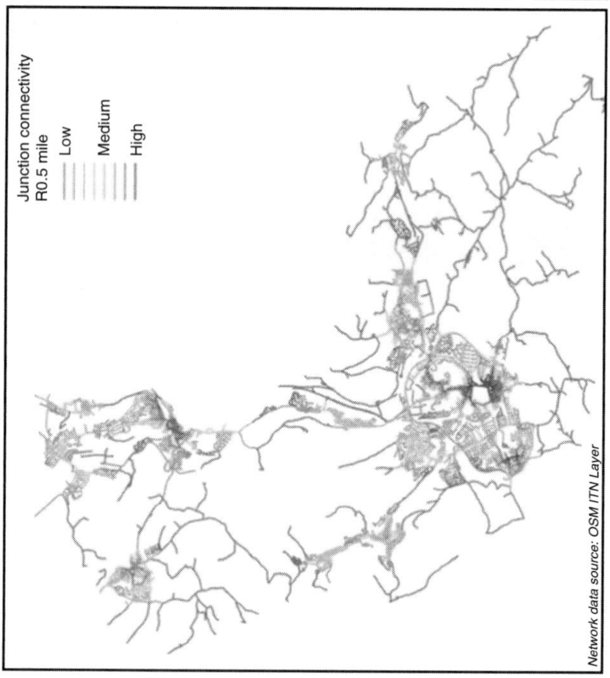
Junction connectivity
R0.5 mile
Low
Medium
High
Network data source: OSM ITN Layer

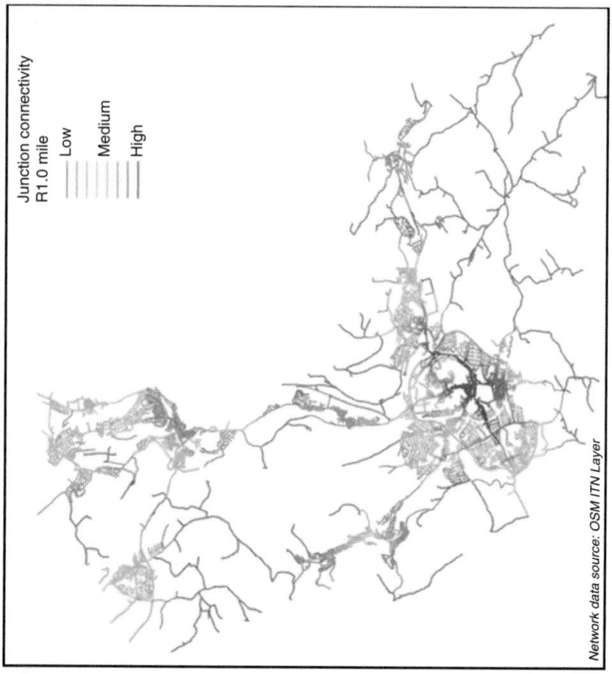
Junction connectivity
R1.0 mile
Low
Medium
High
Network data source: OSM ITN Layer

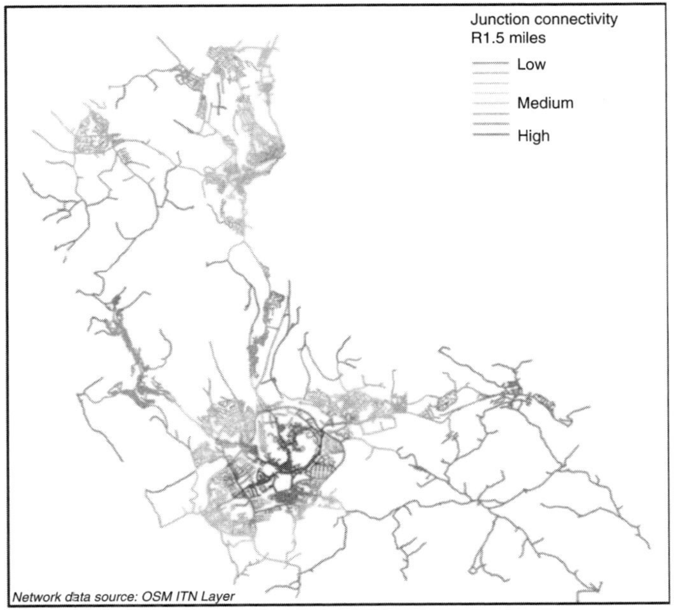

Source: Modelled from UK Ordnance Survey ITN Layer.

Figure 5.14 Analysis of junction connectivity of the street network links at various scales for the study area

pace as a method of quantitative urban analysis and to illustrate the techniques on offer and comment on their relative strengths and weaknesses.

5.3.4 Natural Environment

Natural environment, especially the presence of green spaces, is known to have considerable impact upon health outcomes (see section 4.3.3 of Chapter 4). In the studies reported in the rest of this book, natural environmental measures of slope variability and greenness were included, the former being particularly variable given the geographical location in the Welsh Valleys. Slope raster was processed from a 5 metre resolution Bluesky digital terrain model of the study area in Spatial Analyst, ArcGIS 10.0. The slope model of Caerphilly is shown in Figure 5.15. The degree of variability in slope within an individual's home range was operationalized as the standard deviation of slope in degrees within a 1 kilometre network buffer of an individual's dwelling.

A satellite-derived Normalized Difference Vegetation Index (NDVI) was used as an objective measure of greenness. The NDVI is a unitless index calculated from the reflectance measures in satellite data, comparing the amount of energy absorbed by the chlorophyll in the red portion and the amount scattered by the internal structure of the leaves in the near-infrared region (Jensen, 2005). This contrast has been employed as an estimate for vegetation greenness, as indicated by the following formula:

$$\text{NDVI} = \frac{(\text{NIR} - \text{RED})}{(\text{NIR} + \text{RED})}$$

where RED and NIR stand for the spectral reflectance measurements acquired in the visible (red) and near-infrared regions, respectively. The index ranges between -1 and $+1$, with higher values reflective of healthy green vegetation and vice versa. A 30 metre resolution Landsat 7 satellite data set was employed, and the NDVI index was calculated in Raster Calculator – Spatial Analyst, ArcGIS 10.0. The Landsat satellite Band 3, 630–690 nm, was used as the red region of the electromagnetic spectrum, while Band 4, 760–900 nm, acted as the infrared region, so that the formulae used was NDVI = (Band 4 − Band 3) / (Band 4 + Band 3). The greenness was calculated as the mean NDVI within a 500 metre circular buffer of an individual's dwelling. The NDVI model of Caerphilly is reproduced in Figure 5.16.

5.3.5 Area-Level Deprivation

The Welsh Index of Multiple Deprivation (WIMD) 2005 scores, measured at the level of lower super output area (LSOA) census areas, have been

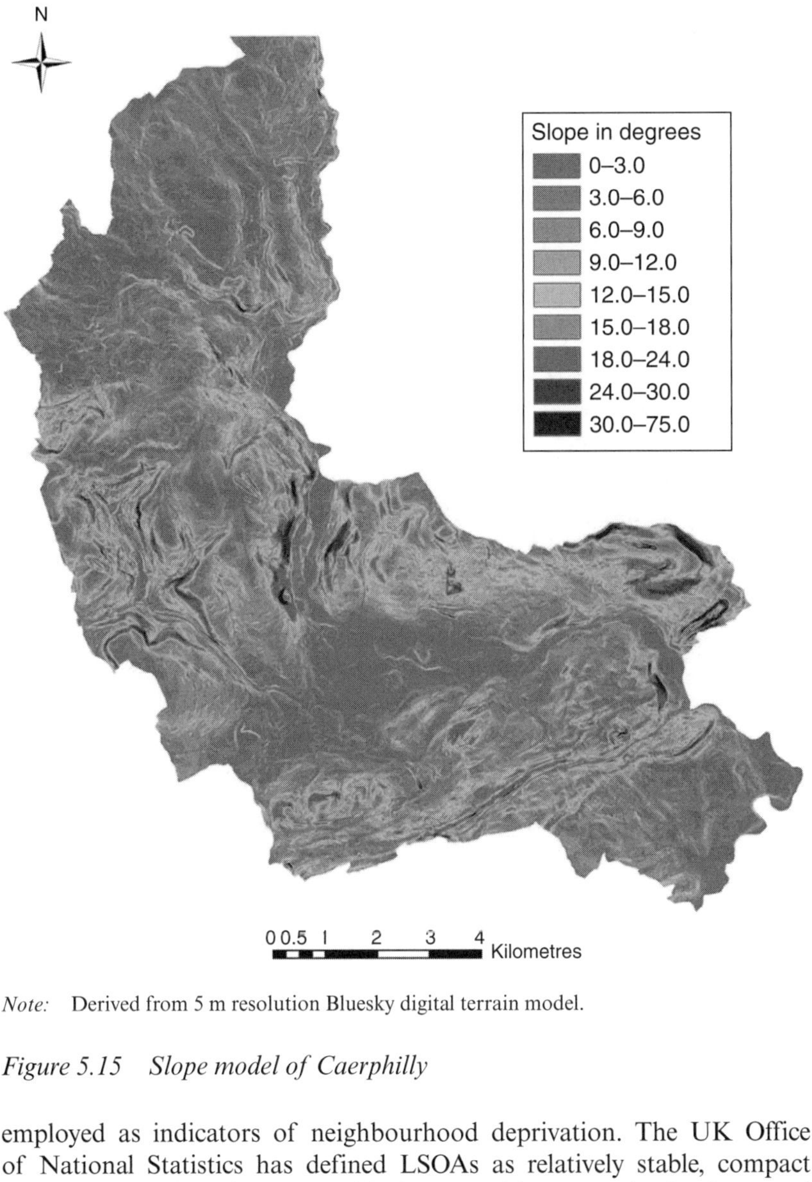

Note: Derived from 5 m resolution Bluesky digital terrain model.

Figure 5.15 Slope model of Caerphilly

employed as indicators of neighbourhood deprivation. The UK Office of National Statistics has defined LSOAs as relatively stable, compact geographical units with reasonable degrees of homogeneity in shape and social composition and an average population of 1500 persons for Wales (D. Martin, 1997, 1998; Bates, 2006; Flowerdew et al., 2008). The WIMD comprises seven unitless indicators of disadvantage (so-called *domain indices*) for income, employment, health, education, housing, physical envi-

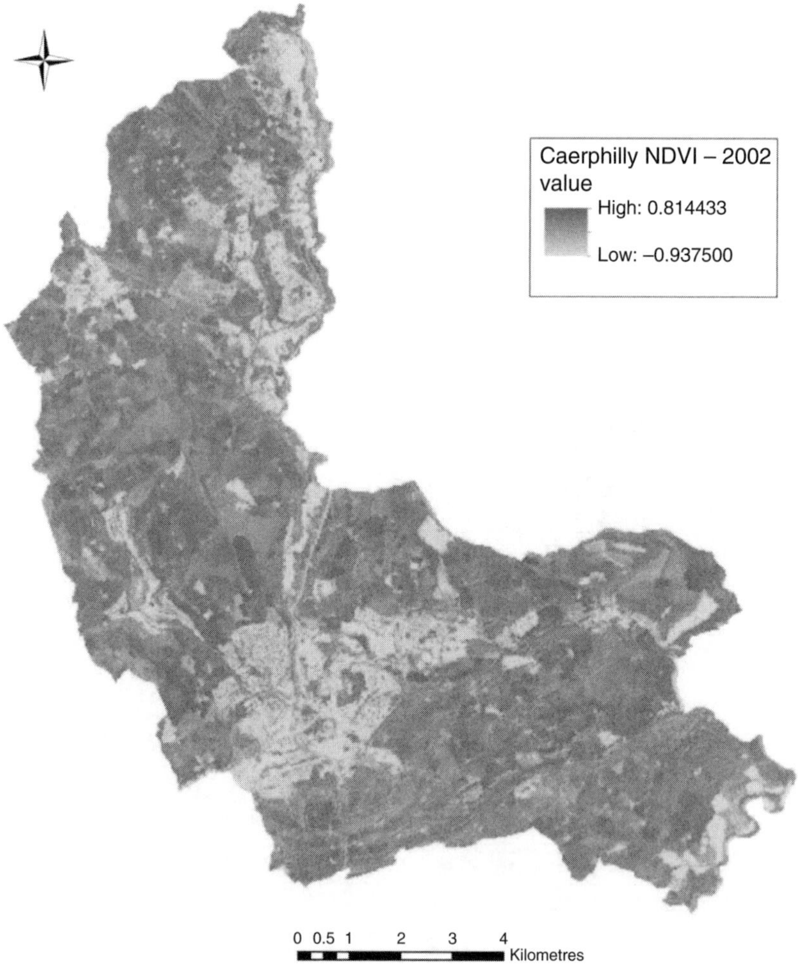

Note: Based on Landsat 7 ETM+ satellite data dated 17 August 2002.

Figure 5.16 NDVI index of greenness for Caerphilly.

ronment and access to services (Welsh Local Government, 2005). The Welsh assembly constituency of Caerphilly comprises 54 LSOAs (Figure 5.17).

5.3.6 Dwelling-Level Morphometrics

These measures were calculated through a set of GIS queries for each respondent's dwelling unit. One is a measure of dwelling type; the other

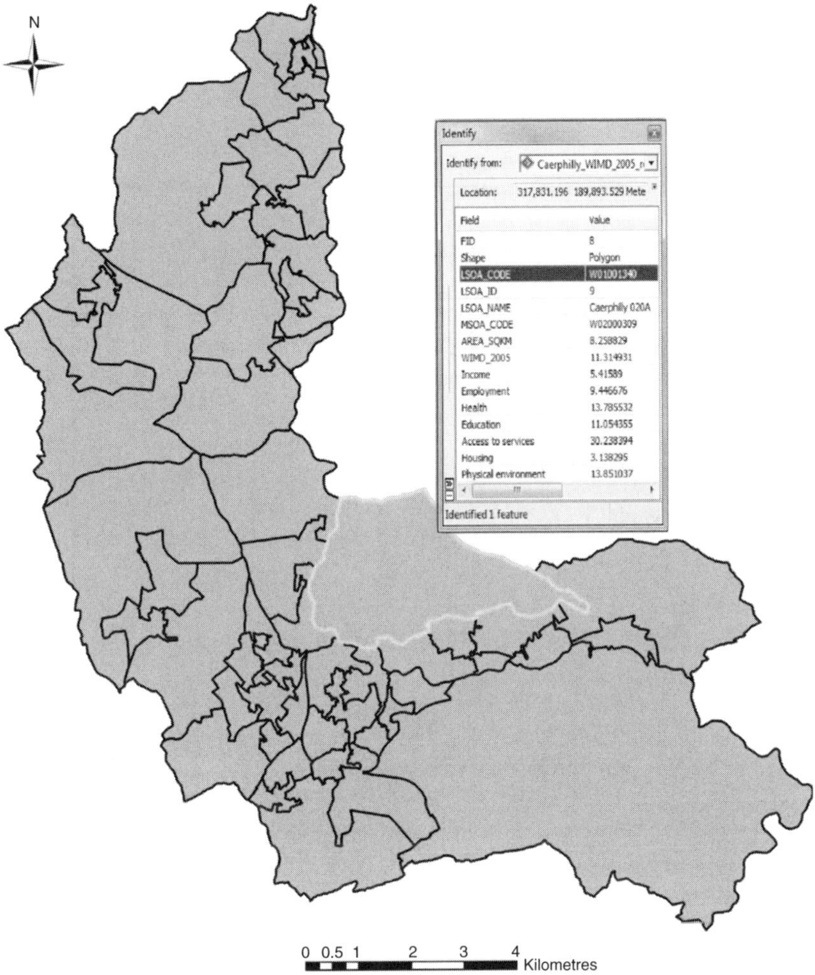

Figure 5.17 Area deprivation measured at the level of lower super output areas (LSOAs)

three are alternative measures of dwelling-centred density, plot exposure, and dwellings per street segment (illustrated in Figure 5.18). Dwelling-centred density refers to the immediate residential density surrounding a dwelling unit and is expressed as the number of dwellings in a 30 metre radius surrounding the dwelling unit. Plot exposure evaluated the number of faces of a dwelling unit exposed to public space and was categorized as 0, 1 and more than 1, with 1 acting as the reference category. Dwelling type

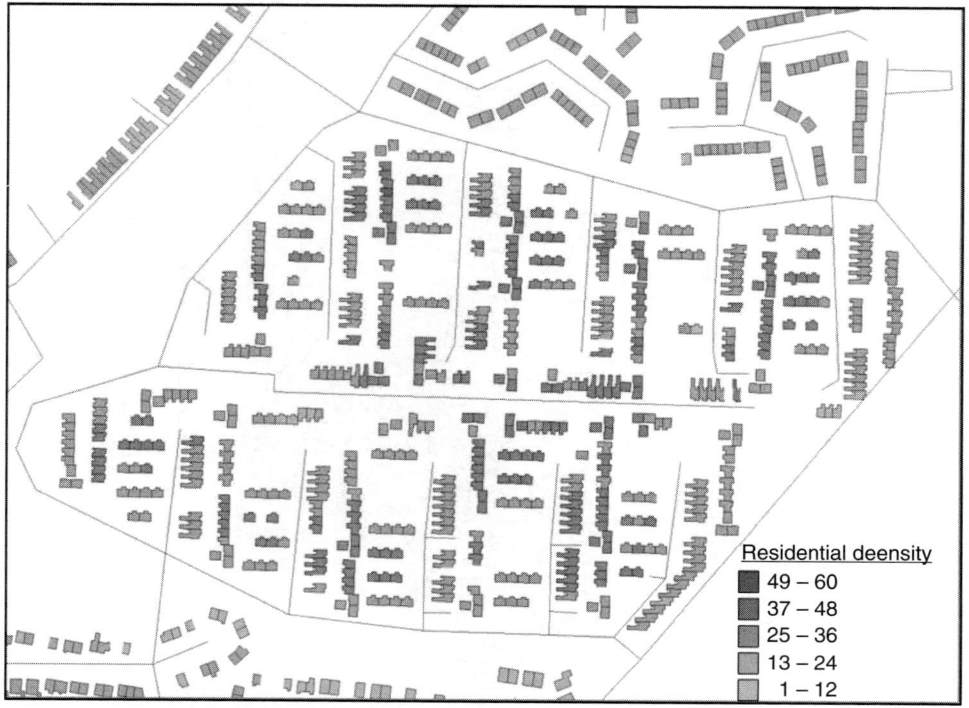

a) Residential density with a 30-metre radius

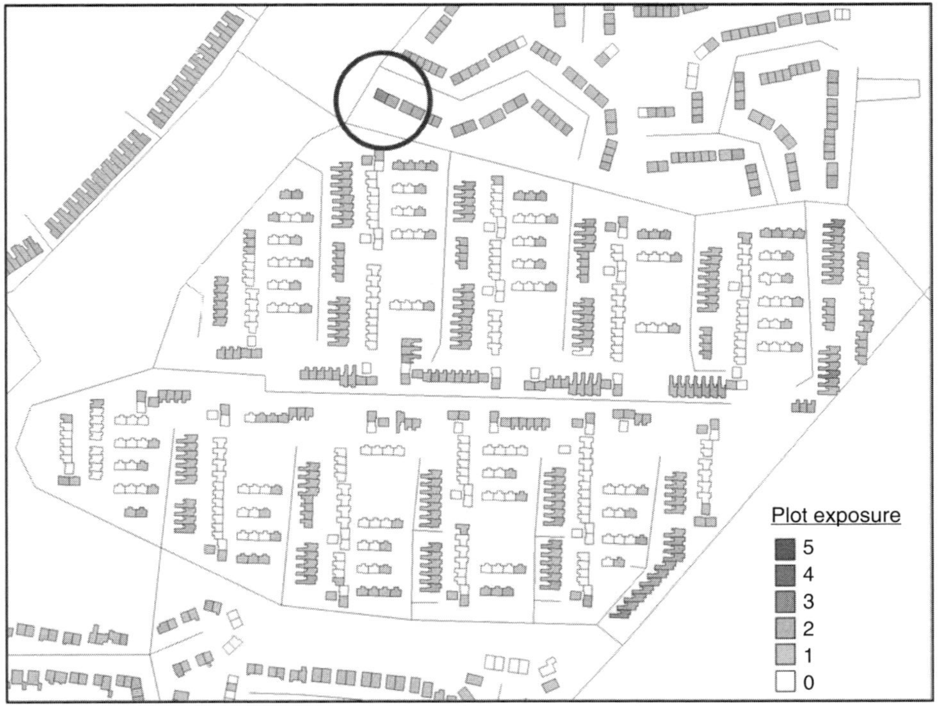

b) Plot exposure

Source: Modelled from UK Ordnance Survey MasterMap layers. © Crown copyright Ordnance Survey. All rights reserved.

Figure 5.18 Dwelling-level morphometrics

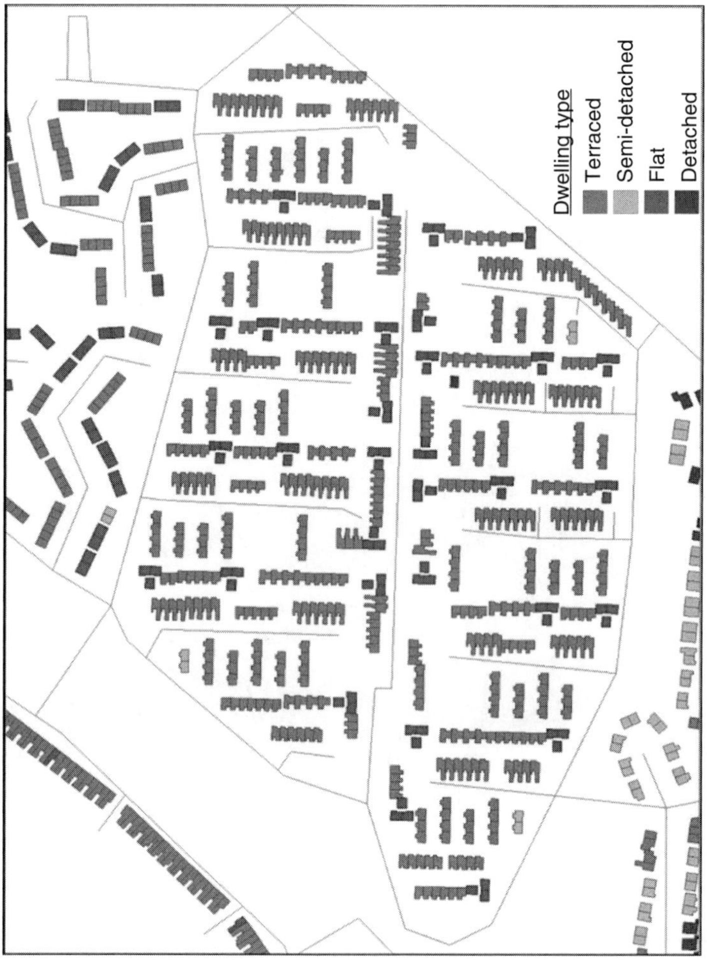

c) Dwelling type

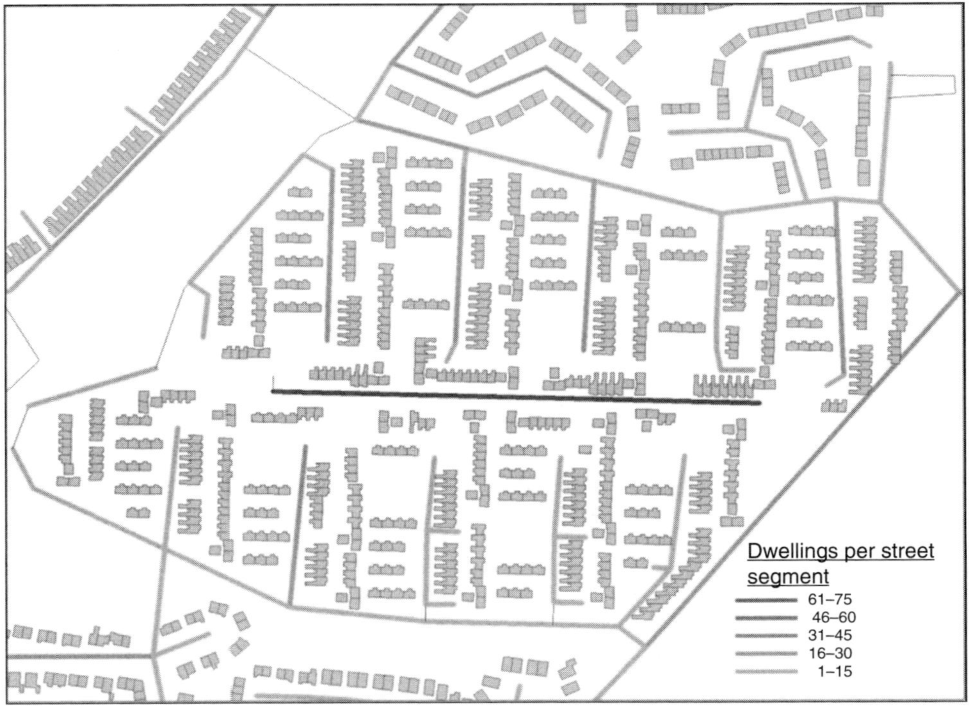

d) Dwellings per street segment

Figure 5.18 (continued)

refers to the type of dwelling unit and consists of four categories: detached, semi-detached, terraced and flats (apartments). Detached dwellings have been defined as having one dwelling per building and with no adjacent neighbour. Semi-detached dwellings have one dwelling per building and with one adjacent neighbour. Terraced houses are those that have one dwelling per building and a neighbour that has more than one neighbour, while flats contain more than one dwelling per building. Dwellings per street segment refers to the number of dwellings connected to each street segment of the route network. A dwelling can be connected to more than one street segment if it has multiple exposures.

5.4 PRELIMINARY EXPLORATORY DATA ANALYSIS

Variables of theoretical importance were first identified from the literature review for inclusion in the statistical models described in Chapters 6–8. The preliminary model-building exercise consisted of a set of the following standard statistical tests for initial screening, iterative grouping and testing for variable selection to obtain a parsimonious model fit:

1. Bivariate correlation analysis was performed to assess the level of correlations between the various built environment parameters.
2. Univariate regression analyses were performed to assess the crude point estimates and level of significance of associations between health outcomes and the various attributes of the built environment to select covariates significantly associated with depression. Key built environment variables including the significant street accessibility betweenness index at specific radii were selected.
3. Built environment variables were included in preliminary multivariate regression models. A stepwise approach was iterated.
4. A subset of built environment explanatory variables were thus identified, and subsequent assessment of variance inflation factors (VIFs) of the explanatory built environment variables in single-level regression further enabled multicollinearity to be avoided. The maximum correlation coefficient observed between the predictors was 0.65, and this was well within the standard rule of thumb for cut-off of 0.7r, indicating sufficient independent variance. All estimated VIFs were less than 5, the cut-off for significant multicollinearity (Kutner et al., 2004).
5. Model statistics in the form of R^2, log likelihood, Akaike information criterion (AIC) and Bayesian information criterion (BIC) were compared between the iterated models so as to select the most stable one.

In Chapters 6–7, the betweenness index of street network accessibility is measured at multiple radii at the local, city and regional scales. The above-mentioned series of statistical iterations enables the identification of three radii, 1200 metres at the local scale, 3000 metres at the city scale, and the global N for the study area. Chapter 8 follows a similar methodology, identifying 0.5 mile (*c.* 800 metres) and 1.0 mile (*c.* 1600 metres) as the significant radii at the local scale. However, as the objective of the experiment was to decipher the potential impacts of the built environment at multiple spatial scales, sDNA metrics at a specific radius were introduced separately in the models.

It must be mentioned that, although the closeness metric was constructed and included in the preliminary analysis, it was dropped from the final list of variables. This was on account of it being mostly non-significant in bivariate models or otherwise being multicollinear with the betweenness index at the corresponding radii. Moreover, as has been highlighted before, the betweenness index has comparatively superior explanatory power, especially in studies associated with individual activity behaviours, as against the closeness index (Crucitti et al., 2006a; Turner, 2007), and hence is conceptually more illuminating in built environment–health models.

5.5 CONCLUSION

A review of the public health literature on the contextual determinants of health indicates that many studies employ self-reported perceived rather than objective measures of the built environment. Such studies fail to fully overcome the inherent weaknesses of the perceptions and judgements of local residents: being weak in validity and reliability (Leslie et al., 2007; Saarloos et al., 2011). In recent years, advances in spatial information sciences, notably the emergence of spatial modelling and network analysis techniques, have provided significant new analytical potential in spatial epidemiology (Macintyre et al., 2002; J. Pearce et al., 2006; Leslie et al., 2007; Ball et al., 2012). Detailed objective assessment of the built environment is a rapidly growing research domain and has the potential to enhance the conceptual and methodological rigour in investigations of built environment–behaviour associations. In order to understand how the built environment variables influence individual behaviours, via physical activity, social capital and mental health, it is necessary to identify and objectively measure specific attributes of the built environment that may promote or inhibit healthy living.

One of the advantages of the present study stems from the fact that a more holistic two-component definition of accessibility has been employed, as advocated by Koenig (1980). Conventionally, the notions of accessibility tend to be expressed as primarily a function of the spatial location of land use destinations (Curtis and Scheurer, 2010). Generally, spatial separation models measure the degree of travel resistance between origins and destinations, expressed as generic distance decay functions, while contour models enumerate the density of destinations within predefined travel-time catchments. In contrast, gravity models explicitly enumerate the actual travel time from an origin and accordingly categorize corresponding accessibility of opportunities in terms of time costs. In this study, in addition to the measures of network distance and density of opportunities which form the *activity element* of accessibility in reference to land use destinations, space syntax-based betweenness constitutes the second component of accessibility, namely the *transport element*. This is based on the widespread realization that accessibility is also a function of the configuration of the intervening spaces between the origins and destinations, which must be traversed. The betweenness is a graphical index of the degree of *centrality* of a street link with respect to the entire street network, simulated as the total sum of through-movement through the street link. More intuitively, the measure enables us to capture the impact of urban topology, form and hence legibility upon travel costs and accessibility. Secondly, such an index is a dynamic one, as enumeration of betweenness at multiple catchment radii enables us to capture the physical street network accessibility at multiple urban spatial scales: local, community and regional.

Many ecological studies have attempted to isolate the effects of built environmental factors upon health. There is a need and a growing ability to empirically test such propositions with the help of objectively measured built environment attributes to which an individual is exposed. We suggest that disaggregated models such as the ones we now demonstrate can contribute more to epidemiological theory than can factorizing models that measure higher-level concepts such as walkability. Our models disaggregate at the level of individual health and individual measures of accessibility, based on the network models described in this chapter. We acknowledge that aggregate and factorized models might sometimes be more useful for policy makers. The primary aim of this book in developing sDNA-UH has been to enable objective assessment of the built environment in public health studies. The subsequent three chapters report studies that employ the morphometrics of sDNA-UH using the accessibility techniques described in this chapter.

6. Urban built environment configuration and psychological distress in later life: cross-sectional results from the Caerphilly Prospective Study (CaPS)

6.1 CONTEXTUAL URBAN ENVIRONMENT AND MENTAL HEALTH

Psychological disorders account for substantial proportions of the burden of disease worldwide. Approximately 14 per cent of the global disease burden has been attributed to neuropsychiatric disorders, mostly depression, alcohol and substance abuse and psychoses, accounting for 28 per cent of all disability-adjusted life-years (Murray and Lopez, 1996; Prince et al., 2007). The World Health Organization (WHO) identified depression as the cause of the greatest proportion of the non-fatal health burden, contributing to almost 12 per cent of total years lived with disability (Üstün et al., 2004). An estimate puts the total cost of adult depression in England at over £9 billion, with £370 million accrued towards direct treatment costs to the NHS (C.M. Thomas and Morris, 2003). The impact of psychological disorder is all the more significant in the case of older adults, for whom cognitive functioning forms the primary determinant of functional capacity and quality of life (Lebowitz et al., 1997).

In recent years, several studies have highlighted the associations between psychological disorders and contextual urban environment characteristics. In addition to the impact of socio-economic inequality and residential stability of urban neighbourhoods (Faris and Dunham, 1939; W.J. Wilson, 1991; Kubzansky et al., 2005; Propper et al., 2005; Fone and Dunstan, 2006; Subramanian et al., 2006; Aneshensel et al., 2007; Wight et al., 2009) upon mental health, myriad built environmental factors have been implicated. Associations have been found between psychological well-being and housing structural attributes (G.W. Evans et al., 2000; G.W. Evans, Kantrowitz et al., 2002; Galea, Ahern et al., 2005), dwelling-level architectural features (Weich et al., 2002; S.C. Brown et al., 2009), observable neighbourhood environmental quality (Araya et al., 2007; H. Thomas et al., 2007), access to facilities and green space (Takano et al., 2002; de Vries et al., 2003; Guite et al., 2006), street quality (Balfour and Kaplan, 2002) and neighbourhood walkability (Berke, Gottlieb et al., 2007; Sallis, Saelens et al., 2009). Most studies have employed either composite (Araya et al., 2007; Berke, Gottlieb et al., 2007; H. Thomas et al., 2007; Sallis, Saelens et al., 2009) or self-reported (Guite et al., 2006; Leslie and Cerin, 2008) measures of the built environment, which often fail to isolate the effects of specific attributes of the built environment upon psychological health in older adults. As far as we can determine, there has been only one study examining the associations between detailed built environmental configuration and psychological health. The study examined the association between objectively measured components of the built environment and mental health, finding higher levels of depression with higher degrees of land use mix and greater retail availability (Saarloos et al., 2011).

In the present study, we hypothesize two underlying mechanisms through which neighbourhood built environment configuration may influence mental health in older adults. Firstly, the configuration of land use (in terms of mix, density and destination accessibility) as well as street networks (connectivity and movement potential) contributes to the supportiveness of the neighbourhood environment by promoting enhanced accessibility to health-promoting community resources (Bernard et al., 2007). This promotes local opportunities for outdoor activities such as utilitarian walking to services, leisure walking, cycling and so on. At the same time, the presence of certain destinations may act as barriers to accessibility and healthy living. The protective effects of neighbourhood walkability and physical activity upon psychological disorder in older adults have been well established (Strawbridge et al., 2002; Bean et al., 2004; Weuve et al., 2004; Berke, Gottlieb et al., 2007; Wiles et al., 2007). Secondly, the residents of a neighbourhood with optimized built environment design have a greater incentive to be outdoors, which in turn will facilitate social inclusion through interactions with friends and neighbours. The positive association between social ties and mental well-being has been well documented (Kawachi and Berkman, 2001; Leyden, 2003; S. Cohen, 2004). These relationships are of particular importance in older adults, whose daily activities tend usually to be confined to the vicinity of their dwelling, making them more sensitive to the health-promoting or -inhibiting attributes of neighbourhood physical configuration (Balfour and Kaplan, 2002; Diez Roux, 2002). We test these hypotheses by examining the independent association of a wide range of morphological metrics (morphometrics) with psychological distress in a population of older men. Furthermore, the natural elements of a neighbourhood environment have been known to influence mental health outcomes (Grahn and Stigsdotter, 2003; Sugiyama et al., 2008), both directly and indirectly in terms of enhanced neighbourhood satisfaction and actual service use (Kaplan, 2001; Ellis et al., 2006). On the contrary, neighbourhood-level deprivation has been shown to exacerbate mental health (Caspi et al., 2000; Stafford and Marmot, 2003). This chapter examines the impact of objectively assessed built environment configuration upon psychological distress and whether this association is moderated by the natural environment and area-level deprivation.

6.2 METHODS

6.2.1 Study Design

The study is based on the fifth phase of the Caerphilly Prospective Study (CaPS), a population-based male cohort in the Welsh assembly constituency of Caerphilly, South Wales, UK. Further details of the CaPS cohort can be found in Chapter 4. Briefly, the fifth examination was conducted during 2002–04 and comprised 1225 surviving cohort members aged 65–84 years. Extensive clinical examinations included anthropometry, assessment of blood pressure, electrocardiogram, and collection of fasting blood samples.

Psychological distress measures and individual-level covariates

Psychological distress was measured employing the 30-item General Health Questionnaire (GHQ-30), a self-completion instrument widely used to rate levels of psychological distress and psychiatric disorders (Goldberg and Williams, 1988). The factors of the 30-item General Health Questionnaire are reproduced in Appendix 1. Individual-level risk factors including age, alcohol consumption and smoking status as well as socio-demographic measures of marital status, social class and educational attainment were collected. The study presented in this chapter also controlled for the existence of vascular morbidities, expressed in terms of prevalence of myocardial infarction, angina, high blood pressure, high cholesterol, diabetes and stroke.

The built environment

The conceptual path model illustrated in Figure 6.1 provides the theoretical framework for the study and guided the formulation and operationalization of a set of robust model variables of built environment configurations and individual-level covariates extracted from the spatial Design Network Analysis for Urban Health (sDNA-UH). A set of built environmental

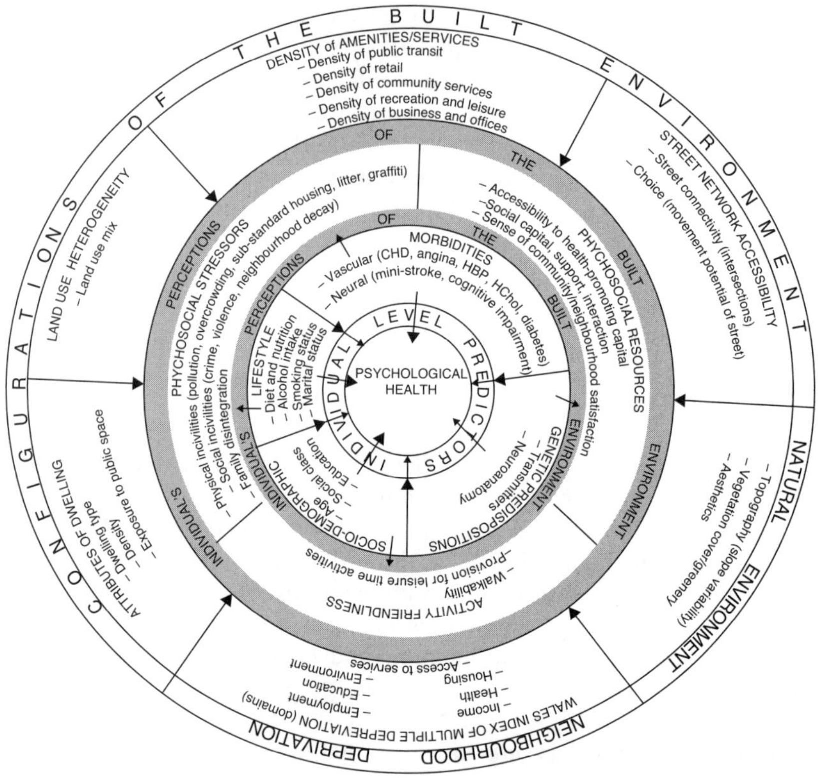

Figure 6.1 Conceptual path model depicting the relationship between the built environment and mental health

factors acting in conjunction with the physical environment, and neighbourhood deprivation have been posited to configure the psychological health of an individual. The built environment provides the activity space wherein people interact and our perceptions of the environment are formed (including perceptions of psychosocial stressors, resources and activity friendliness). Individual-level factors such as socio-demographics, lifestyle, genetics, prevalence of morbidities and levels of cognitive health have the potential to define psychological health directly, as well as indirectly, through their impact upon the perceived mediators. The present study aimed to objectively measure the various facets of built environment configuration and directly establish their potential impact upon psychological health, with the variables of physical environment, neighbourhood deprivation and individual-level factors acting as potential confounders in our statistical models.

Built environment measures from the sDNA-UH were operationalized within a 1 kilometre street network buffer around an individual respondent's dwelling unit. Dwelling-level configurations consisted of plot exposure, dwelling-centred density and dwelling type. Land use configurations were captured through measures of mix and density. A five-category land use mix score was developed consisting of residential dwellings, retail, community services, business and offices, and recreation and leisure facilities. The densities of public transit (bus stops), retail, community services, recreation and leisure, and business and offices were calculated as the number of units divided by the total area within a 1 kilometre street network buffer of a respondent's dwelling unit.

Space syntax modelling was used to measure the physical accessibility of street network segments (Hillier and Hanson, 1984; Hillier et al., 1993; Hillier, 1996; Bafna, 2003; Baran et al., 2008; Hillier, 2012). We employ this technique in the present study to assess the impacts of street-level accessibility on mental health via their influences upon physical activity and social capital. The space syntax model of urban network configuration has its origin in graph theory and quantitatively measures the relational properties of urban space. In an urban space comprising interconnected subspaces, those that are directly linked through better physical connections and longer unhindered fields of visual sight have better syntactic accessibility and hence are associated with higher movement densities and social interactions. To operationalize this, the OSM ITN Layer of Caerphilly was edited, simplified and transcribed into a road centreline map, which is essentially a model of the street network configuration using the simplest set of line segments representing the longest lines of visual sight. This essentially enables us to capture the effects of changes in direction and the presence of intervening streets upon the individual's sense of orientation in an urban space.

As described in Chapter 5, angular segment analysis (Turner, 2007) of the street network was performed on the ITN Layer in Confeego (Gil et al., 2007) to determine two indices of street network accessibility – *connectivity* and *betweenness*. They act as meaningful proxies for the degree of *connectedness* as well as *walkability* of street network segments in the present study. *Connectivity* of a street segment measures the number of segments directly connected to it and is synonymous with the density of street intersections. For older adults, a higher intersection density may inhibit active living on account of higher traffic density and the resulting lack of road safety while crossing streets. *Betweenness*, also sometimes termed *betweenness centrality*, measures the through-movement potential of the street segment. In our models, betweenness was measured for each street segment with reference to networks defined at three spatial scales. The radii were chosen after a series of iterations to attain parsimonious model fit as described in Chapter 5. At a local scale, movement potential was measured at a 1200 metre network catchment (equivalent to a 15-minute stroll), with higher values being synonymous with higher street-level walkability and hence greater pedestrian activity, especially in terms of walking for transport, shopping and recreation. Given the spatial extent of Caerphilly, a radius of 3000 metres was employed to measure city-scale accessibility. Movement potential at this scale represents city-scale accessibility to various service utilities and captures degree of public transport and car usage. At N metres (comprising all network segments in the system), movement potential becomes an index of regional accessibility capturing long-distance transit behaviour. Higher regional-level movement potential such as being located near motorways is generally considered a physical-activity-inhibiting environment, being synonymous with traffic density, congestion and pollution.

Natural environment

Natural environmental measures of slope variability and greenness were included in the models, the former being particularly variable given the geographical location in the Welsh Valleys. Slope variability within an individual's home range was operationalized as the standard deviation of slope in degrees within a 1 kilometre network buffer of an individual's dwelling. Satellite-derived Normalized Difference Vegetation Index (NDVI) was used as an objective measure of greenness, calculated as the mean NDVI within a 500 metre circular buffer of an individual's dwelling.

Area-level deprivation

In order to study the effect of area-level deprivation upon psychological distress, Welsh Index of Multiple Deprivation (WIMD) scores were used, measured at the level of lower super output area (LSOA) census areas. In the present analysis, six of the seven domain indices were included, while the domain 'access to services' was excluded to avoid any potential collinearity.

6.2.2 Statistical Methods

The impact of built environment configuration upon psychological distress was examined through a two-part multi-level regression model, with individual respondents being nested within census-defined LSOAs. It was observed that the GHQ-30 scale was semi-continuous, with a significant proportion of zeros (indicating non-existence of symptoms of psychological distress) and exhibiting a right-skewed distribution (Figure 6.2).

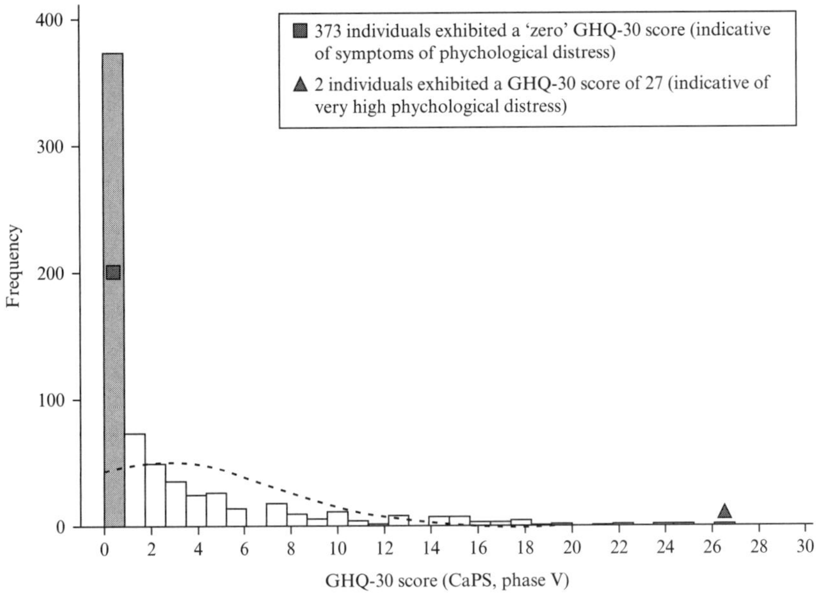

Figure 6.2 Frequency distribution of the GHQ-30 scores of 687 individuals of the fifth phase of the Caerphilly Prospective Study (CaPS)

The prevalence of psychological distress was therefore modelled as a two-level factor (case versus non-case). The conventional GHQ-30 cut-point of a score of 5 or over was employed following a confirmatory validation study conducted in this cohort (Stansfeld et al., 1991). In the first part, two-level logistic mixed effects models with LSOA-level random effects were fitted on the case/non-case binary GHQ scores. A subset of the sample exhibiting a non-zero GHQ-30 score was extracted, and sensitivity analysis was performed to explicitly examine the associations between the intensity of psychological distress (indicated by a non-zero GHQ-30 score) and the characteristics of built environment configurations, without imposition of the case threshold. Hence, the second part of the model comprised a two-level gamma mixed regression model (gamma regression being used to account for the skewed, non-normal distribution of the GHQ-30 scale) with LSOA-level random effects for all the non-zero GHQ-30 scores (indicative of the prevalence of symptoms of psychological distress).

Land use mix was transformed into tertiles (low, medium, high), while standardized z-scores were used for topological accessibility variables to enhance the interpretation of results. For area-level variables, deprivation domain scores ranged between 0 and 100, with higher scores indicating more deprivation and slope variability and NDVI modelled as standardized z-scores.

Age (years) and alcohol consumption (ml/week) were modelled as continuous variables. Social class was expressed in terms of six groups following the Registrar General's occupational classification (Office of Population Censuses and Surveys (OPCS), 1980) and thereafter collapsed into a three-level factor (I/II/III-non-manual, III-manual, IV/V). Marital status was modelled as a three-level factor (married, single, widowed/divorced/separated), as was education (none/apprenticeship, school certificate/higher technical certificate, professional qualification/degree/higher degree). The morbidities of myocardial infarction, angina, high blood pressure, high cholesterol, diabetes and mini-stroke were modelled as two-level factors (present/absent).

Statistical analyses were performed in GLLAMM (GLLAMM, 2010) within the Stata 11.2 (StataCorp, College Station, TX) statistical software package.

6.3 RESULTS

Completed GHQ scores were assessed for 814 men, 745 of whom remained within the geographical boundary of the study area, the rest having migrated. After exclusions for missing data across all categories, the study consisted of 687 valid responses residing within 34 LSOAs. The number of respondents per LSOA ranged from 6 to 47, with a mean of 20.2 (SD = 12.7). The descriptive statistics of the representative sample across the *case* and *no-case* categories as well as the significance of the between-group difference are presented in Table 6.1. The prevalence rate of psychological distress was 19.4 per cent, and the mean age of the sample was 73.5 years (SD = 4.3). Mental health was associated with educational attainment, angina, myocardial infarction, high blood pressure and stroke. The descriptive statistics of environmental variables within the 1 kilometre street buffer employed in the study have been categorized as dwelling-level, land use configuration, topological accessibility of street, natural environment and area-level deprivation variables (Table 6.2).

Table 6.3 presents the results of logistic mixed models to assess the associations between the prevalence of psychological disorders and measurements of built environment configuration, followed by the gamma mixed model for sensitivity analysis. The analytic plan consisted of four analyses. Model 1 examined the associations of psychological distress with the built

Table 6.1 Characteristics of the study sample according to GHQ status

Individual-level confounders	GHQ-30 case		
	Case (n=133) GHQ-30 ≥ 5	No case (n=554) GHQ-30 < 5	p-value of difference
Age: mean (SD)	73.7 (4.3)	73.5 (4.3)	0.549
Alcohol consumption: mean (SD)	49.8 (100.6)	57.5 (96.7)	0.018
Social class (partly skilled/ unskilled): N (%)	25 (18.8)	72 (13.0)	0.085
Educational attainment (none/apprenticeship): N (%)	92 (69.2)	336 (60.6)	0.050
Prevalence of chronic disease:			
Heart attack/coronary thrombosis: N (%)	29 (21.8)	70 (12.6)	0.007
Angina: N (%)	46 (34.6)	105 (19.0)	0.005
High blood pressure: N (%)	72 (54.1)	241 (43.5)	0.027
High cholesterol: N (%)	42 (31.6)	163 (29.4)	0.626
Diabetes: N (%)	22 (16.5)	73 (13.2)	0.313
Stroke: N (%)	23 (17.3)	52 (9.4)	0.006

environment variables, with adjustment for individual-level covariates. Model 2 examined the association of psychological distress with area-level variable (WIMD, slope variability and greenness), also adjusting for individual-level covariates. Model 3 examined the association of psychological distress with both built environment and area-level variables after adjustment for covariates. Apart from these case threshold (GHQ-30 ≥ 5) models, the psychological distress model used non-zero GHQ-30 scores as a continuous variable for sensitivity analysis. Model 4 presents the results of the gamma mixed model performed over a subset of 314 individual men exhibiting a non-zero GHQ-30 score after adjustments for area-level deprivation domain indices, natural environment and covariates.

Analysis of the built environment morphometric variables without adjustment for area-level variables (model 1) found that a higher degree of land use mix was significantly associated with lower odds of psychological distress (OR = 0.54, $p = 0.02$ for the highest tertile). The density of business and offices (OR = 1.02, $p < 0.01$) was associated with higher odds of psychological distress, while density of bus stops was only mildly associated (OR = 1.04, p = 0. 08). Topological accessibility of the street network at a local level, captured by betweenness at a radius of 1200 metres, was associated with lower odds of psychological distress (OR = 0.53, $p < 0.01$). However, regional-level movement potential captured by the global

Table 6.2 Summary of environment variables

Environmental variables	Mean (SD)	Range
Built environment morphometrics		
Dwelling-level variables:[a]		
Dwelling-centred density (within 30 m radius)	14.29 (6.64)	1–40
Dwelling types: N (%):		
Detached	156 (22.70)	
Semi-detached	299 (43.52)	
Terraced	176 (25.63)	
Flats	56 (8.15)	
Plot exposure: N (%):		
No building fronts exposed to public space	76 (11.06)	
One building front exposed to public space	471 (68.56)	
More than one building front exposed to public space	140 (20.38)	
Land use configuration (within 1 km street network buffer):[b]		
Land use mix	0.14 (0.03)	0.03–0.21
Density of bus stops	23.96 (6.00)	7.66–50.46
Density of retail	26.92 (27.58)	1.40–140.7
Density of community services	14.36 (9.93)	1.00–50.95
Density of recreation and leisure facilities	12.91 (5.11)	2.12–34.49
Density of business and offices	30.69 (32.76)	0.87–130.53
Topological accessibility of streets (measured for each street segment at varying radii):[c]		
Betweenness R1200 m	2.40 (0.17)	1.76–2.82
Betweenness R3000 m	3.01 (0.21)	2.40–3.54
Betweenness RNm (all network segments)	3.63 (0.20)	2.92–4.29
Connectivity	3.13 (0.19)	2.66–3.65
Natural environment		
Topography (variability of slope within 1 km street network buffer):[d]		
Neighbourhood slope variability (*mean*)	3.31	0.99–8.04
Greenness (within 500 m airline buffer of dwelling):[e]		
Mean NDVI	0.091	−0.06–0.33
Area-level deprivation		
WIMD 2005 (within census-defined lower super output areas):[f]		
Income domain	24.05 (19.78)	0.34–90.32
Employment domain	25.73 (19.14)	1.00–95.02
Health domain	25.64 (15.71)	1.70–72.3
Education domain	25.82 (16.95)	0.59–62.32

Table 6.2 (continued)

Environmental variables	Mean (SD)	Range
Area-level deprivation		
Housing domain	10.91 (7.44)	0.19–27.23
Physical domain	19.11 (14.63)	1.61–65.4

Notes:
a. Dwelling-level data were extracted from Ordnance Survey Address Layer 2.
b. Land use data were extracted from Ordnance Survey Address Layer 2.
c. Street network was extracted from Ordnance Survey Integrated Transport Network Layer, transformed and subjected to space syntax analysis in Confeego. Measured for each street segment at varying radii to capture the effect of multiple urban scales: regional/city scale (N, 3000 m) and local/walking distance scale (1200 m). Thereafter, connectivity and betweenness were aggregated at the level of a 1 km street network buffer.
d. Slope raster was processed from the Bluesky 5 metre resolution DTM. Measured as the standard deviation of slope in degrees within 1 km street network buffer.
e. Greenness was measured as the Normalized Difference Vegetation Index (NDVI) from the 30 m Landsat data.
f. Area-level deprivation was expressed in terms of the six domain indices of the Welsh Index of Multiple Deprivation, aggregated at the small area level of LSOAs.

betweenness was associated with higher risks of psychological distress (OR = 1.58, $p < 0.01$).

Analysis of the area-level variables, without adjustment for morphometric variables (model 2), found that slope variability was associated with higher odds of psychological distress (OR = 1.38, $p < 0.01$). Greenness measured by the NDVI index was associated with lower risks of psychological distress (OR = 0.76, $p = 0.14$). In terms of the WIMD domains, greater income deprivation was associated with higher odds of psychological distress (OR = 1.03, $p = 0.05$), whilst greater employment deprivation was associated with lower odds of psychological distress (OR = 0.96, $p = 0.02$). Greater physical environment deprivation was associated with increased risks of psychological distress (OR = 1.02, $p < 0.01$).

In the fully adjusted model with both the morphometric and area-level variables together (model 3), higher degrees of land use mix were associated with reduced odds of psychological distress (OR = 0.63, $p = 0.07$ for the middle tertile, and OR = 0.43, $p < 0.01$ for the high tertile). The density of retail or community services or recreation facilities was not related to psychological distress. However, bus stop density (OR = 1.06, $p < 0.\ 01$) and density of business and offices (OR = 1.02, $p < 0.01$) were associated with higher odds of psychological distress. Higher local-level street movement potential captured by betweenness at a radius of 1200 metres was associated with lower odds of psychological distress

Table 6.3 Results of mixed regression with LSOA-level random effects for GHQ-30 case and non-zero GHQ-30 score for the fifth phase of the Caerphilly Prospective Study (CaPS)

Model predictors	Prevalence of psychological distress (logistic model): N=687			Sensitivity analysis (gamma model): N=314
	Model 1†	Model 2†	Model 3†	Model 4‡
	OR (95% CI), p-value	OR (95% CI), p-value	OR (95% CI), p-value	Beta (95% CI), p-value
Built environment morphometrics				
Dwelling-level variables:				
Dwelling-centred density	1.02 (0.97, 1.08), p=0.43		1.02 (0.97, 1.07), p=0.53	0.01 (−0.01, 0.03), p=0.40
Plot exposure (none vs one building face)	0.98 (0.55, 1.73), p=0.94		0.99 (0.57, 1.71), p=0.97	−0.15 (−0.44, 0.13), p=0.30
Plot exposure (more than one building face vs one building face)	0.77 (0.52, 1.14), p=0.19		0.78 (0.53, 1.15), p=0.20	−0.15 (−0.39, 0.09), p=0.23
Dwelling type (semi-detached vs detached)	0.72 (0.41, 1.27), p=0.26		0.74 (0.42, 1.31), p=0.30	−0.06 (−0.33, 0.22), p=0.69
Dwelling type (terraced vs detached)	0.59 (0.26, 1.36), p=0.22		0.48 (0.19, 1.20), p=0.12	−0.28 (−0.61, 0.06), p=0.10*
Dwelling type (flat vs detached)	0.66 (0.20, 2.16), p=0.49		0.75 (0.24, 2.37), p=0.62	0.14 (−0.45, 0.73), p=0.65
Land use configuration:				
Land use mix (z-score):				
T2 vs T1	0.74 (0.44, 1.25), p=0.26		0.63 (0.38, 1.03), p=0.07*	−0.07 (−0.33, 0.19), p=0.62
T3 vs T1	0.54 (0.32, 0.92), p=0.02**		0.43 (0.23, 0.80), p<0.01***	−0.43 (−1.01, 0.15), p=0.15
Density of bus stops	1.04 (1.00, 1.08), p=0.08*		1.06 (1.01, 1.11), p=0.012**	0.03 (0.00, 0.06), p=0.08*

Density of retail	0.99 (0.96, 1.01), p=0.31		0.99 (0.96, 1.03), p=0.70	−0.001(−0.02, 0.02), p=0.93
Density of community services	1.01 (0.96, 1.07), p=0.70		0.99 (0.94, 1.05), p=0.84	−0.01 (−0.04, 0.03), p=0.74
Density of recreation and leisure facilities	0.98 (0.94, 1.02), p=0.38		1.00 (0.95, 1.06), p=0.91	0.004 (−0.02, 0.03), p=0.76
Density of business and offices	1.02 (1.01, 1.03), p<0.01***		1.02 (1.01, 1.04), p<0.01***	0.01 (−0.01, 0.03), p=0.22
Topological accessibility of streets (z-score):				
Betweenness R1200 m	0.53 (0.36, 0.79), p<0.01***		0.41 (0.21, 0.79), p<0.01***	−0.24 (−0.53, 0.05), p=0.10*
Betweenness R3000 m	0.94 (0.63, 1.39), p=0.75		1.70 (0.88, 3.30), p=0.11	0.17 (−0.18, 0.53), p=0.33
Betweenness RNm	1.58 (1.17, 2.12), p<0.01***		1.00 (0.64, 1.56), p=0.94	−0.18 (−0.50, 0.14), p=0.26
Connectivity	1.10 (0.85, 1.40), p=0.47		1.27 (0.97, 1.66), p=0.09*	0.06 (−0.07, 0.19), p=0.34
Natural environment				
Topography (standard deviation in slope)		1.38 (1.11, 1.71), p<0.01***	1.72 (1.18, 2.51), p<0.01***	0.20 (0.04, 0.37), p=0.01**
Greenness (mean NDVI within 500 m)		0.76 (0.58, 0.99), p=0.04**	0.85 (0.58, 1.24), p=0.40	−0.15 (−0.36, 0.07), p=0.18
Neighbourhood deprivation				
Income deprivation		1.03 (1.00, 1.07), p=0.05**	1.02 (0.98, 1.06), p=0.36	0.02 (0.00, 0.04), p=0.10*
Employment deprivation		0.96 (0.93, 0.99), p<0.02**	0.95 (0.92, 0.98), p<0.01***	−0.03 (−0.05, −0.02), p<0.01***
Health deprivation		0.99 (0.98, 1.01), p=0.29	1.00 (0.99, 1.02), p=0.71	0.001 (−0.004, 0.01), p=0.52

Table 6.3 (continued)

Model predictors	Prevalence of psychological distress (logistic model): N=687			Sensitivity analysis (gamma model): N=314
	Model 1†	Model 2†	Model 3†	Model 4‡
	OR (95% CI), p-value	OR (95% CI), p-value	OR (95% CI), p-value	Beta (95% CI), p-value
Education deprivation		1.00 (0.97, 1.03), p=0.84	1.04 (1.00, 1.08), p=0.04**	0.02 (0.00, 0.04), p=0.03**
Housing deprivation		0.99 (0.96, 1.03), p=0.71	0.98 (0.94, 1.02), p=0.35	−0.003 (−0.03, 0.02), p=0.85
Physical environment		1.02 (1.01, 1.04), p<0.01***	1.02 (1.01, 1.04), p<0.01***	0.006 (0.00, 0.02), p=0.18
Individual covariates				
Lifestyle and socio-demographic:				
Age	1.02 (0.97, 1.08), p=0.37	1.02 (0.97, 1.07), p=0.51	1.02 (0.96, 1.08), p=0.56	−0.002 (−0.03, 0.02), p=0.88
Alcohol consumption	1.00 (1.00, 1.00), p=0.84	1.00 (1.00, 1.00), p=0.97	1.00 (1.00, 1.00), p=0.95	−0.0001 (−0.001, 0.001), p=0.79
Smoking status (ex-smoker vs non-smoker)	0.91 (0.50, 1.63), p=0.74	0.90 (0.52, 1.55), p=0.70	0.88 (0.50, 1.57), p=0.67	−0.09 (−0.32, 0.14), p=0.46
Smoking status (current smoker vs non-smoker)	1.47 (0.72, 3.03), p=0.29	1.41 (0.71, 2.79), p=0.33	1.50 (0.72, 3.13), p=0.28	−0.11 (−0.44, 0.22), p=0.50
Marital status (single vs married)	1.01 (0.33, 3.08), p=0.99	1.04 (0.32, 3.39), p=0.95	1.05 (0.34, 3.23), p=0.93	−0.25 (−0.76, 0.25), p=0.33
Marital status (widowed/separated vs married)	0.81 (0.36, 1.81), p=0.61	0.88 (0.42, 1.85), p=0.74	0.90 (0.40, 1.99), p=0.79	0.08 (−0.27, 0.43), p=0.65
Social class (III-manual vs I, II, III-non-manual)	0.97 (0.54, 1.76), p=0.92	0.93 (0.49, 1.75), p=0.81	1.00 (0.52, 1.91), p=0.90	−0.02 (−0.29, 0.26), p=0.91

Social class (IV, V vs I, II, III-non-manual)	1.49 (0.84, 2.64), p=0.17	1.27 (0.71, 2.26), p=0.42	1.59 (0.86, 2.97), p=0.14	0.13 (−0.26, 0.52), p=0.51
Education (school certificates vs none/apprentice)	0.83 (0.48, 1.42), p=0.49	0.89 (0.54, 1.46), p=0.63	0.79 (0.46, 1.38), p=0.41	−0.01 (−0.31, 0.29), p=0.96
Education (degree vs none/apprentice)	0.44 (0.21, 0.94), p=0.04**	0.49 (0.24, 1.03), p=0.06*	0.44 (0.20, 0.98), p=0.05**	−0.21 (−0.70, 0.27), p=0.39
Prevalence of vascular morbidities:				
Heart attack/coronary thrombosis (yes vs no)	1.42 (0.77, 2.62), p=0.26	1.45 (0.82, 2.57), p=0.21	1.55 (0.85, 2.84), p=0.16	0.21 (−0.21, 0.33), p=0.67
Angina (yes vs no)	2.03 (1.06, 3.89), p=0.03**	2.12 (1.16, 3.90), p=0.02**	2.09 (1.07, 4.05), p=0.03**	0.17 (−0.16, 0.49), p=0.32
High blood pressure (yes vs no)	1.66 (1.07, 2.57), p=0.02**	1.55 (0.99, 2.44), p=0.06*	1.71 (1.08, 2.70), p=0.02**	0.27 (0.05, 0.50), p=0.02**
High cholesterol (yes vs no)	0.75 (0.44, 1.27), p=0.29	0.75 (0.46, 1.21), p=0.24	0.76 (0.46, 1.26), p=0.29	−0.12 (−0.40, 0.17), p=0.42
Diabetes (yes vs no)	1.40 (0.85, 2.32), p=0.18	1.32 (0.79, 2.22), p=0.29	1.48 (0.86, 2.54), p=0.16	0.10 (−0.20, 0.39), p=0.52
Stroke (yes vs no)	2.17 (0.99, 4.74), p=0.05**	2.30 (1.10, 4.82), p=0.03**	2.25 (1.030, 4.93), p=0.04**	0.13 (−0.08, 0.34), p=0.22
Model fit				
−2×log likelihood	621.88	624.79	603.99	1650.35

Notes:
Results are expressed as odds ratio, 95% confidence interval and p-value for the logistic regression and beta, 95% confidence interval and p-value for the gamma regression.
T: Tertile (T1, T2, T3 represent the lower, middle and upper tertiles respectively).
* $p<0.10$; ** $p<0.05$; *** $p<0.01$.
† Model 1 consists of built environmental morphometrics. Model 2 includes neighbourhood deprivation captured by six domains of the Welsh Index of Multiple Deprivation and natural environment captured by standard deviation in slope and mean greenness index NDVI. Model 3 indicates the fully adjusted model.
‡ Model 4 represents the results of the fully adjusted gamma regression model for sensitivity analysis.

(OR = 0.41, $p < 0.01$). However, the association of mental health with regional-level street accessibility was lost. Consistent with model 2, hillier topography with higher slope variability was associated with greater psychological distress (OR = 1.72, $p < 0.01$), the effects being more pronounced after adjustments of the built environment. However, the NDVI index of greenness was no longer significant. Amongst the deprivation domains, employment deprivation had a slight protective effect (OR = 0.95, $p < 0.01$), whilst the education and physical environment domains had a slight harmful effect (OR = 1.04, p = 0.04 and OR = 1.02, $p < 0.01$ respectively).

In contrast to the findings for the GHQ-30 case, gamma regression analysis conducted over a subset of individual men exhibiting a non-zero GHQ-30 score (i.e. exhibiting some degree of psychological distress) indicates that none of the built environment variables are significant ($p < 0.05$) (see model 4). However, the slope variability factor ($\beta = 0.20$, p = 0.01) and the employment ($\beta = -0.04$, $p < 0.01$) domain of area deprivation remain statistically significant. The area-level between-LSOA random effects component of the analysis was observed to be very small throughout these models ($\hat{\sigma}_u^2 < 0.10$), indicating negligible heterogeneity between areas.

6.4 DISCUSSION

Consistent with our hypothesis, we have found that a number of land use and street network configuration metrics are significantly associated with levels of psychological distress in a representative sample of older men aged 65–84 years. That the associations were attenuated after adjustments for natural environment, deprivation and individual-level factors emphasizes their importance. Lower odds of psychological distress were associated with greater land use mix and with local-level street accessibility. On the contrary, higher odds of psychological distress were associated with higher density of bus stops and business and office units.

6.4.1 Strengths and Limitations

Strengths of these data lie in the population sample, the detailed assessment of the built environment and the multi-level modelling of putative effects. CaPS has achieved high levels of follow-up throughout, and care has been taken to achieve high levels of case ascertainment. The sample used for this analysis represents a 79 per cent response rate in the most recent (fifth) examination. Although CaPS was considered sufficiently large at conception, the number of men with dementia was only just sufficient for this analysis.

This study explored the association of a wide range of objectively measured robust spatial metrics of land use and street network configurations with psychological health. Several studies have employed composite built environment indices to study their impact upon physical activity (Leslie et al., 2007; Frank et al., 2010; Van Dyck et al., 2010; A.C. King et al., 2011) and mental health (Berke, Gottlieb et al., 2007; Sallis, Saelens et al., 2009). Our study was able to overcome the weaknesses of such composite measures, which often fail to isolate the effects of specific attributes of the built environment upon psychological health. With respect to the street configuration, the street connectivity measure has been employed in health studies to assess the impact of street intersection density upon physical activity (Frank et al., 2004; F. Li et al., 2008; Troped et al., 2010). The application of space syntax-based street network modelling in this book enabled the inclusion of not only street network connectivity, but also the configurational measure of *betweenness* as model predictors (which acted as proxies for accessibility in terms of walkability and social connectivity in this study). Within a space syntax modelling paradigm, street configurational measurements of syntactic accessibility are directly appended to each street segment, thereby enabling the study of potential independent associations between individual health behaviours and street configuration metrics. An inherent advantage of this technique stems from the fact that it enables the analysis of street segments at varying spatial scales, measuring accessibility and movement potential at local, community and regional levels. This allows us to assess the health impacts of accessibility at multiple urban scales. In our models, betweenness of a street segment is proportional to the total simulated counts of passing movements through the segment from and to all the other parts of the network following the shortest angular path heuristic between all pairs of segments. This is supported by evidence that the least angular path analysis is the best predictor of movement (Hillier and Iida, 2005). Thus, the through-movement potential pertaining to each street segment can be enumerated indicating the odds of it being taken while moving through the urban matrix. Modelling the betweenness at multiple radii enabled the assessment of accessibility at multiple urban scales and, by implication, by different modes. These measures add information over and above more established GIS-constructed land use measures of mix and density. In addition, the model used objectively measured natural environment descriptors consisting of slope variability and the NDVI index of greenery. The multi-level analysis, using a random effects model, allowed area-level clustering as well as individual-level variation to be modelled, providing a more accurate analysis.

The two-part modelling provides a rigorous and statistically valid methodology for analysis of the semi-continuous and skewed GHQ-30 scale. A similar two-part approach has been employed for physical activity outcomes (A.H. Lee et al., 2010; A.H. Lee and Xiang, 2011). This could usefully be extended to other psychiatric scales, which often tend to be skewed towards the baseline, thereby overcoming the need for scale transformation and dependence on predetermined cut-points. The random effects logistic component of the two-part model assesses the effects of built environment configuration upon the odds of prevalence of psychological disorders, while, in the second part, the random effects gamma component assesses the effects of built environment configurations upon the intensity of psychological disorders. For non-normal distributions, gamma regression is statistically more accurate in providing realistic estimations for small or moderate sample sizes (compared to standard linear regression).

The cross-sectional design of this analysis limits the confidence with which causal interpretations can be made. The sustained effects of built environment factors upon psychological health through different stages of the life course require further exploration. This can only be achieved through longitudinal analyses. Although adjustment for a wide range of confounders enabled several independent effects of the built environment to be identified, the possibility of residual confounding cannot be excluded. Spatial data were collected as close as possible to the end of CaPS phase V (conducted over the duration of 2002–04) in order to avoid temporal mismatch (Buzzelli and Su, 2006). Nonetheless, limitations owing to this are likely to have been negligible, as the data from Caerphilly County Borough Council indicated relatively stabilized land use and street network characteristics.

6.4.2 Interpretation

Amongst the built environment morphometric results, lower relative odds of psychological disorder with increasing land use mix are consistent with the general hypothesis that higher land use mix is synonymous with enhanced accessibility to health-promoting capital. The effects upon psychological health may manifest themselves along two pathways. The diversity and distribution of community resources may enhance the feeling of neighbourhood satisfaction as well as consolidate social connectivity, thereby adding to social capital (Leslie and Cerin, 2008). On the other hand, a higher land use mix has generally been associated with smaller trip lengths, thereby acting as an incentive for physical activity (Frank et al., 2004; F. Li et al., 2008; Troped et al., 2010). However, it does not confirm the counter-intuitive findings from Saarloos et al. (2011), who found depression to be positively associated with greater land use mix. Saarloos acknowledges his findings require further explanation.

Support for the land use hypothesis in terms of the density of specific land use types was however less clear. No association was found between psychological distress and the density of retail, community services, or leisure and recreation units. This runs contrary to expectations based on the impact of the density of these community resources upon physical activity (Frank et al., 2003; Norman et al., 2006; Diez Roux et al., 2007). These null findings may be due to lack of statistical power. However, the odds ratios are uniformly virtually one, and this does not seem a likely explanation. Alternatively they may be due to over-adjustment, that is, the masking of an association by the inclusion of an index of land use mix in the same model. This possibility was explored by repeating the analysis omitting land use mix. No evidence for an effect of collinearity was found, however. Another possibility is that there was insufficient variation to detect an association, Caerphilly being a relatively homogeneous area. However, at the same time, the study captured the inhibitory effects of specific land uses. That density of business units was inversely related to psychological distress is consistent with one of the study's hypotheses: areas with predominantly commercial or industrial outlook are usually associated with reduced sense of community, typically associated with unwanted social contacts, having large parking spaces and high traffic (Halpern, 1995; Glass and Balfour, 2003; Wood et al., 2010). The positive association of psychological distress with increasing density of bus stops was not anticipated. Although this may be a chance effect, it may be that the availability of public transport reduces walking behaviour in older men and this has implications for psychological well-being. Density of bus stops may be associated with reduced sense of traffic safety among older adults, as well as higher levels of noise pollution. Alternatively, higher density of public transport routes may in this community be a proxy variable for aspects of social deprivation that were not captured through the WIMD. Larger concentrations of lower-priced properties in certain locations, for example, have a high propensity for subletting and thus a greater tendency for the formation of clusters of vulnerable adults living in low-income and supported housing.

The space syntax metrics enabled the study to capture the configuration and design of urban form at multiple spatial scales (Kashef, 2011). Throughout the models, no significant association between psychological distress and street connectivity could be established. Higher local-level street betweenness (measured within a radius of 1200 metres) was associated with lower odds of psychological disorders in all models, controlling for all other variables. This is of specific importance, as higher local-level betweenness of destinations may help create a walkable, well-integrated community with enhanced accessibility to health-promoting capital. These findings underscore the positive influence of community-level street network accessibility upon psychological health and the need for optimizing urban design in this respect. Higher regional-level street movement potential was associated with increased odds of psychological distress (model 1). This might have been attributed to living in the vicinity of major roads, generally associated with traffic density, pollution and reduced perception of safety from traffic, especially among older adults. However, this association was attenuated, no longer being significant in our fully controlled model (model 3) after the introduction of natural environment and area-level deprivation variables. This was indicative of the moderating effects of natural environment. The slope variability factor introduces the terrain-induced disincentive to going out for longer trips, especially in older adults. Furthermore, the beneficial effect of natural greenness in diluting traffic-related pollution and stress is well known. These findings underscore the positive influence of community-level street network accessibility upon psychological health and the need for optimizing urban design in this respect.

Among the natural environment variables, slope variability was consistently associated with psychological distress irrespective of the built environment as well as in the fully adjusted model. This may be attributed to reduced physical capacity and mobility of the elderly in a hilly terrain. In a study conducted by Wood et al. (2010), perception of steep hills was reported to be associated with a 3.36 per cent decrease in the sense of community. That none of the built environment variables were significantly associated with the non-zero GHQ-30 score model in a subset population exhibiting symptoms of psychological distress is of interest. On the one hand, in the case/non-case threshold model, the hypothesis is that higher slope variability combined with the built environment attributes acts as a disincentive to 'go out' among the psychologically distressed compared to the non-cases. On the other hand, among the non-zero GHQ population, slope variation alone has an influence on the variation in psychological distress level. It seems that the terrain-induced disincentive to 'go out' kicks in for the population subset exhibiting symptoms of psychological distress, thereby rendering them insensitive to built environmental factors.

A statistically significant association between the beneficial effects of greenness and psychological health was also observed to be independent of the built environment; however, the association became null after the inclusion of built environmental configurational measures. This is fascinating, since it suggests that network configuration may be more important than proximity to green space per se.

In the models, income, employment and physical environment domains of area-level deprivation were found to be associated with psychological distress, ignoring built environment patterns (model 2). LSOAs having higher deprivation with respect to income and physical environment deprivation domains were associated with higher odds of psychological distress. The physical environment domain index operationalizes environment deprivation through indicators of air quality, air emissions, proximity to waste disposal and industrial sites, and flood hazard. However, higher employment deprivation was associated with lower odds of psychological distress in the elderly. An explanation of this might be that the employment deprivation index is reflective of social security and benefits, measuring the proportion of working-age people claiming out-of-work benefits and consisting of indicators of claimants of unemployment benefits, incapacity benefit, severe disability allowance and so on. Since the study cohort is largely beyond the legal working age, the presence of unemployed family and community members entitled to benefits may constitute a socially supportive and cohesive environment, having a positive impact upon the psychological health of elderly people.

After the inclusion of built environment parameters in the model, only the employment and education domains of deprivation indictors remained significant. LSOAs with higher educational deprivation were associated with higher prevalence of psychological distress. Since employment effects are controlled for, this might indicate an improved ability to cope with psychological distress with increasing levels of educational attainment.

CaPS is a cohort of middle-aged and older men; hence, one must be cautious in generalizing the nature of associations to other sections of the population, particularly on account of differences in individual risk factor profiles between populations, for example in older women or in younger men. Nevertheless CaPS may be considered a reasonably representative population sample, and the data are highly informative for this demographic group. It is important to recognize that the influence of different components of land use configuration on mental health is likely to be complex and may vary not only according to mix and density but also according to the natural and economic environment. For example, CaPS is situated in the South Wales Valleys, where there is high slope variability and an ongoing post-industrial transition of land use. Under such circumstances it is important to consider the level of generalizability of the observed associations. It may be, for example, that the benefit to mental health of higher local area street accessibility is more widely generalizable than the inverse association of bus stop density with mental health. Only further research can address these issues.

6.5 CONCLUSIONS

The evidence from the study supports the hypothesis that variation in the way the built environment is configured (by design or evolution) has an impact upon the psychological health of older adults. The exact causal mechanisms linking built and natural environments with mental health emerge over time as a result of complex interactions and are likely to be age specific. This necessitates a replication of the present study through a robust prospective design operating at a much larger scale with diverse age groups.

There has been substantial ongoing debate about the implications of sound urban planning and design upon preventive health management. The objective measurements of built and natural environment factors produce much-needed scientific tests in support of evidence-based research into holistic public health planning such as urban design and retrofitting of the built environment in pursuit of health-sustaining communities. Consequently, the study has specific relevance in local authority planning decisions with respect to optimizing the neighbourhood activity space so as to promote healthy activity behaviour. So the distribution and siting of the health-promoting community resources in the urban matrix may be planned so as to make them more accessible to dwelling locations. Similarly, street segments associated with high local-scale syntactic accessibility and, hence, a higher potential to support pedestrian density may be specifically targeted for further improvements with an aim to enhance neighbourhood walkability and social connectivity. In this regard, retrofitting with improved design features and pedestrian infrastructure including nature and quality of sidewalks, a high proportion of dwelling block faces exposed to sidewalks, the presence of traffic-calming features and speed impediments, and enhancements in aesthetic aspects may all have positive effects upon healthy activity behaviour. As a preventive approach to geriatric psychological health, care homes for the vulnerable old and handicapped should be planned in optimized locations, with a view to encouraging healthy activity behaviour and social connectivity as well as creating an improved perception of community satisfaction. Thus, optimizing urban planning and design at a community level may contribute towards devising effective intervention strategies in preventive health. Large-scale studies are required for gathering further evidence to support informed planning decisions.

7. Built environment configuration and change in body mass index: the Caerphilly Prospective Study (CaPS)

7.1 PHYSICAL INACTIVITY AND THE EPIDEMIC OF OBESITY: PUBLIC HEALTH IMPACTS

Physical activity has emerged as one of the key determinants of public health in our modernized technology-based society. Technological innovations have mechanized most of our daily routine tasks, resulting in sedentary lifestyles and unhygienic food habits (such as increased dependence on inexpensive, calorie-dense foods and beverages). The past three decades have witnessed a twofold increase in the prevalence of obesity (Caballero, 2007), posing serious public health risks. In 2008, approximately 34 per cent of adults (1.46 billion) worldwide were overweight, with a body mass index (BMI) of 25 kg/m^2 or more, of which 502 million were obese, with a BMI of 30 kg/m^2 or more (Kimokoti and Millen, 2011). Current trends project 65 million more obese adults in the USA and 11 million more obese adults in the UK by 2030 (Y. Claire Wang et al., 2011).

In the UK, 7.3 per cent of all disability-adjusted life-years (DALYs) are directly attributable to overweight and obesity, accounting for 66 737 directly related deaths. The direct annual health costs of overweight and obesity to the NHS have been estimated to be around £3.23 billion, while a separate study attributed £1.06 billion towards the costs of physical inactivity (Allender and Rayner, 2007; Allender et al., 2007). In England, obesity levels increased from 13.2 per cent in 1993 to 24 per cent in 2008 in men, and from 16.4 per cent to 25 per cent in women over the same period. A greater proportion of men than women (42 per cent compared with 32 per cent) in England were classified as overweight in 2008 (BMI 25 to less than 30 kg/m^2). In the case of adolescents, 16.8 per cent of boys aged 2–15 years, and 15.2 per cent of girls in this age group were classed as obese. Statistics on self-reported measures of physical activity indicate that only 39 per cent of men and 29 per cent of women met the recommended levels of at least 30 minutes of moderate-intensity activity at least five times a week in 2008 (Eastwood, 2010). Data from the 2004 Canadian Community

Health Survey indicate that the national prevalence of overweight and obesity among Canadian adults was 36 per cent and 23 per cent respectively (Canadian Institute for Health Information, 2006). The direct and indirect medical costs associated with overweight and obesity in Canada in 2001 were estimated at C$1.6 billion and C$2.7 billion, respectively, accounting for 2.2 per cent of total health care costs (Katzmarzyk and Janssen, 2004; Pouliou and Elliott, 2010). Australian statistics indicate that only 46.1 per cent of adults and about 45.5 per cent of women were active at moderate to vigorous levels for at least 30 minutes per day on a minimum of five days a week (Bauman et al., 2001). A similar trend has been projected for the non-industrialized countries, with an estimation that three-quarters of the obese population worldwide will belong to the non-industrialized countries by 2025 (WHO, 2005b). Ziraba et al. (2009) studied demographic and health survey data (collected 1992–2005) from seven African countries and concluded that the prevalence of obesity increased by approximately 35 per cent during the same period. Cross-country analysis of data on overweight children and childhood obesity indicates an increasing trend (Youfa Wang and Lobstein, 2006).

The bulk of epidemiological evidence highlights the fact that physical inactivity has a significant association with weight gain and obesity (Summerbell et al., 2009). This primarily results from the simultaneous increased calorific intake and decreased calorific expenditures leading to a *positive* energy balance. Physical activity has been known to play a defensive role, offsetting a number of chronic diseases, both independently and via its effects on weight gain and obesity (Miles, 2007). Obesity is associated with increased risk of vascular, metabolic, neoplastic and mental health outcomes (USDHHS, 1996; W.P. James, 1998; Kopelman, 2000; Pi-Sunyer, 2002; Warburton et al., 2006; Flegal et al., 2007; Ogden et al., 2007; Wiles et al., 2007; Haskell et al., 2009).

Although the impact of obesity on mortality is smaller in the oldest old (85-plus years), obesity remains an important predictor of all causes of mortality in older people, being a particularly strong predictor of vascular mortality (Stevens et al., 1998). The projected doubling (11 per cent to 22 per cent) of the older adult population (60-plus years) by 2050 will, therefore, likely exacerbate the global obesity problem (WHO, 2007). Furthermore, the health risks posed by obesity are significantly exacerbated by the compositional changes occurring in the body with the ageing process. There is a progressive increase in body fat mass, which usually peaks at the age of 65 years in men and later in women. This is accompanied by a simultaneous loss of muscle mass and decline in muscle strength. This is often termed *sarcopenic obesity*, a condition that increases the risk of physical disability, morbidity and mortality (Roubenoff, 2004; Zamboni et al., 2008).

7.2 THE ROLE OF THE BUILT ENVIRONMENT

In addition to the inherent physiological, lifestyle and socio-demographic factors, the built environment has been implicated in explaining the sharp rise in obesity as well as its socio-spatial distribution. The constituent components of the built environment, especially its design and the configuration of land use and street networks, govern the distribution of resources and services, configure the neighbourhood activity space, and thereby influence individual physical activity behaviour and weight outcomes. Enhanced accessibility to health-promoting community resources improves local opportunities for physical activity, walking and social interactions and has been linked to reduced body weight (J. Pearce et al., 2006; Bernard et al., 2007). In a review of several studies that try to assess the associations between physical environment variables and individuals' propensity to use walking and cycling for transport, Saelens, Sallis and Frank (2003) quantified the extent of association from a physical activity and health perspective. They estimated the mean difference between high- and low-walkable neighbourhoods in terms of approximately one to two walking trips per week, which converts to 1–2 kilometres, or about 15–30 minutes' more walking per week for each resident in high-walkable neighbourhoods. This amounted to energy expenditure in the range of 3000–6000 kcal, or about 0.85–1.75 lb (0.39–0.79 kg) for any 150 lb (68 kg) person. Van Dyck et al. (2010) provided an even higher estimate in European cities: living in a neighbourhood with a high-walkability configuration is associated with 80 minutes/week more walking for transport, 40 minutes/week more cycling, 20 minutes/week more recreational walking and 35 minutes/week less motorized transport.

Recent research has highlighted the positive influences of mixed land use (Saelens, Sallis, Black et al., 2003; Frank et al., 2004), green spaces and recreational facilities (Norman et al., 2006; Diez Roux et al., 2007; Nielsen and Hansen, 2007; Björk et al., 2008; Wolch et al., 2011), transit stops (Bassett et al., 2008; B.B. Brown and Werner, 2008; R.D. Edwards, 2008), supermarkets (Inagami et al., 2006; Morland et al., 2006; Black et al., 2010) and sports facilities (Giles-Corti et al., 2003; Rutt and Coleman, 2005) upon individual weight outcomes. In contrast, street network segments associated with higher connectivity and higher global accessibility are generally synonymous with higher traffic density and speed, increasing levels of pollution and reduced perception of safety; hence they are associated with higher odds of obesity under the hypothesis that these factors deter walking (Timperio et al., 2005; Norman et al., 2006; Boer et al., 2007; Jerrett et al., 2010). Several measures have been developed to quantify salient parameters of the built environment factors. Cervero and Kockelman (1997) introduced the 3Ds – density, diversity and pedestrian-oriented designs – as measures of the built environment that have a statistically significant influence upon walking and physical activity. Subsequently, two more Ds – destination accessibility and distance to transit stops – were added, to make it 5Ds (Ewing and Cervero, 2001). C. Lee and Moudon (2006a) were able to isolate a statistically significant subset of built environment correlates of walking, which were grouped as destination, distance, density and route, that is, 3D + R. To underscore the importance of these effects of the built environment, the term *neighbourhood walkability* has emerged in recent years, which may be conceptualized as the degree to which the attributes of the built environment may promote or inhibit walking and physical activity behaviour (Leslie et al., 2007).

The facilitative role of the built environment in influencing weight outcomes is arguably particularly important in older adults. Although they may have more time for leisure activity, they are also likely to have reduced physical capability. Consequently, built environment factors that promote physical activity, especially design, configuration of land uses, the presence of walkable destinations in the form of service utilities, aesthetics and safety, may have an enhanced influence on weight outcomes in the elderly. Several cross-sectional studies have highlighted the positive association between physical activity levels and accessibility to facilities, parks and green spaces, safety, aesthetics, mixed land uses, traffic volume and street connectivity for older adults (Humpel et al., 2002; Patterson and Chapman, 2004; F. Li, Fisher, Brownson et al., 2005; Berke, Koepsell et al., 2007; Nagel et al., 2008; Frank et al., 2010; Gómez et al., 2010). Other studies have established a direct association between obesity and built environmental attributes like land use mix and density of fast-food outlets (F. Li et al., 2008), aesthetics and pedestrian-friendly design (Boehmer et al., 2007), and neighbourhood psychosocial hazards (Glass, Rasmussen et al., 2006). Even though these studies provide evidence of association, their cross-sectional designs mean that the cumulative effect of the built environment upon weight outcomes may be underestimated and the possibility of reverse causation cannot be discounted. There exist no long-term longitudinal studies assessing BMI trends of older adults in relation to the built environment. Only one short-term study has been reported. F. Li, Harmer, Cardinal, Bosworth et al. (2009) followed 1145 men and women aged 50–75 years for one year, finding that both weight and waist circumference increase according to frequency of visiting fast-food restaurants.

The hypothesis driving the present study in this chapter is that the various attributes of the built environment influence patterns of individual physical activity behaviour, thereby affecting adiposity in older adults. We test this hypothesis using longitudinal data from the Caerphilly Prospective

Study (CaPS), which has repeatedly measured obesity (body mass index) over a 12-year period. We test the association of these measurements with a broad range of objectively measured built environmental factors.

7.3 METHODS

7.3.1 Study Design

The study was constituted by the living members of the CaPS who had participated in the third, fourth and fifth phases of examination and resided within the study area. The third phase of examination (1989–93) was employed as a baseline, while the latest follow-up (2002–04) comprised 1225 surviving men aged 65–84 years. Longitudinal BMI data over the period of study were available for 912 individual respondents. However, 70 lived outside the study area, 96 had observations missing on individual-level morbidities, and a further 62 individuals had observations missing across lifestyle and socio-demographic variables. Eventually, the study cohort was limited to 684 valid responses distributed over the three time points, across 35 census-defined lower super output areas (LSOAs).

7.3.2 Individual-Level Variables

Each phase of the study involved an extensive clinical examination including anthropometry, assessment of blood pressure, electrocardiogram and collection of fasting blood samples. Obesity was assessed in terms of body mass index, calculated as body weight in kilograms divided by height in metres squared. Height was measured in bare feet using a Holtain stadiometer and weight in light clothes was measured using standard scales. Lifestyle, socio-demographic and vascular risk factors were identified from the literature. Occasion-specific lifestyle risk factors included age, alcohol consumption and smoking status. Alcohol consumption was expressed as a continuous variable and measured in ml/week over each time point. Smoking status at each time point was modelled as a three-level factor (non-smoker, ex-smoker and current smoker). Socio-demographic factors consisted of marital status, education and social class. Marital status was modelled as a three-level factor (married, single or divorced/separated/widowed), whilst education was modelled as a three-level factor (none/apprenticeship, school certificate/higher technical certificate, professional qualification/degree/higher degree). Social class was assessed using the Registrar General's occupational classification (Office of Population Censuses and Surveys (OPCS), 1980) and was modelled as a two-level factor (manual, non-manual). This was preferred to the more recent National Statistics socio-economic classification given the pre-2001 baseline of the present study as well as the predominantly elderly composition of the respondents beyond retirement age. The study further controlled for the impact of six vascular risk factors, as assessed in the most recent examination (myocardial infarction, angina, high blood pressure, high cholesterol, diabetes and mini-stroke).

7.3.3 Built Environment Variables

The theoretical foundations and the variable selection process in the study were guided by epidemiological research evidence relating to the built environment, walking behaviour and obesity (C. Lee and Moudon, 2006a; Papas et al., 2007; Saelens and Handy, 2008; Brownson et al., 2009; Feng et al., 2010). The built environment measures from the spatial Design Network Analysis for Urban Health (sDNA-UH) were operationalized within a 1 kilometre street network buffer around an individual respondent's dwelling unit. The initial model-building exercise included iteration and testing for variable selection to obtain a parsimonious model fit using variables of theoretical importance (described in Chapter 5). The following five sets of 16 built environment morphometrics were included in the finally selected models.

Land use morphometrics

Land use mix evaluated the degree of heterogeneity of land uses within a defined buffer of 1 kilometre. A five-category land use mix consisting of residential dwellings, retail, community services, business and offices, and recreation and leisure was enumerated within each buffer using a method proposed by Frank et al. (2004, 2006). The densities of walkable service destinations, bus stops, retail, churches, community services, and recreation and leisure amenities were also measured within each buffer.

Destination accessibility

This was operationalized in terms of network distances to the nearest green space, facility for physical activity and sports, and health care facilities. It was thereafter divided into three categories, namely 0–50 percentile, 51–75 percentile and 76–100 percentile. The bottom 50 percentile of network distance was employed as the reference category in the regression analyses.

Topological accessibility of the street network

We posit that in an urban space, in addition to the location and density of services, the configuration of the street network determines individual behavioural and cognitive abilities to identify locations and navigate to the services, thus shaping walking, transit behaviour and eventually the accessibility and the social interactions therein. Following Hillier and colleagues, the geometry of urban space can be thought of as comprising three typologies: the linear space in the form of street segments through which people move, the convex space consisting of squares and public spaces through which they interact, and the ever changing visual field through which they perceive the surroundings as they move within space. As discussed in Chapter 5, Hillier proposed the space syntax modelling technique wherein the continuous urban space is configured into a set of discrete interconnected units (subspaces) and the topological connectivity and accessibility of these subspaces govern individuals' movement within them (Hillier and Hanson, 1984; Hillier et al., 1993; Hillier, 1996; L. Vaughan, 2007; Baran et al., 2008; Cutumisu and Spence, 2009). Behaviourally meaningful subtleties in street network topology may thus act as a proxy of walking and transit behaviour, eventually influencing body weight and other health outcomes. As has been reported in Chapter 5, to produce a space syntax model, the OSM ITN Layer of Caerphilly was first edited and further simplified to produce a road centreline map, and angular segment analysis (Turner, 2007) was then performed in Confeego (Gil et al., 2007). As with the study in Chapter 6, two graphical measures of topological accessibility – connectivity and betweenness – have been employed in the present study to act as a proxy for the degree of walkability of each street network segment. Betweenness was measured for each street segment with reference to networks defined at multiple catchment radii. After model testing for the study area, three varying radii RN (the longest distance between two street segments in the spatial model, in other words encompassing the entire network), R3000 and R1200 metres, representing the movement potential at spatial scales of regional, town and local walkable distances respectively, were employed. At a local scale of 1200 metres radii betweenness captures the pedestrian flows (behaviour), street segments with a higher value of betweenness being more likely to be used by pedestrians, while at scales of N, and 3000 metres, the betweenness index becomes an indicator of transit behaviour, high betweenness being synonymous with increased traffic density and congestion.

Topography

On account of the geographical location of the study area in the Welsh Valleys, a slope variability factor was tested for its influence on BMI, either as an inhibitor of weight gain or as an inhibitor of walking (exacerbating weight gain). The degree of variability in slope within an individual's home range was operationalized as the standard deviation of slope in degrees within a 1 kilometre network buffer of an individual's dwelling.

Dwelling-level morphometrics

Dwelling-level variables consisted of the two measures of dwelling-centred density and dwelling type.

7.3.4 Data Analysis

A three-level mixed effect longitudinal model was adopted. A longitudinal analysis gives due credence to the dual components of clustering, namely time and area clustering effects, to obtain realistic estimates (Allman-Farinelli et al., 2009). Time-level within-individual clustering in the BMI data arises as a result of repeated measures taken at subsequent time points. In addition, there is an area-level clustering, which reflects the contextual effects. Level 1 was measurement occasion (time), level 2 was the individual participant, and level 3 was the lower layer super output area (LSOA). The study examined the impact of built environment morphometrics upon the repeated measures of BMI over three time points encompassing a period of 12 years. Phase III of CaPS was the baseline point, with phases IV and V the subsequent time points in the study. Adjustment was made on each measurement occasion for socio-economic and lifestyle factors. The UK Census has defined LSOAs as relatively stable, compact zonal systems with reasonable degrees of homogeneity in shape and social composition. We have therefore taken the LSOAs as the areal units for studying the potential contextual variations in BMI (Bates, 2006). Between-LSOA-level clustering in the BMI of individuals residing in the same LSOA may originate on account of sharing a similar set of socio-economic and built environmental conditions. In the analysis the independent effect of the built environment was characterized by the effect of the LSOA after adjustment for socio-economic and lifestyle factors and vascular morbidities.

The fixed component of the model assessed the magnitude, direction and significance of the relationship between the built environment variables and BMI as well as confounders, while the random component measures the inherent correlations in the observations within levels, separating these into individual-level and LSOA-level random effects. Measurement occasions were nested within individuals, and individuals were nested within LSOAs. This class of model therefore estimates the individual changes in BMI by partitioning the variance in BMI into three components: between-individual variance, between-occasions variance and between-LSOA variance.

Standard data quality checks described in Chapter 5 were performed for all variables before their inclusion in the multi-level framework to ensure parsimonious model fit. These included removal of extreme outliers and running the regression diagnostics plots to access the need for data transformations. Standardized z-scores were used for land use mix and topological accessibility variables to enhance the interpretation of results. Model coefficients (beta), robust standard errors, 95 per cent confidence intervals and significance tests were derived for each independent variable. An additional precaution for parsimonious fit was ensured by adjusting the standard errors using the Huber–White sandwich estimator, which is a robust estimator of the variance–covariance matrix of the regression parameters (Williams, 2000; C.J.M. Maas and Hox, 2004). All analyses were conducted using GLLAMM (GLLAMM, 2010) within the Stata 11.2 statistical software package.

7.4 RESULTS

The study cohort reported 2052 observations at three time points for 684 individuals distributed over 35 LSOAs. The descriptive statistics of the individual-level variables are presented in Table 7.1. Mean BMI in the third, fourth and fifth phases of examination was 26.89, 27.15 and 27.82 kg/m^2 respectively, while the prevalence of obesity was 16.81, 18.86 and 26.61 per cent respectively. The spatial location of the CaPS respondents and their weight outcomes are shown in Figure 7.1.

The mean age of the cohort during the third, fourth and fifth phases was 61.52, 65.18 and 73.22 years respectively. There was a moderate change in lifestyle factors over the period of study. Alcohol consumption reduced from 15.82 ml/week in the third phase to 5.66 ml/week in the fifth phase. Current smokers constituted 27.63 per cent of the population in the third phase, but 25 per cent in the fourth phase and 17.54 per cent in the fifth phase. The level of vascular morbidity in the latest follow-up was 13 per cent having experienced a heart attack, 20 per cent with angina, 45 per cent with high blood pressure, 30 per cent with high cholesterol, 14 per cent with diabetes, and 10 per cent having had a mini-stroke.

The description of the built environment predictors included in the model and their basic statistics have been presented in Table 7.2. The study area manifests marked heterogeneity with respect to the built environment, ranging from urban characteristics in the town centre to rural in the periphery. A respondent's dwelling located in a typical urban area with high land use mix near the town centre is shown in Figure 7.2a, while a typical dwelling in a predominantly rural area with low mix is shown in Figure 7.2b. The standard deviation in slope, in degrees experienced

Table 7.1 Descriptive statistics for individual-level variables

Variable name	Mean (SD) or frequency (%)		
	Third examination	Fourth examination	Fifth examination
Weight outcomes:			
BMI in kg/m^2 (mean, SD)	26.89 (3.45)	27.15 (3.50)	27.82 (3.97)
Normal (BMI $\leq$ 25 kg/m^2)	203 (29.7%)	170 (24.9%)	155 (22.7%)
Overweight (25 kg/m^2 $\leq$ BMI $\leq$ 30 kg/m^2)	366 (53.5%)	385 (56.3%)	347 (50.7%)
Obese (BMI $\geq$ 30 kg/m^2)	115 (16.8%)	129 (18.8%)	182 (26.6%)
Occasion-specific risks:			
Age (mean, SD)	61.5 (4.2)	65.2 (4.2)	73.2 (4.0)
Alcohol consumption (mean, SD)	15.82 (19.66)	13.47 (16.93)	5.66 (9.45)
Smoking status:			
Non-smoker	151 (20.1%)	153 (22.4%)	187 (27.3%)
Ex-smoker	344 (50.3%)	360 (52.6%)	377 (55.1%)
Current smoker	189 (27.6%)	171 (25.0%)	120 (17.6%)
Socio-demographic variables:			
Marital status (N, %):			
Married	618 (90.4%)		
Single	26 (3.8%)		
Separated/divorced/ widowed	40 (5.8%)		
Social class (N, %):			
Non-manual	256 (37.4%)		
Manual	428 (62.6%)		
Education (N, %):			
None/apprenticeship	416 (60.8%)		
School certificate/higher technical certificate	186 (27.2%)		
Professional qualification/ degree/higher degree	82 (12.0%)		
Occurrence of vascular morbidities (N, %):			
MI			91 (13.3%)
Angina			139 (20.3%)
Diabetes			95 (13.9%)
Transient ischaemic attack (TIA)/mini-stroke			67 (9.8%)
Hypertension			309 (45.2%)
High cholesterol			202 (29.5%)

Note: N = 684.

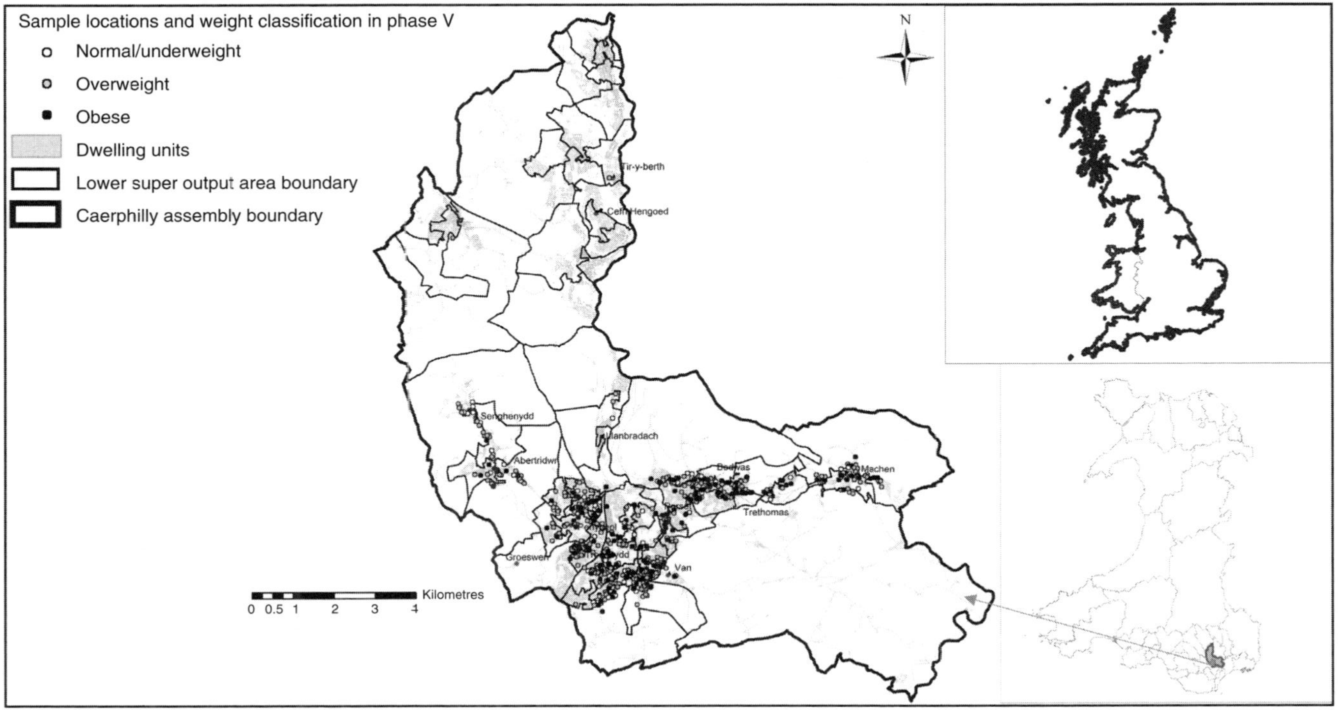

Figure 7.1 Spatial location of participants and their 12-year follow-up weight outcome

Table 7.2 Built environment predictors included in the model

Built environment morphometrics	Mean (SD)	Range
Land use morphometrics (per 1 km street network buffer):*		
Land use mix density	0.160 (0.035)	0.053–0.229
Retail	28.583 (28.725)	1.405–139.090
Church	2.653 (2.116)	0–12.284
Community services	11.982 (8.389)	0.997–43.570
Recreation and leisure facilities	12.698 (5.074)	2.007–34.495
Business and offices	32.643 (33.776)	0.908–129.036
Destination accessibility (street network distance in metres from dwelling):**		
Green space	504.079 (352.274)	8.511–1939.012
Sports facilities	577.212 (314.736)	10.317–1648.040
Health care facilities	568.236 (297.749)	21.028–2015.920
Topological accessibility of streets (measured for each street segment at varying radii):***		
Connectivity	2.020 (0.172)	1.629–2.411
Betweenness RNm (all networks)	3.623 (0.191)	2.919–4.228
Betweenness R3000 m	3.008 (0.208)	2.365–3.540
Betweenness R1200 m	2.406 (0.175)	1.732–2.823
Topography (variability of slope within 1 km street network buffer):****		
Neighbourhood slope variability	3.26	0.996–7.362
Dwelling-level morphometrics (within 30 m kernel of dwelling):*****		
Dwelling-centred density	14.149 (6.738)	0–48
Dwelling types:		
Detached	155 (22.66 %)	
Semi-detached	299 (43.71 %)	
Terraced	182 (26.61 %)	
Apartments	48 (7.02 %)	

Notes:
* Land use data were extracted from Ordnance Survey Address Layer 2.
** Spatial location of destinations was extracted from Ordnance Survey Address Layer 2.
*** Street network was extracted from Ordnance Survey Integrated Transport Network Layer, transformed and subjected to space syntax analysis in Confeego. Measured for each street segment at varying radii to capture the effect of multiple urban scales: city scale (N, 3000 m) and local/walking-distance scale (1200 m). Thereafter, connectivity and route betweenness were aggregated at the level of a 1 km street network buffer.
**** Slope raster was processed from the Bluesky 5 metre resolution DTM. Measured the standard deviation of slope in degrees within a 1 km street network buffer.
***** Dwelling-level data extracted from Ordnance Survey Address Layer 2. Dwelling-centred density surrounding the dwelling unit was measured within a 30 m kernel.

within 1 kilometre of the individual's dwelling, ranged from 0.996 to 7.362, reflecting the unevenness of the topography.

The results of a sequence of the three-level mixed effects linear regression with individual- and LSOA-level random effects for BMI are presented in Table 7.3. Fixed effects are presented in the top half of the table, followed by the random effects. Model fit was assessed by −2×log likelihood, with smaller values indicating a better fit. For the purpose of comparison, model 0 represents the baseline model with no built environment and individual-level predictors (see note to Table 7.3). In model 1 all five sets of built environment morphometrics predictors are present, while in model 2 adjustments were made for age and socio-demographic (marital status, social class and education) as well as lifestyle (alcohol consumption and smoking) factors. Finally, in model 3, further adjustment was made for the prevalence of vascular morbidities.

The random effects components of the analysis found there to be negligible and non-significant heterogeneity between areas once the built environment variable had been added ($\hat{\sigma}_u^2$<0.001), although a high degree of heterogeneity between individuals was retained after adjustment for other covariates ($\hat{\sigma}_u^2 = 9.956$). The fixed-effects component of the model found that the occasion-specific variance ($\hat{\sigma}_e^2$) in the BMI varied from 1.971 (0.352) in model 0 to 1.958 (0.351) in model 3. An occasion-specific intra-class correlation coefficient of 0.164 in the final model implies that 16.4 per cent of the variance in BMI is occasion-specific, attributed to the time interval of 12 years. Furthermore, the increments in BMI over the three time points were consistently significant throughout the four models.

In model 1, seven of the 16 built environment morphometrics were observed to be significantly associated with BMI. Higher land use mix was significantly associated with increasing BMI levels ($\beta_1 = 0.402$, $p = 0.044$). The density of the amenities was observed to be inversely associated with BMI levels: density of retail ($\beta_1 = -0.033$, $p = 0.014$), churches ($\beta_1 = -0.315$, $p = 0.009$), recreation and leisure facility ($\beta_1 = -0.086$, $p = 0.007$). Higher city-scale route betweenness at 3000 m was associated with improved BMI outcomes ($\beta_1 = -1.197$, $p < 0.001$), while local-scale betweenness at 1200 m was associated with poorer weight outcomes ($\beta_1 = 0.849$, $p = 0.022$). The slope variability factor played a significant role in predicting BMI levels; a higher standard deviation in slope within the defined buffer was associated with improved BMI levels ($\beta_1 = -0.327$, $p = 0.019$). Further adjustments for socio-demographic and lifestyle factors found BMI to be associated with alcohol consumption ($\beta_2 = 0.006$, $p = 0.021$), smoking ($\beta_2 = -0.810$, $p < 0.001$) and social class ($\beta_2 = 0.579$, $p = 0.038$), but these made very little material difference to associations of BMI with the built environment (model 2). Subsequent adjustments for

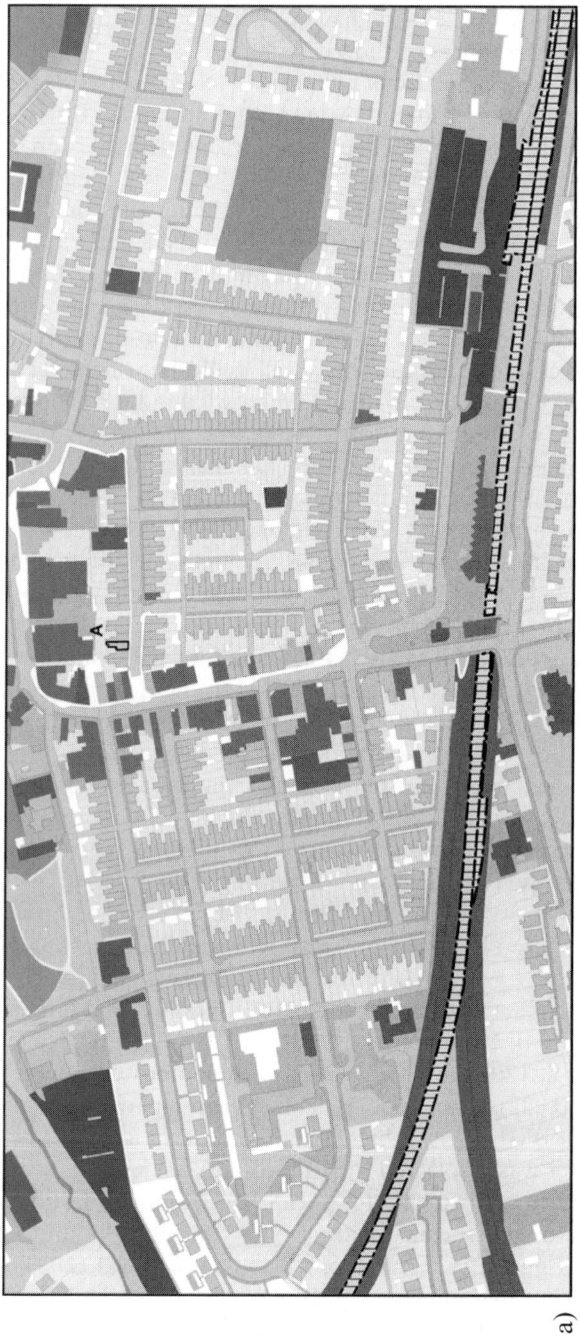

a)

b)

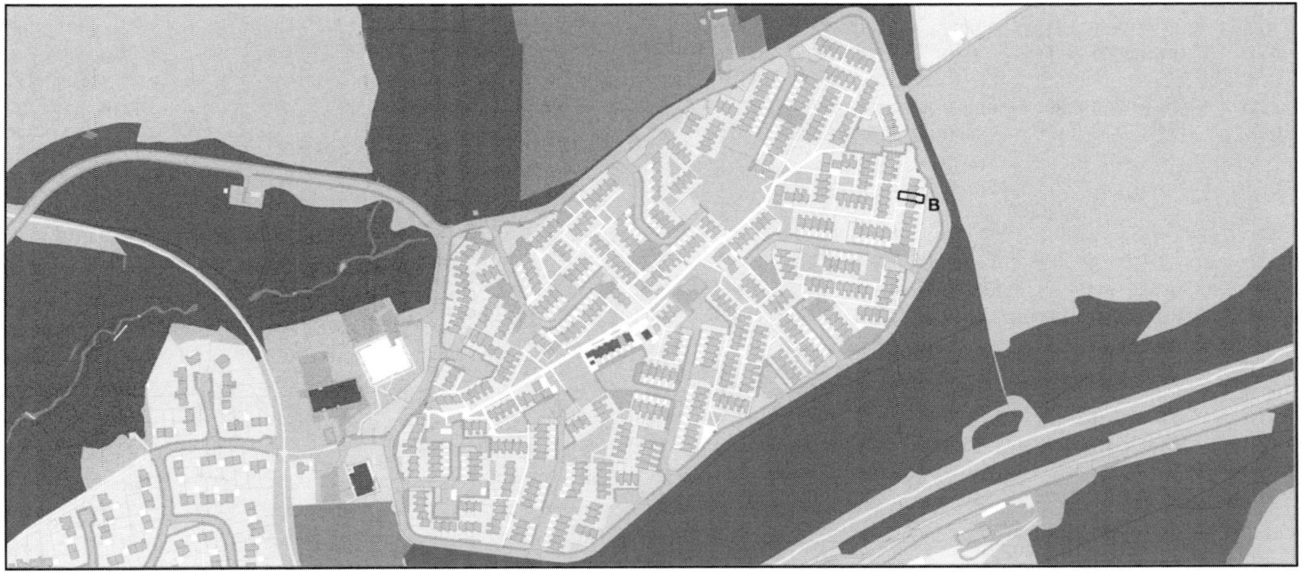

Source: Derived from UK Ordnance Survey supplied Topographic Layer and Address Layer 2.

Figure 7.2 Contrasting neighbourhood built environments of Caerphilly
a) Dwelling A located in an urban neighbourhood characterized by high density and mix in the town centre
b) Dwelling B located in a rural neighbourhood with a residential outlook located at the town periphery with adjoining agricultural land

Table 7.3 *Results of three-level mixed effects linear regression with individual- and LSOA-level random effects for BMI in 684 older men in 35 LSOAs*

Variable	Model 0		Model 1		Model 2		Model 3	
	β_0 (95% CI)	p	β_1 (95% CI)	p	β_2 (95% CI)	p	β_3 (95% CI)	p
FIXED EFFECTS								
Intercept	26.897 (26.56, 27.23)	<0.001	28.751 (26.72, 30.79)	<0.001	28.800 (24.38, 33.23)	<0.001	28.172 (24.20, 32.15)	<0.001
Land use morphometrics:								
Land use mix (z-score)			0.387 (0.01, 0.76)	0.044	0.358 (−0.01, 0.72)	0.05	0.348 (0.02, 0.68)	0.038
Bus stop density			0.052 (−0.02, 0.12)	0.14	0.049 (−0.02, 0.12)	0.15	0.047 (−0.02, 0.12)	0.18
Retail density			−0.033 (−0.06, −0.07)	0.014	−0.036 (−0.06, −0.01)	0.006	−0.033 (−0.06, −0.08)	0.010
Church density			−0.315 (−0.55, −0.08)	0.009	−0.337 (−0.58, −0.09)	0.007	−0.356 (−0.57, −0.14)	0.001
Community service density			0.079 (−0.03, 0.19)	0.15	0.088 (−0.02, 0.20)	0.12	0.088 (−0.01, 0.19)	0.09
Recreation and leisure density			−0.086 (−0.15, −0.02)	0.007	−0.083 (−0.15, −0.02)	0.012	−0.083 (−0.14, −0.02)	0.009
Destination accessibility: Network distance to:								
Green space								
50–75% vs 0–50%			−0.095 (−0.74, 0.55)	0.77	−0.049 (−0.68, 0.58)	0.88	0.085 (−0.57, 0.74)	0.80
75–100% vs 0–50%			−0.347 (−1.13, 0.44)	0.39	−0.316 (−1.08, 0.49)	0.42	−0.108 (−0.82, 0.61)	0.77
Sports facility:								
50–75 % vs 0–50%			−0.315 (−0.94, −0.31)	0.33	−0.290 (−0.86, 0.28)	0.32	−0.348 (−0.83, 0.14)	0.16
75–100 % vs 0–50%			−0.592 (−1.32, 0.14)	0.11	−0.683 (−1.40, 0.03)	0.06	−0.815 (−1.45, −0.18)	0.012

Topological accessibility of streets (z-score):						
Connectivity	0.240 (−0.13, 0.61)	0.20	0.238 (−0.12, 0.59)	0.19	0.144 (−0.20, 0.49)	0.41
Betweenness RNm	0.329 (−0.17, 0.83)	0.20	0.273 (−0.21, 0.76)	0.27	0.229 (−0.29, 0.75)	0.38
Betweenness R3000 m	−1.197 (−1.77, −0.62)	<0.001	−1.132 (−1.73, −0.53)	<0.001	−1.113 (−1.73, −0.49)	<0.001
Choice R1200 m	0.849 (0.12, 1.58)	0.022	0.864 (0.15, 1.58)	0.018	0.857 (0.19, 1.53)	0.012
Topography:						
Standard deviation in slope	−0.327 (−0.60, −0.05)	0.019	−0.324 (−0.60, −0.05)	0.019	−0.325 (−0.60, −0.05)	0.021
Dwelling-level morphometrics:						
Dwelling-centred density	0.017 (−0.03, 0.06)	0.45	0.019 (−0.03, 0.06)	−0.41	0.021 (−0.02, −0.06)	0.32
Detached vs semi-detached	−0.147 (−0.73, 0.44)	0.62	−0.121 (−0.74, 0.50)	0.70	0.096 (−0.49, 0.69)	0.75
Terraced vs semi-detached	−0.024 (−0.80, 0.75)	0.95	0.0002 (−0.75, 0.75)	1.00	0.027 (−0.67, 0.72)	0.94
Apartment vs semi-detached	−0.648 (−1.75, 0.46)	0.25	−0.528 (−1.61, 0.56)	0.34	−0.653 (−1.81, 0.51)	0.27
Individual confounders:						
Age and lifestyle:						
Age			−0.006 (−0.062, 0.050)	0.84	−0.007 (−0.056, 0.041)	0.77
Alcohol consumption			0.006 (0.001, 0.012)	0.021	0.007 (0.001, 0.012)	0.015
Smoking status (ex- vs non-smoker)			−0.088 (−0.395, 0.218)	0.57	−0.114 (−0.408, 0.181)	0.45

Table 7.3 (continued)

Variable	Model 0		Model 1		Model 2		Model 3	
	β_0 (95% CI)	p	β_1 (95% CI)	p	β_2 (95% CI)	p	β_3 (95% CI)	p
Smoking status (current vs non-smoker)					−0.810 (−1.188, −0.432)	<0.001	−0.797 (−1.148, −0.447)	<0.001
Socio-demographic factors:								
Marital status:								
Single vs married					−0.772 (−1.695, 0.150)	0.10	−1.060 (−2.000, −0.120)	0.027
Widowed/separated vs married					−0.124 (−1.158, 0.909)	0.81	−0.206 (−1.052, 0.640)	0.63
Social class:								
Manual vs non-manual					0.579 (0.031, 1.126)	0.038	0.629 (0.154, 1.105)	0.009
Educational qualifications:[a]								
None/apprentice vs school certificates					0.331 (−0.178, 0.839)	0.20	0.293 (−0.227, 0.813)	0.27
None/ apprenticeship vs degree					0.567 (−0.185, 1.319)	0.14	0.385 (−0.505, 1.274)	0.40
Vascular morbidities:								
Myocardial infarction (yes vs no)							−0.160 (−0.717, 0.396)	0.57
Angina (yes vs no)							0.580 (−0.211, 1.372)	0.15

High blood pressure (yes vs no)							1.113 (0.665, 1.562)	<0.001
High cholesterol (yes vs no)							−0.526 (−1.161, 0.110)	0.11
Diabetes (yes vs no)							1.688 (0.848, 2.529)	<0.001
Mini-stroke (yes vs no)							−0.052 (−0.991, 0.887)	0.91
Time point:								
Phase IV vs Phase III	0.252 (0.172, 0.333)	<0.001	0.252 (0.172, 0.333)	<0.001	0.269 (0.046, 0.491)	0.018	0.276 (0.078, 0.475)	0.006
Phase V vs Phase III	0.922 (0.722, 1.122)	<0.001	0.922 (0.722, 1.122)	<0.001	0.975 (0.332, 1.618)	0.003	0.999 (0.441, 1.557)	<0.001
Between-occasion variance (SE):	1.971 (0.352)	–	1.971 (0.352)	–	1.958 (0.351)	–	1.958 (0.351)	–
RANDOM EFFECTS								
Between-individual variance (SE)	11.201 (0.807)	–	10.964 (0.760)	–	10.600 (0.739)	–	9.956 (0.711)	–
Between-LSOA variance (SE)	0.114 (0.099)	–	<0.001 (0.000)	–	<0.001 (0.000)	–	<0.001 (0.000)	–
MODEL FIT STATISTIC								
−2×log likelihood	9200.037	–	9180.476	–	9149.967	–	9109.145	–

Notes:
[a] Education is modelled as: 1: none/apprenticeship; 2: school certificate/higher technical certificate; and 3: professional qualification/degree/higher degree.
Model 0: Unconditional null model.
Model 1: Model with only built environment variables (with no level-specific predictors).
Model 2: Model with built environment variables adjusted for age, socio-economic and lifestyle factors.
Model 3: Model with built environment variables adjusted for age, socio-economic and lifestyle factors, as well as prevalence of vascular morbidities.

vascular morbidities in model 3 found BMI to be significantly associated with high blood pressure ($\beta_3 = 1.113$, $p < 0.001$) and diabetes ($\beta_3 = 1.688$, $p < 0.001$). These associations had a mild impact on associations of BMI with the built environment, with the exception that BMI was now found to be associated with network distance to a sports facility ($\beta_3 = -0.815$, $p = 0.012$).

7.5 DISCUSSION

In a representative population sample of older men, a range of built environment morphometrics have been shown in this study to be associated with a change in BMI over 12 years. This is the first long-term longitudinal evidence relating the built environment to a change in obesity in older people. The built environment factors identified included the walkability of street segments and the street gradient variability.

7.5.1 Strengths and Limitations

Strengths of the present study include its longitudinal design, innovative assessment of diverse facets of the built environment captured through a set of objectively measured robust morphometrics, and the use of a multi-level analysis which enables the assessment of area, individual and chronologically dependent variances. The objective of the study was to analyse the role of sustained exposure to a set of persistent built environmental factors that could plausibly influence weight outcomes with the ageing process, and a longitudinal design diminished the possibility of selection bias, which commonly plagues cross-sectional studies. Selective migrations by the CaPS residents to neighbourhoods that promote physical activity within the study area may have been a possibility. Longitudinal design, encompassing a period of 12 years, and the extensive adjustments for confounding at multiple levels diluted the problem of migration/reverse causality in respect of the confounding factors. Space syntax modelling enabled the inclusion of street movement potential and walkability in addition to measures of mix, amenity density and network proximity. This addition is of particular importance in studies of older adults, in whom physical capacity declines with age. A range of covariates were examined in the analysis to reduce the likelihood of confounding and reverse causation.

Limitations include the assumption that environment conditions had changed little over the study period. We regard this as a relatively unimportant potential source of error, however, because of the stability of built environmental parameters over this period of time. Although we acknowledge that several of the built environmental parameters may have changed slightly over this period, data from the Caerphilly County Borough Council indicate that most of the LSOAs had been well settled and relatively stabilized over the three phases of the study, in terms both of land uses and of street network characteristics. Recently, longitudinal studies with similar designs have been reported (F. Li, Harmer, Cardinal, Bosworth et al., 2009; Jerrett et al., 2010; Wolch et al., 2011). Nevertheless, an improvement for future studies would be to overcome the bottleneck of detailed historic land use data sets and look at the effects of changes in built environment parameters over time.

Although we considered a street network buffer of 1 kilometre to represent the local home range for this age group, there is no standard definition of local home range. Nagel et al. (2008) have considered buffers of 0.25 and 0.5 mile radius; F. Li, Fisher, Brownson et al. (2005) employed 0.5 mile buffers; Berke, Koepsell et al. (2007) used circular buffers of 100, 500 and 1000 metres; W.C. King et al. (2005) used 1500 metre network buffers; and F. Li et al. (2008) took census-defined spatial aggregates as proxies for neighbourhoods. The use of a 1 kilometre network buffer in our study was a compromise which took account of the change in age of the cohort during the period of the study.

Although we adjusted for a range of potential confounders, we cannot exclude the possibility of some residual confounding. That the study is limited to men is a legacy of its initial focus on heart disease. Nevertheless, these finding are likely to be indicative of associations that might be found in older women.

That a set of built environment morphometrics related to neighbourhood walkability remained significant subsequent to individual-level adjustments is indicative of a physical-activity-related mechanism involved in obesity causation. Nonetheless, specific temporal hierarchies and causal pathways of the longitudinal effect of the built environment in conjunction with individual-level risk factors still remain to be identified. One of the major methodological constraints in the demonstration of such a causal link in built environment research arises on account of the fact that many of the individual-level socio-economic and obesity risk factors may in reality play a mediatory role rather than being confounders of built environment effects. Future study designs should attempt to capture cross-level interactions that may moderate or exacerbate the effects of neighbourhood accessibility (Diez Roux, 2002, 2004a; F. Li, Fisher, Bauman et al., 2005). The causal processes through which the built environmental factors affect health can be drawn from evidence of long-term public health and planning interventions and natural experiments such as the longitudinal health effects of large-scale regeneration programmes as well as retrofitting the built environment at community and city levels.

7.5.2 Interpretation

The results of the study reported in this chapter are consistent with the hypothesis that the built environment affects adiposity in later life. Several built environment morphometrics considered to be associated with walkability and physical activity were significantly related to individual-level variations in BMI. After controlling for individual-level lifestyle factors, socio-demographic confounders and morbidities, higher densities of retail land use, churches and recreation and leisure facilities in the vicinity were more likely to lower BMI. The negative association between retail use and BMI levels is consistent with the principles of walkability, as retailing acts as an attractor in the built environment, generating more movement (Frank et al., 2003). Similar results have been reported by Norman et al. (2006) and Sallis, Bowles et al. (2009). Our study not only corroborates these previous findings, but also provides a more detailed analysis of the built environment features that co-vary with BMI.

In the case of the density of recreational and leisure facilities, the results were consistent with previous findings that BMI is inversely associated with accessibility to such facilities (Giles-Corti et al., 2003) and that physical activity is positively associated with the density of recreational facilities (Norman et al., 2006; Diez Roux et al., 2007). The density of churches in the defined buffer was included in the model on the assumption that churches have a positive effect upon social capital as well as perceptions of neighbourhood satisfaction. They may also capture aspects of land use pattern centrality not captured in the other measures (it is well known that historical churches form the centres of very long-lived clusters of human activity in Europe).

That higher levels of land use mix were associated with increased levels of BMI appears contrary to the general understanding that a heterogeneous neighbourhood acts as a generator of physical activity leading to reduced BMI (Saelens, Sallis, Black et al., 2003; Frank et al., 2004; F. Li et al., 2008). However, B.B. Brown et al. (2009) concluded that the presence of walkable destinations may be more important in influencing healthy weight outcomes than land use mix per se, while Rutt and Coleman (2005) and Forsyth et al. (2008) report findings similar to ours, with increasing land use mix associated with higher levels of BMI and obesity. Our findings may be explained by the underlying negative association between sense of community and land use mix reported in certain Australian studies (Wood et al., 2008, 2010). This is more relevant given that Caerphilly is a semi-urban commuting town characterized by a fairly low mix and dwelling density.

Accessibility to green space and health care facility destinations measured by network distance exhibited no significant association with BMI levels. Network distance to sports facilities was significant only with full adjustment (model 3). However, the association was counter-intuitive: subjects living at locations in the top 25 percentile of network distance had significantly lower BMI compared to those in the bottom 50 percentile. These findings contradict the general expectation that a non-obesogenic neighbourhood should have a dense network of sports and recreational facilities in its vicinity. In another study, Jilcott et al. (2007) could not establish any significant relationship between network distance to physical activity resource and levels of activity among low-income middle-aged women. The classification of sports facility in our study included fitness club, club house, golf, golf range, leisure centre, snooker, stables, tennis courts, playing field, sports pavilion, and sports viewing facilities. The direction of observed association may be a manifestation of the fact that the facilities are localized at specific parts of the town and the usage of a particular type of facility is governed primarily by the intrinsic affinity of an individual towards a particular type of sports facility rather than by the network proximity factor. In other words, we hypothesize that older men, at least, are relatively insensitive to distance to local facilities, and that they include recreation in their time budgets and walk to their chosen facility regardless of distance (clearly within a maximum walking time or distance). The result is that men living at greater distances tend, *ceteris paribus*, to have a lower BMI. This is a controversial finding particularly worthy of further testing.

Space syntax metrics have long been used to capture configuration and design parameters of urban form (Kashef, 2011). In this study we apply them to understanding health outcomes. Higher local-scale betweenness was associated with poorer weight outcomes, while higher city-scale route choice was associated with improved weight outcomes. Route betweenness at a local scale of 1200 metres may act as proxy for pedestrian movement and street-level crowding. Even though very well connected, streets with high pedestrian density may be associated with a feeling of lack of safety and possibly uncleanliness associated with high pedestrian flows. Furthermore, high local betweenness is associated with a highly gridded street pattern with high intersection density, which in turn may act as a potential inhibitor of strolling for older people on account of the traffic risk at the street crossings. On the other hand, betweenness at a city-scale radius of 3000 metres captures overall city-level accessibility to various attractive destinations. This may mean that elderly men living in such locations perceive a wider range of accessible destinations than those in other locations and are more likely to take walks as a result. A cross-sectional study conducted in the city of Glasgow, United Kingdom could not establish any evidence of street network connectivity, body mass index and obesity (Ball et al., 2012). The application of space syntax modelling allows the measurement of street network configuration in greater detail. In addition to the conventional connectivity measures, space syntax models can capture the simulated (implied) counts of movement potential through street segments, thus providing a more realistic prediction of individual activity behaviour.

With respect to topography, higher slope variability was associated with improved weight outcomes, indicating that individuals indulging in walks expend more calories in an uneven topography. Two previous studies have considered the impact of slope on BMI (Rutt and Coleman, 2005) and walkability (C. Lee and Moudon, 2006a), but the present one is the first study to report a significant association, possibly because of the greater slope variance in the study area.

7.6 CONCLUSIONS

There is an urgent need to trace the nature of relationships between BMI and the built environment over the life course in order to guide effective intervention strategies for controlling obesity and related morbidities. This study provides the evidence for the hypothesis that, in older persons, the built environment can contribute to better weight outcomes. The detailed analysis of the built environment used in this study enabled a finer granularity of built environment classification than has been previously possible in population-based studies. This highlights the necessity for large-scale population studies in order to be able to influence urban design in a way that optimizes the built environment for the community as a whole. Of particular interest is identifying the impact of the built environment on specific physical activities for particular age groups, allowing the integration of urban planning and public health initiatives.

8. Does accessibility to health-promoting services affect self-perceived health and HADS anxiety and depression? Findings from a multi-level analysis of older men in Caerphilly

8.1 INTRODUCTION

As we have demonstrated in the previous chapters of this book, in the recent discourses on *place effects on health* several studies have established the facilitative role of accessibility in urban space in influencing individual behaviour and health (J. Pearce et al., 2006; Bernard et al., 2007). In one of the earliest studies of the impact of physical accessibility on individual behaviour, Horton and Reynolds (1971) conceptualized the notion of *action spaces* and stressed that the formation of individual action space is governed by socio-economic factors, travel preferences, home locations, cognitive image of the urban environment, duration of residence at a specific area, and the objective spatial configuration of the micro-level activity spaces and city as a whole, that is, a locus of all urban destinations perceived and visited by an individual as a result of day-to-day activities. In another study of four neighbourhoods of Glasgow differing in socio-economic profile, Macintyre et al. (2002) proposed that one of the key reasons for health inequalities originates as a result of differential accessibility to neighbourhood opportunity structures, expressed in terms of access to material and infrastructural resources, which included: (1) physical attributes of the environment to which residents of the area are exposed, such as quality of air, drinking water and so on; (2) the presence of health-promoting domestic and occupational environments; and (3) publicly or privately provided services to support daily lives. More recently, Bernard et al. (2007) defined the neighbourhood sociologically in terms of both availability of and access to health-relevant resources, while neighbourhood opportunity space emerges in a way that is described using

Giddens's structuration theory (1984). The neighbourhood opportunity space has been conceived by Bernard as an environment for accessing resources and emerges as a result of reciprocal interactions between existing social structure and individual residents who act as agents. On the one hand, individual residents act as agents whose diurnal activities produce discernible social structures, while these social structures provide opportunities as well as enforce constraints upon individuals' activity behaviour. According to this model, access to resources in a neighbourhood physical and social environment is governed by four sets of rules encompassing five mutually interactive domains, which in turn influence individual health and health inequalities. The *physical domain* constitutes the physical environment and governs the proximity to both positive and negative resources of the built and natural environment. The social environment is constituted by: the *economic domain*, which governs price; the *institutional domain*, which regulates entitlement to resources; and the *local sociability domain* and *community organization domain*, which are governed by bonds of informal reciprocity and valued relationships formed between individuals and communities.

As reviewed in Chapter 4 and 5, a series of empirical studies assessing the effects of accessibility to health-promoting or -inhibiting neighbourhood resources on health have generally tended to parameterize accessibility in terms of indices of density, diversity, destination proximity and street-level connectivity (C. Lee and Moudon, 2006a; Diez Roux et al., 2007; Leslie et al., 2007; F. Li et al., 2008). In older adults, the health benefits of improved accessibility to health-defining neighbourhood resources have been known to originate on account of enhanced levels of mobility and physical activity (Strawbridge et al., 2002; Weuve et al., 2004; Berke, Gottlieb et al., 2007; Berke, Koepsell et al., 2007), as well as the corresponding enhanced degrees of participation in social and productive activities (Bassuk et al., 1999; F. Baum et al., 2000; F. Baum and Palmer, 2002; Pollack and von dem Knesebeck, 2004; Glass, De Leon et al., 2006; Richard et al., 2009).

In Chapter 5, we noted that the process of urbanization entails a reconfiguration of unstructured, or primitively structured, *space* into *urban places* characterized by discrete interconnected and contested subspaces, wherein people reside and conduct their daily activities. The urban built environment has a specific design and configuration, each element being characterized by its inherent identity, continuity and enclosure, quality of public realm, ease of movement, legibility, adaptability and diversity (CABE, 2000). The urban places that emerge by design or evolution can be thought of as comprising *linear subspaces* in the form of street segments through which people move, *convex spaces* consisting of squares and public spaces through which they interact, and the dynamic visual field through which they perceive their surroundings (Hillier and Hanson, 1984; Hillier et al., 1993; Hillier, 1996). In the present study we propose that the spatial built environment may be hypothesized as an activity plane – a collection of configured health-promoting community resources and opportunity structures with which an individual resident associates information and subjective utility. In response to this information and the values attached, the individual's activity behaviour is influenced. In other words, the distribution of health-promoting community resources and opportunity structures produces a differential social, economic and accessibility gradient between individuals, resulting in differential behavioural patterns in terms of levels of physical activity, walking, social interactions, and so on. The first objective of the present study is to examine the effects of a broad set of built environmental factors on general and psychological health in older adults. Secondly, any systematic study of the effects of attributes of the built environment on health should entail a detailed examination of the effects of differential accessibility at multiple spatial scales. To the present knowledge of the author, there is no published feasible analytical methodology to capture the chronological and simultaneous impacts of a wide range of urban morphological health correlates at multiple spatial scales. In most studies, built environment attributes are measured for census-defined spatial units such as wards, counties and output areas and, consequently, underestimate the effects of detailed spatial variations in services and hence the effects of differential accessibility of an individual's dwelling with respect to multiple service and facility catchments at multiple spatial scales. The present study thus aimed to assess the potential health effects of differential accessibility at multiple spatial scales. The manner in which neighbourhood-level deprivation may potentially moderate the association between built environment factors and health outcomes is also investigated. With this objective in mind, the present chapter measures both service accessibility and street network accessibility at two specific network catchment radii of 0.5 and 1.0 mile.

8.2 METHODS

8.2.1 Study Design

The Caerphilly Prospective Study (CaPS) has been following up on the health of a population-based male cohort in the Welsh assembly constituency of Caerphilly, South Wales for the past 25 years. Further details of the CaPS cohort can be found in Chapter 5. The present analysis is based on the most recent, that is, the fifth, phase of examination of the CaPS study, which occurred between September 2002 and June 2004. This consisted of two pre-clinic questionnaires sent out to the 1225 men remaining in the study and aged 65–84 years, subsequently followed up at an appointment which also included extensive clinical examinations.

8.2.2 Health Measures and Individual-Level Covariates

Self-reported measures of health consisted of perceived general health, long-standing disability and HADS anxiety and depression. Respondents were asked to rate their health status on a five-point scale, comprising categories of 'excellent', 'good', 'fair', 'poor' and 'very poor'. The respondents were asked if they suffered from any long-standing illness or disability. The symptoms of anxiety and depression were assessed with the help of the Hospital Anxiety and Depression Scale (HADS), a 14-item self-administered standard psychological instrument (Zigmond and Snaith, 1983). The HADS comprises seven anxiety (HADS-A) and seven depression (HADS-D) component items, each of which is rated on a four-point scale and summed up to form the respective sub-scales (as indicated in Appendix 2). The scores can range from 0 to 21, with higher scores indicative of more severe psychological disorder. Individual-level socio-demographic covariates consisted of age, marital status, social class and educational attainment.

8.2.3 Assessment of the Built Environment

The spatial Design Network Analysis for Urban Health (sDNA-UH) model described in detail in Chapter 5 acted as a source of a set of robust variables of built environment configurations and individual-level covariates. With an objective to assess the impact of accessibility at varying spatial scales, in the present experiment the built environment measures from sDNA-UH were measured within 0.5 mile and 1 mile street network catchments around an individual respondent's dwelling unit. Dwelling-level configurations consisted of dwelling-centred density, plot exposure and dwelling type. Land use configurations were expressed in terms of density of health-defining services. The densities of public transit (bus stops), retail, community services, recreation and leisure, and business and offices were calculated as the number of units divided by the total area within 0.5 mile and 1 mile street network buffers respectively.

With an objective to incorporate the effects of varying degrees of street network accessibility to health-specific destinations, the network distances to the nearest green space, facility for physical activity and sports, health care facility, food takeaway shop and allotment were included in the analyses.

To assess the effects of multi-scalar street network configuration and accessibility upon health outcomes, the spatial Design Network Analysis (sDNA) software described in Chapter 5 was employed. This software became available at a later stage of writing this book, and it was therefore thought appropriate to test it in this chapter, both to add to the novelty of the book and to explore the method's performance in this kind of application. The OSM ITN Layer of Caerphilly was subjected to network analysis in the sDNA software. As mentioned in Chapter 5, sDNA uses the OSM ITN network links as the fundamental unit of computation in the graphical analyses, thereby improving upon the reliability of the measurements as a result of having an improved and industry-standard underlying data structure. Minimum data preparation and a faster algorithm enable faster processing of large-scale urban networks (http://www.cardiff.ac.uk/sdna). In the present study, three indices of street network accessibility, namely betweenness, hull area and junction connectivity, were modelled within catchments of 0.5 and 1.0 mile. Betweenness measures the through-movement potential, hull area measures the network area encompassing all the constituent origin–destination links, and junction connectivity is synonymous with the number of street intersections within a defined catchment.

The composite score of the Welsh Index of Multiple Deprivation (WIMD) for 2005, measured at the level of lower super output areas (LSOAs), was employed as a proxy for LSOA-level deprivation.

8.2.4 Statistical Methods

Perceived general health was modelled as a two-level factor. The five-point scale was dichotomized in our analyses into 'fair/poor/very poor' versus 'excellent/good'. Long-standing illness/disability was modelled as a two-level factor (presence versus absence). The prevalence of anxiety and depression was also modelled as a two-level factor (case versus non-case) using the cut-point of 8 or more, which has been confirmed by previously conducted cohort studies in the UK (Gale et al., 2011).

The individual-level covariates of age (years) were employed as a continuous variable. Social class was expressed in terms of six groups following the Registrar General's occupational classification (Office of Population Censuses and Surveys (OPCS), 1980) and thereafter collapsed into a three-level factor (I/II/III-non-manual, III-manual, IV/V). Marital status was modelled as a three-level factor (married, single, widowed/divorced/separated). Educational attainment was also modelled as a three-level factor (none/apprenticeship, school certificate/higher technical certificate, professional qualification/degree/higher degree).

Multicollinearity between the built environment variables was checked with the *collin* command for logistic regression in Stata, as well as through prior assessment of variance inflation factors (VIFs) before their incorporation into the multi-level modelling framework. sDNA-measured betweenness scores were log-transformed using the zero-skewness log transform option in Stata. The area-level variable of WIMD was converted into quartiles, with the first quartile (corresponding to least deprived LSOAs) taken as the reference category.

The presence of hierarchically clustered data with individuals nested within census-defined LSOAs enabled the assessment of the impact of built environment configuration upon general and psychological health through a series of multi-level logistic regression models. Two-level logistic mixed effects models with LSOA-level random effects were fitted on the health indicators of perceived general health, long-standing disability, anxiety and depression. The analysis comprised four models. Model 1 examined the associations of psychological distress with the built environment variables measured within a 0.5 mile network buffer. Model 2 examined the association of psychological distress with the built environment variables measured within a 0.5 mile network buffer subsequent to adjustments for area-level deprivation. Model 3 examined the association of psychological distress with the built environment variables measured within a 1.0 mile network buffer. Model 4 considered the further effects of adjustments for area-level deprivation. Fixed effects were assessed through the odds ratio, 95 per cent credible intervals and the level of statistical significance (α) at p, while model fit was expressed in terms of the Bayesian deviance information criterion. Statistical analyses were performed with the user-written *runmlwin* command within Stata 11.2 (Leckie and Charlton, 2011). The command fits multi-level models from within the MLwiN v.2.25 package using the Markov Chain Monte Carlo (MCMC) simulation (W.J. Brown, 2012).

8.3 RESULTS

For the 1127 men who responded to the latest follow-up of CaPS, completed data across all the variables were available for 807 men in the analysis of perceived general health and long-standing illness or disability. The analysis of HADS was possible for 677 men after excluding missing responses on each of the model variables. These men were distributed across 33 census-defined LSOAs of Caerphilly assembly constituency.

The prevalence rate of diminished perceived general health was 47.21 per cent, while 64.06 per cent reported a long-standing illness or disability. The prevalence rates of anxiety (HADS-A $\geq$ 8) and depression (HADS-D $\geq$ 8) were 13.15 per cent and 8.86 per cent respectively. The descriptive statistics of the representative sample including the built environment variables incorporated in the analysis are presented in Table 8.1.

The results of two-level mixed effects models for perceived general health and long-standing illness/disability are shown in Table 8.2. Among the dwelling-level variables, a higher dwelling-centred density was consistently associated with better health in the analyses within 0.5 and 1.0 mile catchments ($OR_{0.5mi} = 0.956$, $p = 0.001$ and $OR_{1.0mi} = 0.962$, $p = 0.006$ for perceived general health and $OR_{0.5mi} = 0.973$, $p = 0.030$ and $OR_{1.0mi} = 0.977$, $p = 0.058$ for long-standing illncss/disability). Residents of flats (apartments) had a higher propensity to report poor health as compared to those living in detached dwellings ($OR_{0.5mi} = 2.198$, $p = 0.016$ and $OR_{1.0mi} = 2.214$, $p = 0.019$ for perceived general health and $OR_{0.5mi} = 1.737$, $p = 0.081$ for long-standing illness/disability). However, in the analysis that used a 1.0 mile buffer, this was no longer significant in the case of long-standing illness/disability. None of the variables of destination accessibility exhibited significant association ($p < 0.05$) with either perceived general health or long-standing illness/disability. However, there was a mild association between proximity to green space and propensity to report poor perceived health ($OR_{0.5mi} = 0.999$, $p = 0.097$ and $OR_{1.0mi} = 0.999$, $p = 0.059$ for perceived general health). Among the variables of service density, the density of community services was beneficially associated with long-standing illness/disability only in the analysis using a 0.5 mile radius ($OR_{0.5mi} = 0.991$, $p = 0.047$) in model 1. However, adjusting for neighbourhood-level deprivation in the model diluted the level of significance ($OR_{0.5mi} = 0.992$, $p = 0.069$) in model 2. The density of recreation and leisure was negatively associated with perceived general health only in the analysis using a 1.0 mile radius ($OR_{1.0mi} = 1.026$, $p = 0.041$) in model 3; however, it was no longer significant subsequent to the adjustment for neighbourhood-level deprivation. In the case of long-standing illness/disability, a similar trend of negative associations was observed in models without neighbourhood-level deprivation at both 0.5 and 1.0 mile buffer radii ($OR_{0.5mi} = 1.008$, $p = 0.065$ in model 1 and $OR_{1.0mi} = 1.028$, $p = 0.023$ in model 3 respectively). Among the variables for street network accessibility, higher levels of betweenness at both 0.5 and 1.0 mile catchment radii were beneficially associated with perceived general health ($OR_{0.5mi} = 0.795$, $p = 0.007$ in model 2 and $OR_{1.0mi} = 0.785$, $p < 0.001$ in model 4 respectively). The network hull area was mildly associated with perceived general health only after adjustments for area-level

Table 8.1 Descriptive statistics of variables employed in the mixed effects analysis

Variable name	Mean (SD) or frequency (%)	Range
Health measures:		
Perceived general health, n (%) (N=807):		
Excellent	39 (4.8%)	
Good	387 (48.0%)	
Fair	301 (37.3%)	
Poor	68 (8.4%)	
Very poor	12 (1.5%)	
Long-standing illness/disability, n (%) (N=807):		
No case	290 (35.9%)	
Case	517 (64.0%)	
HADS, mean (SD) (N=677):		
HADS – Anxiety	3.67 (3.57)	0–19
HADS – Depression	3.08 (2.86)	0–15
Socio-demographics:		
Age, mean (SD)	73.3 (4.1)	65.2–83.3
Marital status, n (%):		
Married	728 (90.2%)	
Single	30 (3.7%)	
Separated/divorced/widowed	49 (6.1%)	
Social class, n (%):		
I, II, III-non-manual	293 (36.3%)	
III-manual	395 (48.9%)	
IV, V	119 (14.7%)	
Educational attainment, n (%):		
None/apprenticeship	501 (62.1%)	
School certificate	213 (26.4%)	
Degree	93 (11.5%)	
Built environment variables:		
Dwelling-level variables:		
Dwelling-centred density, mean (SD)	14.3 (6.8)	1–48
Plot exposure, n (%):		
None	88 (10.9%)	
One building face	560 (69.4%)	
More than one building face	159 (19.7%)	
Dwelling type, n (%):		
Detached	173 (21.4%)	
Semi-detached	352 (43.6%)	
Terraced	220 (27.3%)	
Flat	62 (7.7%)	

Table 8.1 (continued)

Variable name	Mean (SD) or frequency (%)	Range
Network distance to nearest services, mean (SD):		
Green space	528.1 (307.6)	1.7–1654.1
Sports facility	612.4 (318.6)	6.9–1652.2
Health care facility	560.4 (296.4)	2.8–1584
Takeaway	1353.8 (1212.2)	34.2–5559.5
Allotment	627.4 (391.4)	4.5–1968.9
Service density, mean (SD):		
Bus stops 0.5 mile	68.6 (20.9)	14.6–138.5
Bus stops 1.0 mile	55.6 (13.5)	20.4–85.8
Retail 0.5 mile	74.3 (89.6)	0–461.1
Retail 1.0 mile	60.2 (43.6)	9.2–186
Community services 0.5 mile	39.5 (31.1)	0–150.1
Community services 1.0 mile	31.6 (14.5)	5.6–74.2
Recreation and leisure facilities 0.5 mile	35.9 (18.1)	0–96
Recreation and leisure facilities 1.0 mile	29.2 (8.5)	6.4–74
Business and offices 0.5 mile	79 (94.1)	0–430.5
Business and offices 1.0 mile	74.5 (55.6)	2.3–308.2
Topological accessibility of streets, mean (SD):		
Betweenness R0.5 mile	4.81E+6 (5.82E+6)	2.27E+4–3.29E+7
Betweenness R1.0 mile	3.19E+7 (5.10E+7)	1.59E+5–2.96E+8
Hull area R0.5 mile	1.9 (2.2)	0.0–127
Hull area R1.0 mile	1.3 (0.3)	0.3–2.0
Junction connectivity R0.5 mile	74.8 (36.3)	5.0–192.0
Junction connectivity R1.0 mile	250.3 (113.9)	31.0–585.0
LSOA level deprivation, mean (SD):		
WIMD scores†	23.2 (13.5)	5.2–67.1
Q1 (most affluent)	9.1 (1.7)	5.1–11.3
Q2	17.3 (2.5)	11.9–19.5
Q3	26.8 (5.0)	20.1–34.2
Q4 (most deprived)	42.9 (7.7)	34.4–67.1

Note: † Q: Quartile (Q1, Q2, Q3 and Q4 represent the lower, lower-middle, upper-middle and upper quartiles respectively).

deprivation. The analysis at 0.5 mile indicated that the association was beneficial ($OR_{0.5mi} = 0.925$, $p = 0.08$ in model 2), while at a scale of 1.0 mile the association was negative ($OR_{1.0mi} = 1.966$, $p = 0.09$ in model 4). However, neither betweenness nor hull area was significantly associated with long-standing illness/disability. The effects of junction connectivity

Table 8.2 Results of two-level mixed effects models for perceived general health and long-standing illness/disability in 807 older men across 33 LSOAs

Predictors	Perceived general health				Long-standing illness/disability			
	0.5 mile network buffer		1.0 mile network buffer		0.5 mile network buffer		1.0 mile network buffer	
	Model 1*	Model 2**	Model 3***	Model 4****	Model 1*	Model 2**	Model 3***	Model 4****
	OR (95% Cred.I), p	OR (95% Cred.I), p	OR (95% Cred.I), p	OR (95% Cred.I), p	OR (95% Cred.I), p	OR (95% Cred.I), p	OR (95% Cred.I), p	OR (95% Cred.I), p
Dwelling-level variables:								
Dwelling-centred density	0.956 (0.928, 0.985), p=0.001	0.956 (0.927, 0.984), p=0.001	0.963 (0.934, 0.992), p=0.007	0.962 (0.934, 0.992), p=0.006	0.974 (0.946, 0.999), p=0.04	0.973 (0.945, 0.997), p=0.030	0.977 (0.949, 1.004), p=0.054	0.977 (0.948, 1.006), p=0.058
Plot exposure (one building face vs none)	1.127 (0.686, 2.042), p=0.272	1.142 (0.714, 2.047), p=0.250	1.230 (0.752, 2.162), p=0.187	1.213 (0.737, 2.118), p=0.204	1.332 (0.830, 2.367), p=0.10	1.350 (0.831, 2.345), p=0.104	1.422 (0.872, 2.499), p=0.071	1.384 (0.858, 2.454), p=0.085
Plot exposure (more than one face vs none)	1.155 (0.658, 2.256), p=0.274	1.161 (0.678, 2.248), p=0.245	1.175 (0.681, 2.229), p=0.253	1.158 (0.672, 2.209), p=0.267	0.968 (0.564, 1.811), p=0.495	0.948 (0.547, 1.792), p=0.502	0.944 (0.545, 1.773), p=0.478	0.916 (0.535, 1.733), p=0.447
Dwelling type (semi-detached vs detached)	1.260 (0.837, 2.043), p=0.117	1.199 (0.798, 1.931), p=0.174	1.308 (0.873, 2.100), p=0.089	1.228 (0.809, 1.984), p=0.156	0.892 (0.592, 1.416), p=0.353	0.845 (0.561, 1.330), p=0.257	0.838 (0.554, 1.324), p=0.249	0.798 (0.528, 1.277), p=0.191
Dwelling type (terraced vs detached)	1.302 (0.798, 2.341), p=0.133	1.264 (0.768, 2.292), p=0.164	1.298 (0.795, 2.355), p=0.130	1.251 (0.737, 2.246), p=0.182	1.175 (0.717, 2.094), p=0.233	1.083 (0.661, 1.967), p=0.327	1.037 (0.633, 1.853), p=0.385	1.011 (0.610, 1.823), p=0.432
Dwelling type (flat vs detached)	2.303 (1.127, 5.384), p=0.011	2.198 (1.072, 5.154), p=0.016	2.280 (1.130, 5.528), p=0.012	2.214 (1.047, 5.257), p=0.019	1.972 (0.914, 4.656), p=0.04	1.737 (0.792, 4.170), p=0.081	1.641 (0.807, 3.909), p=0.082	1.530 (0.706, 3.634), p=0.138

Network distance to nearest services:								
Green space	0.998 (0.999, 1.000), p=0.078	0.999 (0 999, 1.000), p=0.097	0.999 (0.995, 0.999), p=0.041	0.999 (0.999, 1.000), p=0.059	1.000 (0.999, 1.000), p=0.163	1.000 (0.999, 1.000), p=0.291	0.999 (0.999, 1.000), p=0.038	0.999 (0.999, 1.000), p=0.147
Sports facility	1.000 (0.999, 1.000), p=0.239	0.999 (0.999, 1.000), p=0.165	1.000 (0.999, 1.000), p=0.227	1.000 (0.999, 1.000), p=0.27	1.0001 (0.999, 1.001), p=0.431	1.000 (0.999, 1.001), p=0.467	1.0001 (1.000, 1.001), p=0.333	1.000 (1.000, 1.001), p=0.370
Health care facility	1.001 (1.000, 1.001), p=0.138	1.0004 (1.000, 1.001), p=0.151	1.001 (1.000, 1.002), p=0.070	1.001 (1.000, 1.002), p=0.061	1.000 (0.999, 1.001), p=0.41	1.000 (0.999, 1.001), p=0.422	1.000 (0.999, 1.001), p=0.417	1.000 (0.999, 1.001), p=0.440
Takeaway	0.999 (0.999, 1.000), p=0.370	1.000 (1.000, 1.001), p=0.435	1.000 (1.000, 1.001), p=0.086	1.000 (1.000, 1.001), p=0.102	1.000 (1.000, 1.0002), p=0.478	1.000 (0.999, 1.000), p=0.381	1.000 (0.999, 1.000), p=0.227	1.000 (0.999, 1.000), p=0.353
Allotment	1.000 (0.999, 1.000), p=0.208	0.999 (0.999, 1.000), p=0.247	1.000 (0.999, 1.000), p=0.198	1.000 (0.999, 1.000), p=0.223	1.0003 (1.000, 1.001), p=0.158	1.0003 (1.000, 1.001), p=0.127	1.0002 (1.000, 1.001), p=0.252	1.0002 (1.000, 1.001), p=0.258
Service density:								
Density of bus stops	1.004 (0.994, 1.014), p=0.206	1.003 (0.994, 1.014), p=0.252	1.002 (0.975, 1.026), p=0.475	0.996 (0.970, 1.021), p=0.343	1.001 (0.992, 1.011), p=0.396	1.002 (0.991, 1.012), p=0.384	1.017 (0.993, 1.040), p=0.081	1.017 (0.992, 1.042), p=0.096
Density of retail	0.998 (0.993, 1.005), p=0.318	0.999 (0.992, 1.006), p=0.379	1.008 (0.989, 1.036), p=0.183	1.012 (0.990, 1.039), p=0.129	1.000 (0.994, 1.006), p=0.493	0.999 (0.992, 1.005), p=0.346	1.003 (0.983, 1.027), p=0.440	1.006 (0.984, 1.027), p=0.315
Density of community services	0.995 (0.986, 1.005), p=0.186	0.995 (0.984, 1.006), p=0.185	0.973 (0.929, 1.018), p=0.106	0.977 (0.933, 1.019), p=0.143	0.991 (0.982, 0.998), p=0.047	0.992 (0.981, 1.003), p=0.069	0.976 (0.935, 1.017), p=0.127	0.976 (0.936, 1.015), p=0.119
Density of recreation and leisure facilities	1.006 (0.995, 1.017), p=0.142	1.003 (0.991, 1.015), p=0.303	1.026 (1.002, 1.064), p=0.041	1.022 (0.989, 1.059), p=0.100	1.008 (0.998, 1.019), p=0.065	1.006 (0.994, 1.017), p=0.170	1.028 (1.001, 1.056), p=0.023	1.019 (0.987, 1.048), p=0.125

Table 8.2 (continued)

Predictors	Perceived general health				Long-standing illness/disability			
	0.5 mile network buffer		1.0 mile network buffer		0.5 mile network buffer		1.0 mile network buffer	
	Model 1*	Model 2**	Model 3***	Model 4****	Model 1*	Model 2**	Model 3***	Model 4****
	OR (95% Cred.I), p	OR (95% Cred.I), p	OR (95% Cred.I), p	OR (95% Cred.I), p	OR (95% Cred.I), p	OR (95% Cred.I), p	OR (95% Cred.I), p	OR (95% Cred.I), p
Service density:								
Density of business and offices	1.001 (0.996, 1.005), p=0.368	1.001 (0.996, 1.006), p=0.286	0.996 (0.983, 1.006), p=0.217	0.995 (0.984, 1.007), p=0.213	1.0003 (0.996, 1.005), p=0.457	1.002 (0.997, 1.007), p=0.230	1.001 (0.989, 1.011), p=0.490	1.000 (0.989, 1.011), p=0.460
Topological accessibility of streets:								
Betweenness	0.804 (0.687, 0.964), p=0.014	0.795 (0.673, 0.967), p=0.007	0.795 (0.715, 0.886), p<0.001	0.785 (0.692, 0.875), p<0.001	1.007 (0.829, 1.160), p=0.453	1.000 (0.825, 1.156), p=0.536	0.948 (0.871, 1.054), p=0.162	0.945 (0.852, 1.040), p=0.122
Hull area	0.922 (0.825, 1.032), p=0.082	0.925 (0.829, 1.033), p=0.08	1.616 (0.638, 5.286), p=0.142	1.966 (0.705, 7.237), p=0.09	0.931 (0.844, 1.044), p=0.10	0.936 (0.847, 1.042), p=0.118	1.342 (0.602, 4.165), p=0.211	1.515 (0.670, 4.576), p=0.130
Junction connectivity	1.010 (1.002, 1.017), p=0.006	1.008 (1.001, 1.017), p=0.014	1.000 (0.996, 1.004), p=0.442	1.000 (0.995, 1.004), p=0.444	1.004 (0.996, 1.011), p=0.191	1.003 (0.995, 1.010), p=0.210	0.997 (0.994, 1.001), p=0.059	0.997 (0.994, 1.003), p=0.060

Socio-demographics:								
Age	1.033 (1.003, 1.066), p=0.014	1.036 (1.001, 1.069), p=0.021	1.039 (1.015, 1.069), p=0.004	1.041 (1.017, 1.068), p<0.001	1.004 (0.976, 1.040), p=0.411	1.002 (0.979, 1.038), p=0.369	1.007 (0.985, 1.028), p=0.266	1.005 (0.979, 1.030), p=0.343
Single vs married	0.610 (0.272, 1.482), p=0.153	0.595 (0.272, 1.485), p=0.143	0.585 (0.262, 1.437), p=0.134	0.601 (0.268, 1.480), p=0.148	0.731 (0.342, 1.688), p=0.245	0.702 (0.332, 1.692), p=0.232	0.666 (0.316, 1.568), p=0.193	0.702 (0.323, 1.623), p=0.212
Widowed/ separated vs married	1.181 (0.650, 2.364), p=0.250	1.177 (0.648, 2.373), p=0.251	1.223 (0.685, 2.437), p=0.217	1.236 (0.679, 2.455), p=0.217	0.790 (0.441, 1.576), p=0.275	0.791 (0.436, 1.532), p=0.257	0.789 (0.443, 1.581), p=0.276	0.769 (0.434, 1.548), p=0.262
Social class (III-manual vs I, II, III-non-manual)	1.390 (1.003, 2.049), p=0.035	1.329 (0.928, 1.971), p=0.057	1.428 (1.005, 2.120), p=0.024	1.344 (0.989, 2.018), p=0.052	1.193 (0.843, 1.795), p=0.141	1.187 (0.829, 1.777), p=0.158	1.233 (0.862, 1.855), p=0.117	1.192 (0.833, 1.773), p=0.154
Social class (IV, V vs I, II, III-non-manual)	1.903 (1.192, 3.289), p=0.004	1.756 (1.093, 3.072), p=0.010	1.839 (1.151, 3.173), p=0.006	1.700 (1.063, 3.003), p=0.014	1.252 (0.775, 2.130), p=0.162	1.190 (0.752, 2.087), p=0.209	1.219 (0.771, 2.135), p=0.179	1.190 (0.738, 2.048), p=0.223
Education (school cert vs none/ apprentice)	0.702 (0.494, 0.998), p=0.035	0.700 (0.494, 0.999), p=0.040	0.706 (0.499, 0.999), p=0.043	0.696 (0.490, 0.997), p=0.036	1.008 (0.714, 1.494), p=0.434	1.024 (0.722, 1.525), p=0.401	1.022 (0.719, 1.518), p=0.407	1.014 (0.711, 1.518), p=0.427
Education (degree vs none/ apprentice)	0.360 (0.206, 0.660), p<0.001	0.357 (0.200, 0.666), p<0.001	0.366 (0.210, 0.679), p<0.001	0.352 (0.200, 0.664), p<0.001	0.926 (0.564, 1.675), p=0.458	0.955 (0.573, 1.706), p=0.487	0.942 (0.580, 1.685), p=0.474	0.943 (0.565, 1.684), p=0.469
LSOA-level variables:								
WIMD scores†								
WIMD (Q2 vs Q1)		1.220 (0.742, 2.354), p=0.209		1.179 (0.669, 2.469), p=0.277		1.237 (0.777, 2.125), p=0.164		1.143 (0.720, 1.954), p=0.260

Table 8.2 (continued)

Predictors	Perceived general health				Long-standing illness/disability			
	0.5 mile network buffer		1.0 mile network buffer		0.5 mile network buffer		1.0 mile network buffer	
	Model 1*	Model 2**	Model 3***	Model 4****	Model 1*	Model 2**	Model 3***	Model 4****
	OR (95% Cred.I), p	OR (95% Cred.I), p	OR (95% Cred.I), p	OR (95% Cred.I), p	OR (95% Cred.I), p	OR (95% Cred.I), p	OR (95% Cred.I), p	OR (95% Cred.I), p
LSOA-level variables:								
WIMD (Q3 vs Q1)		1.812 (1.082, 3.478), p=0.014		2.116 (1.149, 4.502), p=0.007		1.255 (0.771, 2.142), p=0.159		1.234 (0.768, 2.189), p=0.173
WIMD (Q4 vs Q1)		1.417 (0.839, 2.693), p=0.089		1.534 (0.812, 3.363), p=0.090		1.631 (1.003, 2.911), p=0.028		1.567 (1.001, 2.984), p=0.047
Bayesian deviance information criterion	1087.35	1088.08	1087.05	1085.57	1083.18	1085.45	1082.01	1085.55

Notes:
Results are expressed as odds ratio, 95% credible interval (Cred.I) and p-value for the mixed effects logistic regression with the MCMC method.
† Q: Quartile (Q1, Q2, Q3 and Q4 represent the lower, lower-middle, upper-middle and upper quartiles respectively).
* Model 1: Consists of analysis with built environmental morphometrics with 0.5 mile catchment and adjustments for individual-level socio-demographics.
** Model 2: Consists of analysis with built environmental morphometrics with 0.5 mile catchment and adjustments for individual-level socio-demographics and neighbourhood-level deprivation.
*** Model 3: Consists of analysis with built environmental morphometrics with 1.0 mile catchment and adjustments for individual-level socio-demographics.
**** Model 4: Consists of analysis with built environmental morphometrics with 1.0 mile catchment and adjustments for individual-level socio-demographics and neighbourhood-level deprivation.

were detrimental to health at a 0.5 mile catchment, but beneficial with a 1.0 mile catchment. In the case of perceived general health, the association was negative and significant at 0.5 mile ($OR_{0.5mi}$ = 1.010, p = 0.006 in model 1 and $OR_{0.5mi}$ = 1.008, p = 0.014 in model 2). However, it was positively associated at a 1.0 mile catchment for long-standing illness/disability ($OR_{1.0mi}$ = 0.997, p = 0.059 in model 3 and $OR_{1.0mi}$ = 0.997, p = 0.06 in model 4).

Table 8.3 presents the results of two-level mixed effects models for HADS anxiety and depression. Among the dwelling-level variables, residents of dwellings having one building face exposed to public space consistently had higher odds of anxiety in reference to those with no building face exposed to public space, at both 0.5 and 1.0 mile catchment analyses ($OR_{0.5mi}$ = 2.577, p = 0.027 and $OR_{1.0mi}$ = 2.684, p = 0.017 in models 2 and 4 respectively). However, no significant association was reported with depression. None of the destination accessibility measures were observed to be significantly associated with HADS anxiety and depression. Among the variables measuring service density, the density of bus stops was associated with higher odds of depression only in the analysis using a 0.5 mile catchment ($OR_{0.5mi}$ = 1.020, p = 0.036 and $OR_{0.5mi}$ = 1.021, p = 0.018 in models 1 and 2 respectively). The density of recreation and leisure facilities was also associated with higher odds of depression, but only in the analysis using a 1.0 mile catchment ($OR_{1.0mi}$ = 1.046, p = 0.048 and $OR_{1.0mi}$ = 1.041, p = 0.074 in models 3 and 4 respectively). Among the variables of street network accessibility, higher levels of betweenness at the 1.0 mile catchment radius were associated with lower odds of anxiety ($OR_{1.0mi}$ = 0.858, p = 0.041 and $OR_{1.0mi}$ = 0.858, p = 0.059 in models 3 and 4 respectively), while in the case of depression the association was beneficial with both 0.5 and 1.0 mile buffer radii ($OR_{0.5mi}$ = 0.744, p = 0.035 and $OR_{1.0mi}$ = 0.693, p = 0.002 in models 2 and 4 respectively).

Higher LSOA-level deprivation measured by the Welsh Index of Multiple Deprivation was consistently associated with poorer health outcomes. In reference to the deprivation scores in the lowest quartile (most affluent LSOAs), residents of LSOAs that fall in the third quartile have a higher propensity to report poor perceived general health ($OR_{0.5mi}$ = 1.812, p = 0.014 and $OR_{1.0mi}$ = 2.116, p = 0.007), while those in the fourth quartile have a higher propensity to report long-standing illness/disability ($OR_{0.5mi}$ = 1.631, p = 0.028 and $OR_{1.0mi}$ = 1.567, p = 0.047). Those residing in LSOAs that fall in the second quartile reported significantly higher levels of anxiety in the 0.5 mile buffer analysis ($OR_{0.5mi}$ = 1.944, p = 0.054). However, higher levels of depression were reported in residents of LSOAs that fall in the second ($OR_{0.5mi}$ = 3.878, p = 0.026 and $OR_{1.0mi}$ = 2.456, p = 0.066) as well as the third quartile ($OR_{0.5mi}$ = 4.865, p = 0.01 and $OR_{1.0mi}$ = 4.155, p = 0.011).

Table 8.3 Results of two-level mixed effects models for HADS anxiety and depression in 677 older men across 33 LSOAs

Predictors	HADS – Anxiety				HADS – Depression			
	0.5 mile network buffer		1.0 mile network buffer		0.5 mile network buffer		1.0 mile network buffer	
	Model 1*	Model 2**	Model 3***	Model 4****	Model 1*	Model 2**	Model 3***	Model 4****
	OR (95% Cred.I), p	OR (95% Cred.I), p	OR (95% Cred.I), p	OR (95% Cred.I), p	OR (95% Cred.I), p	OR (95% Cred.I), p	OR (95% Cred.I), p	OR (95% Cred.I), p
Dwelling-level variables:								
Dwelling-centred density	1.002 (0.956, 1.054), p=0.442	1.003 (0.956, 1.052), p=0.442	1.005 (0.958, 1.052), p=0.427	1.005 (0.959, 1.055), p=0.411	0.962 (0.904, 1.024), p=0.118	0.966 (0.906, 1.031), p=0.153	0.965 (0.907, 1.025), p=0.129	0.969 (0.910, 1.029), p=0.154
Plot exposure (one building face vs none)	2.616 (1.052, 7.747), p=0.019	2.577 (1.014, 7.885), p=0.027	2.708 (1.073, 8.009), p=0.017	2.684 (1.071, 8.242), p=0.017	0.975 (0.419, 2.886), p=0.469	1.060 (0.422, 2.870), p=0.451	1.234 (0.516, 3.589), p=0.302	1.165 (0.516, 3.569), p=0.309
Plot exposure (more than one face vs none)	1.996 (0.676, 6.177), p=0.115	2.072 (0.664, 6.768), p=0.114	1.817 (0.615, 5.727), p=0.145	1.872 (0.648, 6.171), p=0.132	0.678 (0.228, 2.252), p=0.296	0.756 (0.237, 2.425), p=0.319	0.648 (0.215, 2.255), p=0.259	0.677 (0.230, 2.371), p=0.291
Dwelling type (semi-detached vs detached)	0.876 (0.462, 1.79), p=0.393	0.899 (0.468, 1.901), p=0.424	0.871 (0.465, 1.785), p=0.386	0.899 (0.482, 1.909), p=0.442	1.154 (0.526, 3.189), p=0.309	1.109 (0.47, 2.876), p=0.401	1.302 (0.584, 3.334), p=0.246	1.123 (0.493, 3.041), p=0.337
Dwelling type (terraced vs detached)	0.607 (0.258, 1.564), p=0.163	0.597 (0.258, 1.521), p=0.150	0.570 (0.245, 1.399), p=0.112	0.576 (0.242, 1.455), p=0.131	0.583 (0.18, 1.936), p=0.198	0.545 (0.161, 1.706), p=0.144	0.524 (0.162, 1.663), p=0.137	0.446 (0.139, 1.535), p=0.110
Dwelling type (flat vs detached)	0.664 (0.188, 2.252), p=0.277	0.661 (0.189, 2.247), p=0.262	0.642 (0.189, 2.099), p=0.240	0.663 (0.189, 2.234), p=0.267	1.835 (0.459, 7.007), p=0.188	1.596 (0.361, 6.46), p=0.276	2.010 (0.526, 8.149), p=0.151	1.795 (0.430, 7.463), p=0.206

Network distance to nearest services:								
Green space	1.000 (0.999, 1.001), p=0.477	1.000 (0.999, 1.001). p=0.425	0.999 (0.999, 1.001), p=0.477	0.999 (0.998, 1.001), p=0.158	1.000 (0.998, 1.001), p=0.370	1.000 (0.998, 1.001), p=0.334	0.999 (0.998, 1.001), p=0.177	0.999 (0.998, 1.001), p=0.180
Sports facility	1.0001 (0.999, 1.001), p=0.425	1.000 (0.999, 1.001), p=0.475	1.000 (0.999, 1.001), p=0.425	1.0003 (0.999, 1.001), p=0.280	1.0002 (0.999, 1.002), p=0.436	1.000 (0.998, 1.001), p=0.462	1.001 (0.999, 1.002), p=0.216	1.001 (0.999, 1.002), p=0.195
Health care facility	0.999 (0.998, 1.001), p=0.127	0.999 (0.998, 1.001), p=0.136	0.999 (0.998, 1.001), p=0.127	0.999 (0.998, 1.001), p=0.116	0.999 (0.997, 1.001), p=0.118	0.999 (0.997, 1.001), p=0.136	0.999 (0.998, 1.001), p=0.224	0.999 (0.998, 1.001), p=0.277
Takeaway	1.0001 (1.000, 1.001), p=0.335	1.0001 (1.000, 1.001), p=0.221	1.0001 (1.000, 1.001), p=0.335	1.000 (0.999, 1.001), p=0.239	1.000 (0.999, 1.000), p=0.265	1.000 (0.999, 1.000), p=0.356	1.000 (0.999, 1.000), p=0.061	1.000 (0.999, 1.000), p=0.086
Allotment	1.001 (1.000, 1.001), p=0.141	1.001 (1.000, 1.001), p=0.132	1.0004 (1.000, 1.001), p=0.141	1.0005 (1.000, 1.001), p=0.169	1.0002 (0.999, 1.001), p=0.325	1.0002 (0.999, 1.001), p=0.303	1.000 (0.999, 1.001), p=0.477	1.000 (0.999, 1.001), p=0.462
Service density:								
Density of bus stops	1.009 (0.993, 1.027), p=0.127	1.012 (0.996, 1.029), p=0.065	1.005 (0.969, 1.042), p=0.388	1.003 (0.969, 1.038), p=0.420	1.020 (1.001, 1.039), p=0.036	1.021 (1.004, 1.043), p=0.018	1.009 (0.963, 1.054), p=0.353	1.000 (0.955, 1.054), p=0.491
Density of retail	1.003 (0.993, 1.012), p=0.308	1.004 (0.993, 1.015), p=0.244	1.002 (0.967, 1.035), p=0.463	0.996 (0.961, 1.033), p=0.430	1.000 (0.985, 1.015), p=0.490	0.999 (0.984, 1.016), p=0.497	0.995 (0.952, 1.04), p=0.392	0.994 (0.949, 1.053), p=0.438
Density of community services	0.999 (0.982, 1.015), p=0.437	0.993 (0.976, 1.012), p=0.226	0.992 (0.931, 1.058), p=0.407	1.000 (0.942, 1.068), p=0.484	1.001 (0.979, 1.022), p=0.469	0.997 (0.974, 1.020), p=0.409	0.986 (0.912, 1.070), p=0.380	0.995 (0.902, 1.078), p=0.448
Density of recreation and leisure facilities	0.993 (0.974, 1.010), p=0.227	0.992 (0.972, 1.011), p=0.203	1.029 (0.987, 1.077), p=0.087	1.028 (0.98, 1.073), p=0.128	1.002 (0.979, 1.026), p=0.429	0.997 (0.971, 1.021), p=0.391	1.046 (1.001, 1.109), p=0.048	1.041 (0.986, 1.108), p=0.074
Density of business and offices	0.997 (0.990, 1.005), p=0.248	0.997 (0.989, 1.005), p=0.264	1.001 (0.982, 1.02), p=0.478	1.003 (0.983, 1.022), p=0.360	0.994 (0.982, 1.006), p=0.152	0.996 (0.982, 1.007), p=0.231	1.001 (0.975, 1.024), p=0.467	1.005 (0.974, 1.029), p=0.402

Table 8.3 (continued)

Predictors	HADS – Anxiety				HADS – Depression			
	0.5 mile network buffer		1.0 mile network buffer		0.5 mile network buffer		1.0 mile network buffer	
	Model 1*	Model 2**	Model 3***	Model 4****	Model 1*	Model 2**	Model 3***	Model 4****
	OR (95% Cred.I), p	OR (95% Cred.I), p	OR (95% Cred.I), p	OR (95% Cred.I), p	OR (95% Cred.I), p	OR (95% Cred.I), p	OR (95% Cred.I), p	OR (95% Cred.I), p
Topological accessibility of streets:								
Betweenness	0.858 (0.666, 1.059), p=0.082	0.830 (0.662, 1.087), p=0.084	0.858 (0.731, 0.999), p=0.041	0.858 (0.732, 1.038), p=0.059	0.787 (0.566, 0.998), p=0.046	0.744 (0.564, 0.995), p=0.035	0.691 (0.588, 0.883), p=0.002	0.693 (0.565, 0.838), p=0.002
Hull area	2.169 (0.313, 9.664), p=0.442	1.814 (0.398, 8.550), p=0.465	2.086 (0.441, 11.079), p=0.180	1.882 (0.423, 8.750), p=0.189	1.968 (0.375, 4.880), p=0.281	1.945 (0.302, 5.987), p=0.373	2.130 (0.460, 4.791), p=0.120	2.005 (1.006, 5.353), p=0.047
Junction connectivity	1.003 (0.986, 1.018), p=0.383	1.004 (0.986, 1.020), p=0.338	0.998 (0.992, 1.004), p=0.244	0.998 (0.992, 1.004), p=0.213	1.003 (0.982, 1.023), p=0.397	0.999 (0.977, 1.021), p=0.462	0.997 (0.989, 1.005), p=0.241	0.995 (0.988, 1.003), p=0.119
Socio-demographics:								
Age	0.982 (0.948, 1.025), p=0.225	0.986 (0.941, 1.033), p=0.233	0.980 (0.944, 1.023), p=0.185	0.983 (0.936, 1.021), p=0.177	1.021 (0.977, 1.07), p=0.191	1.020 (0.967, 1.067), p=0.232	1.026 (0.976, 1.076), p=0.153	1.017 (0.979, 1.069), p=0.226
Single vs married	0.911 (0.202, 3.411), p=0.503	0.964 (0.210, 3.524), p=0.488	0.800 (0.172, 2.934), p=0.402	0.782 (0.169, 3.023), p=0.417	0.473 (0.01, 2.589), p=0.176	0.487 (0.014, 2.827), p=0.198	0.384 (0.011, 2.071), p=0.129	0.350 (0.012, 2.33), p=0.155

Widowed/separated vs married	1.483 (0.616, 3.679), p=0.160	1.485 (0.616, 3.595), p=0.161	1.605 (0.677, 3.936), p=0.120	1.619 (0.686, 3.963), p=0.115	0.364 (0.049, 1.507), p=0.090	0.373 (0.05, 1.526), p=0.090	0.380 (0.048, 1.522), p=0.092	0.358 (0.048, 1.491), p=0.086
Social class (III-manual vs I, II, III-non-manual)	1.010 (0.597, 1.930), p=0.412	1.036 (0.594, 2.031), p=0.394	1.011 (0.591, 1.916), p=0.431	1.004 (0.576, 1.96), p=0.432	1.304 (0.653, 3.122), p=0.199	1.210 (0.581, 2.923), p=0.284	1.475 (0.724, 3.429), p=0.136	1.299 (0.635, 3.137), p=0.218
Social class (IV, V vs I, II, III-non-manual)	1.110 (0.534, 2.485), p=0.342	1.087 (0.498, 2.486), p=0.390	1.058 (0.496, 2.364), p=0.403	1.023 (0.481, 2.401), p=0.417	1.390 (0.556, 3.969), p=0.21	1.188 (0.461, 3.346), p=0.335	1.469 (0.581, 4.036), p=0.195	1.186 (0.473, 3.379), p=0.323
Education (school cert vs none/ apprentice)	0.771 (0.437, 1.429), p=0.232	0.776 (0.439, 1.456), p=0.244	0.778 (0.438, 1.432), p=0.237	0.768 (0.436, 1.433), p=0.233	0.421 (0.183, 0.987), p=0.024	0.408 (0.177, 0.950), p=0.018	0.387 (0.173, 0.907), p=0.013	0.351 (0.155, 0.858), p=0.010
Education (degree vs none/apprentice)	0.627 (0.265, 1.630), p=0.197	0.662 (0.274, 1.722), p=0.232	0.695 (0.297, 1.742), p=0.253	0.721 (0.300, 1.781), p=0.270	0.720 (0.003, 0.576), p=0.003	0.680 (0.003, 0.582), p=0.004	0.780 (0.003, 0.594), p=0.004	0.710 (0.003, 0.584), p=0.004
LSOA-level variables:								
WIMD scores†								
WIMD (Q2 vs Q1)		1.944 (0.868, 4.596), p=0.054		1.299 (0.643, 2.998), p=0.204		3.878 (1.005, 15.669), p=0.026		2.456 (0.757, 8.581), p=0.066
WIMD (Q3 vs Q1)		1.421 (0.631, 3.649), p=0.184		1.128 (0.501, 2.763), p=0.340		4.865 (1.272, 20.338), p=0.010		4.155 (1.188, 14.169), p=0.011

Table 8.3 (continued)

Predictors	HADS – Anxiety				HADS – Depression			
	0.5 mile network buffer		1.0 mile network buffer		0.5 mile network buffer		1.0 mile network buffer	
	Model 1*	Model 2**	Model 3***	Model 4****	Model 1*	Model 2**	Model 3***	Model 4****
	OR (95% Cred.I), p	OR (95% Cred.I), p	OR (95% Cred.I), p	OR (95% Cred.I), p	OR (95% Cred.I), p	OR (95% Cred.I), p	OR (95% Cred.I), p	OR (95% Cred.I), p
LSOA-level variables:								
WIMD (Q4 vs Q1)		1.052 (0.431, 2.751), p=0.439		0.876 (0.369, 2.194), p=0.425		2.683 (0.652, 11.058), p=0.093		2.208 (0.618, 7.845), p=0.115
Bayesian deviance information criterion	566.26	569.23	565.93	570.39	410.76	410.04	411.12	410.92

Notes:
Results are expressed as odds ratio, 95% credible interval (Cred.I) and p-value for the mixed effects logistic regression with the MCMC method.
† Q: Quartile (Q1, Q2, Q3 and Q4 represent the lower, lower-middle, upper-middle and upper quartiles respectively).
* Model 1: Consists of analysis with built environmental morphometrics with 0.5 mile catchment and adjustments for individual-level socio-demographics.
** Model 2: Consists of analysis with built environmental morphometrics with 0.5 mile catchment and adjustments for individual-level socio-demographics and neighbourhood-level deprivation.
*** Model 3: Consists of analysis with built environmental morphometrics with 1.0 mile catchment and adjustments for individual-level socio-demographics.
**** Model 4: Consists of analysis with built environmental morphometrics with 1.0 mile catchment and adjustments for individual-level socio-demographics and neighbourhood-level deprivation.

The random effects component measuring between-LSOA variance consistently indicated small and non-significant heterogeneity in all the health outcomes across the LSOAs.

8.4 DISCUSSION

In a population sample of elderly men the study found that perceived general health and long-term illness/disability and HADS anxiety and depression were significantly associated with certain specific attributes of the built environment. The study also found that the associations were moderated by varying the spatial scales at which they were measured as well as by including a measure of neighbourhood-level deprivation (the Welsh Index of Multiple Deprivation).

8.4.1 Strengths and Limitations

The main strengths of the present study include detailed and objective assessment of the built environment, application of multi-level modelling, and the application of a population sample with a high response rate (CaPS). In order to examine the effects of varying degrees of land use and street network accessibility on health, the built environment was measured at network 'influence catchments' of 0.5 and 1.0 mile. The inclusion of the LSOA-level Welsh Index of Multiple Deprivation enabled the potential moderating effects of neighbourhood-level deprivation to be studied.

The study was able to employ a combination of self-perceived measures of health as well as a standard psychometric instrument of psychological health and examine their association with various facets of the built environment. The models used to measure general health and long-term illness/disability assessed individuals' perception about their health, while HADS is a screening test to assess the presence of clinically significant degrees of anxiety and depression employed on patients both in and outside hospital care.

As Chapter 4 discusses, previous studies have employed measures of street connectivity mostly expressed in terms of street intersection density to assess the impact of street-level accessibility on health outcomes, especially obesity and physical activity behaviours (F. Li et al., 2008; Troped et al., 2010). Many other studies have employed composite indices of neighbourhood walkability (Berke, Gottlieb et al., 2007; Leslie et al., 2007; Van Dyck et al., 2010; Frank et al., 2010) and street-level connectivity (Ball et al., 2012) which fail to isolate the effects of specific facets of the built environment. To our knowledge this (as well as Chapter 6) is the first study examining in detail the effects of various facets of street network accessibility on the psychological health of older adults. The application of the state-of-the-art sDNA model for generating street network accessibility indices of betweenness, hull area and junction connectivity enabled more accurate assessment of street-level accessibility (Chiaradia, Hillier et al., 2012). The sDNA network model employs the OSM ITN street links as the fundamental unit of computation. One of the potential advantages of employing standardized ITN street links is that this is able to overcome the so-called *network distortions* or *noise* often present in the angular segment analysis used in the space syntax analysis and employed in the street network analysis in Chapters 6 and 7.

Limitations of the study include its cross-sectional design, which hinders any exploration of causal association, as well as temporal variation in health outcomes. CaPS is a cohort of older men; hence one should be cautious in generalizing the results to other sections of the population of different age group and sex. The study has limited geographical reach constrained to the LSOAs within the Caerphilly assembly constituency, a semi-urban commuting town with low mix and dwelling density located north of Cardiff. It must be stressed that a much stronger effect of urban spatial scales upon health outcomes is expected in more highly urbanized areas.

8.4.2 Interpretation

Of the dwelling-level variables, the positive association between perceived health and dwelling-centred density may be explained via physical activity and social capital mechanisms. Previous studies have consistently established the beneficial effects of dwelling-level density upon outcomes of physical activity (F. Li, Fisher, Brownson et al., 2005; C. Lee and Moudon, 2006b; Troped et al., 2010), obesity (Pouliou and Elliott, 2010; Burgoine et al., 2011) and walkability (Saelens, Sallis, Black et al., 2003). Higher suburban density may also be associated with enhanced density of acquaintanceship, community ties and neighbourhood satisfaction (Talen, 1999). Living in flats has been generally associated with poorer health, especially mental health (Fanning, 1967; Wilkinson and Britain, 1998; G.W. Evans et al., 2003). In the present study, the negative association between flats and poorer perceived health in older adults may be interpreted in terms of lack of access to shared outdoor areas, including opportunities to visit the gardens and enjoy the natural views they may afford, as well as reduced mobility and resulting social isolation. The negative association between number of building faces exposed to public space and HADS anxiety may be attributed to the unwanted social interactions and lack of privacy in buildings having more exposures to adjacent streets. That no association was found with HADS depression suggests that the association with HADS anxiety is unlikely to be due to confounding. This is a novel finding not reported elsewhere. In fact, as far as the authors are aware, this association has not been measured in any published study.

The positive association between a reduced propensity to report longstanding illness/disability and density of community services is along the expected lines. The density of community services may act as a proxy of social care and support. However, the negative association between density of recreation and leisure facilities with self-reported health and with HADS depression is counter-intuitive and may be a chance effect, particularly as depression is associated with poor self-reported health. As observed in Chapter 6, the negative association between density of bus stops and HADS depression was unanticipated. Higher density of public transport routes may act as a proxy for socially deprived micro-scale housing clusters not captured by the WIMD score.

Among the street network accessibility variables, sDNA-measured betweenness is a significant predictor of perceived general health and of HADS anxiety and depression. The associations remained mostly beneficial at scales of 0.5 and 1.0 mile. This is equivalent to the results obtained in the case of GHQ-30 in Chapter 6. Such an association may be explained via physical activity and social capital mechanisms. High betweenness accessibility at the fairly local scales of 0.5 and 1.0 mile is synonymous with high movement potential and consequent increased walkability to local services. This may well promote enhanced social connectivity and mutual support amongst the elderly. Network hull area at 0.5 mile was beneficially associated with perceived general health only after controlling for neighbourhood deprivation, but the association was negative at 1.0 mile. This may highlight the importance of close-knit and compact community morphology with high local-level street accessibility. The negative association between junction connectivity and perceived general health within a catchment of 0.5 mile underscores the negative effects of street intersections on the elderly with respect to traffic density, lack of safety while crossing the streets and the propensity to walk around one's neighbourhood when elderly.

The results of controlling for area-level deprivation indicate that higher levels of deprivation are associated with poorer health outcomes, as expected. That the associations between the various attributes of the built environment and health outcomes are slightly affected (both in point estimates and in level of significance) points towards a moderating effect of neighbourhood-level deprivation. In the models of psychological distress measured by HADS, the beneficial effects of social support and networking in high-betweenness areas are further reinforced by simultaneously being in a more deprived area.

The observed differences in point estimates and level of significance when comparing the two scales (0.5 and 1.0 mile) of catchment areas measured point to the health impacts of differential accessibility. Such impacts may originate from both differential physical accessibility and differential perceptions of accessibility to health-promoting capital. For example, if the density of a specific important health-promoting resource is high within a 0.5 mile buffer, the physical accessibility to it is enhanced. The same may be the case for perceived accessibility, as residents are likely to hold a positive image of the neighbourhood environment. The physical and perceived factors together may contribute to resource utilization within the 0.5 mile buffer and corresponding health benefits. In such a case any increment in the density of the particular service between 0.5 and 1.0 mile catchments may no longer be important, thereby rendering the density measured at the 1.0 mile catchment non-significant. Several examples of this phenomenon can be isolated from the statistical models presented. The density of community services within a 0.5 mile catchment remains significantly associated with lower odds of reporting long-standing illness/disability, but the association is no longer significant in the analysis using a 1.0 mile catchment. Another example is the case of the association between junction connectivity and odds of reporting long-standing illness/disability. Using a 0.5 mile catchment buffer, junction connectivity is related to higher odds of long-standing illness/disability, but the association is not significant. In the analysis using a 1.0 mile buffer, higher junction connectivity is, however, significantly associated with lower odds of long-standing illness/disability. This may be attributed to the fact that, at a scale of 0.5 mile, junction connectivity acts as a proxy variable for street-level safety and crowding; however, at the level of a 1.0 mile catchment, it may measure for degree of street-level integration in the neighbourhood (i.e. measuring greater perceived access to walkable opportunities).

8.5 CONCLUSION

The final study of this book has demonstrated associations between objectively assessed built environment measures and mental health for a specific demographic in a specific location. Findings both confirm and elaborate the findings of other studies reviewed in Chapter 4. At least one novel finding has emerged – the link between anxiety in elderly men and living in a home that has at least one face abutting public open space. Future studies need to be conducted on a more heterogeneous population in order to explore this and the other effects reported across diverse age groups and among women. The impact of accessibility to health-promoting or -inhibiting resources at multiple urban scales needs to be assessed in areas with varying degrees of 'urbanness', especially in large cities and high-density inner-city areas. Evidence gathered from this and similar studies is potentially of great use in optimizing the configuration, design and management of built environments to encourage mobility, physical activity and social connectivity and thereby foster physical and mental health.

9. Conclusion

We have presented in this book much of the mounting research evidence that now exists of the significant associations between urban morphology and public health. This was a relationship that began to be explored scientifically in earnest from the second half of the nineteenth century, and it was a key driver in shaping the modern urban planning movement and profession. For much of the twentieth century, city planners in the West had lost touch with their public health roots. That is now changing, as we have traversed a full circle, with among other things an epidemic of obesity and cardiovascular problems endemic to sedentary urban lifestyles and a demographic health care time bomb that amplifies the problems.

It is now widely recognized that health outcomes as well as the success of clinical interventions are shaped by *context*; more precisely by the attributes of socio-economic, built and natural environments. This book endeavours to examine the basic question: how do physiological, socio-demographic, built and natural environmental factors combine to produce specific socio-spatial distributions of health in a city? More specifically, does the city's built environment – its configuration and design as well as the distribution of services within it – influence our cognition, behaviour and lifestyle and thereby the health of its citizens?

In the early chapters of the book, we conceptualize what we have termed the *urban health niche* as a novel holistic and spatially explicit paradigm for articulating public health and urban planning analysis and interventions. The health niche model of a healthy city can be used both descriptively and prescriptively: for framing empirical studies of the associations between urban form and health performance; and then using this analysis to suggest how to improve, or even optimize, urban performance on various health-related dimensions. The book focuses on the descriptive use of the model as a starting point in the bigger project that we and similar groups of researchers are currently engaged in. Looking forward, we anticipate two types of prescriptive use being made of this body of work. First, as the results of empirical work in this crossover field become more widely known by both urban planning and public health practitioners, we would expect professional doctrines, practices and policies to reflect some of the stronger findings. This is already starting to happen, with for example the doctrines of mixed land use and densification becoming widely accepted in urban planning. We would hope that this book and the other attempts to disseminate the evidence base for such doctrines would lead to refinements of such doctrines. Looking beyond this loose coupling of evidence and practice, we anticipate that, before long, it should be possible to develop more sophisticated decision support tools such as Bayesian network models of public health that add built environment context into probabilistic models of diagnosis as well as prognosis, thereby enabling determination of causal inferences. With this in mind, we are currently working with the UK Biobank to create built environmental metrics for the Biobank's 500 000 cohort members.

We also provide an overview of the scientific research evidence relating built environment attributes to health outcomes. These lay the foundation for the empirical chapters of the book and help establish baseline knowledge for researchers and practitioners. Demonstrating how the urban health niche paradigm may be implemented to investigate analysis of multi-scale built environmental effects, multi-level data sets pertaining to health and the socio-economic, built and natural environment have been developed and integrated to constitute a high-resolution health niche database: spatial Design Network Analysis for Urban Health (sDNA-UH). Three empirical studies consisting of multi-level cross-sectional and longitudinal models have been presented, which examine the association between specific attributes of a built environment and health outcomes.

9.1 RECAPITULATION

Chapter 1 lays a foundation for the book by reviewing the argument that public health concerns need to be reintroduced into urban planning. City designers, planners and managers seek to optimize their designs and plans according to multiple social and private objectives. Theoretically, the task is to configure a city in such a way as to optimize the net agglomeration benefits (the benefits of many people living together minus the costs). At various times and in various parts of the world, different performance dimensions have dominated the optimization calculus. In contemporary China, for example, officials have set explicit urban gross domestic product (GDP) targets and municipal income targets, and this more or less single-dimensionally determines the pace and shape of city building. In the West, for the past 100 years, housing construction (in Britain after the war, for example), economic growth (1960s and 1980s Britain), and urban compaction in pursuit of travel and energy reduction (2000s) have driven urban planning. Public health drove the slum clearance of Britain in the late nineteenth and early twentieth centuries and drives contemporary slum clearance in many cities of the developing world. The simple model of urban costs and benefits in Chapter 1 illustrates the possibility of optimal city sizes of various kinds. It makes the simple point that, if poor health is taken as a source of agglomeration benefit reduction and health care costs as a source of rising costs of supporting an agglomeration of people, then both become an important consideration in urban planning. Put another way, an economically sustainable city is one that is able to reproduce its main factor of production, namely labour, and this means that it should support the health of its population and various sub-populations. Ideally, the health-supporting effects of a city should yield more than the health subsistence of its labour force: it should yield a 'health surplus', that is, health gains that enhance the quality of life. This will help make cities more attractive and contribute to their growth. Large cities in the industrial and pre-industrial periods typically did not do this, with mortality rates in the urban areas much higher than in rural areas. At the present time, there is a new mood and will to configure cities via urban planning and public health interventions to further enhance the urban health surplus. The purpose of this book has been to extend and test new scientific tools in pursuit of this goal.

Chapter 2 traces the evolving relationship between urban planning and public health. It describes the evolution of the modern disciplines of town planning, public health and epidemiology in response to the complexities and challenges of urban health originating from the industrialization and urbanization during the pre- and post-war eras. The chapter begins by describing early-nineteenth-century Britain, characterized by the advent of industrialization and urbanization, often resulting in high-density settlements with endemic problems of overcrowding, pollution and lack of basic hygiene and sanitation. Significantly higher mortality from infectious diseases in cities than in the rural areas triggered the onset of urban public health as a modern governance and scientific concern. Sanitarians and city planners of the age forged a strong strategic collaboration focusing primarily on preventive population-level interventions for better hygiene. The chapter goes on to describe the subsequent era of germ theory, which focused on individualistic clinical interventions in the form of vaccines and antibiotics for epidemic control. However, it was around this time that the alliance between public health and urban planning was severed. With the increased pace of urban expansion, the twentieth century witnessed significant transformations in economic and social landscapes. Public transport systems evolved and brought with them urban sprawl. Planning concepts including garden cities, the Broadacre City, and land use zoning emerged during the period as means to offset the negative health impacts of urban life, especially those pertaining to high density and pollution from industry and traffic. Spatial delineation of neighbourhoods and road hierarchies attempted to engineer better access to basic services and segregate residential areas from sources of pollution. Post-Second World War, the economic and social developments as well as advances in epidemiology and clinical medicine meant that the aetiology of disease shifted from *infectious* to *chronic*, characterized by longer latency and multiple causality. The chapter then describes the evolving epidemiological paradigms that have attempted to explain complex disease causality, including chronic disease epidemiology, molecular epidemiology and social epidemiology. The necessity of a more holistic and integrated paradigm for explaining disease aetiology is highlighted in the chapter by the description of contemporary more holistic eco-epidemiological frameworks. The chapter concludes that urban life in the present century has contributed to unhealthy and sedentary lifestyles, often manifested by increasing incidences of obesity, cardiovascular disease and psychological disorders. They all point to the so-called *miasma* of the built environment (a public health concept first popularized in the nineteenth century) and call for an effective re-engagement between the disciplines of public health and urban planning.

In recognition of the increasing calls for a holistic approach to health highlighted in Chapter 2, Chapter 3 conceptualizes the notion of the *urban health niche* as an all-encompassing epidemiological planning paradigm that links individual, population, spatial and temporal dimensions. The urban health niche is a hypothetical hypervolume that encompasses the epidemiologic triad of person, place and time. Health is thus considered a function of the spatio-temporal variations in an urban health niche wherein the multiple multi-level causal factors and processes are active over space–time coordinates. With the objective of unravelling the black box of *contextual* determinants of health, such a framework essentially incorporates the role of contextual social, built and natural environmental factors of disease causation. Drawing upon diverse strands of research, the health niche framework integrates three basic epidemiological principles: (1) the multi-level spatial scales (micro, meso and macro scales) at which the health-defining processes function; (2) the multiple levels of aggregation at which health is produced, distributed and studied; and (3) the temporal dynamism in disease aetiology from life stage to life course. Such a framework not only integrates the various sub-disciplines of epidemiology but also enables identification of causation by capturing the dynamic interactions from micro via meso to macro scales. Subsequently, the chapter illustrates the effectiveness of the concept of the urban health niche with the help of a bottom-up model of the healthy city. It is based on the assumption that the socio-spatial distribution of health in a city is self-organized as a result of complex dynamic interactions between multiple, multi-level causal variables. The objective of such a model is to highlight the integrating links between epidemiological research evidence and its dissemination through effective planning and policy interventions.

Following the proposed urban health niche framework, in Chapter 4 we conduct a systematic review of epidemiologic literature on the built environment and health. Determinants of health at the housing and neighbourhood levels are discussed in fine detail. Discussion of housing-level determinants of physical health include the impacts of cold and damp, mould, overcrowding, disrepair, pest infestation, indoor air pollution, lighting and noise. Housing type and floor level, housing quality and overcrowding have been identified as the key built environment correlates or determinants of mental health. Neighbourhood-level determinants of health include indices of density/intensity, diversity, destination accessibility (expressed as accessibility to retail, green space, recreational facilities, physical activity resources and local food environments), street network morphology and connectivity, access to public transit and active transport, and pedestrian-oriented design. The association between health outcomes and composite measures to capture walkability and environmental quality are also discussed in this chapter.

Chapter 5 presents the specific hypothesis of the book, that the configuration of the city, especially the distribution of land uses and design of street networks, defines physical connectivity and accessibility to health-promoting community resources and thereby influences health variation. Physical access structures, it is hypothesized, influence an individual's activity patterns and mental and behavioural responses, as well as social interactions, and thereby are associated with health outcomes. Street network configuration matters. With the objective of operationalizing the spatial elements of the urban health niche model in Chapter 3, this chapter describes in detail what we call *spatial Design Network Analysis for Urban Health* (sDNA-UH), a high-resolution GIS model comprising sophisticated built environment morphological metrics (morphometrics). This has been developed for one of the UK's most closely studied public health laboratories: the assembly constituency of Caerphilly in South Wales, UK (83 600 inhabitants over 114.54 square kilometres, with a density of 727 inhabitants per square kilometre). A systematic methodology was adopted in the construction of sDNA-UH. The choice of metrics was guided by the extensive review of published epidemiological studies on the association between the built environment and health (Chapter 4), and multi-level data were integrated together along the micro, meso and macro scales as defined by the urban health niche paradigm of Chapter 3. The Caerphilly Prospective Study (CaPS) constituted the source of anonymized individual health and socio-demographic data. The respondents who participated in the third, fourth and fifth phases of examination and resided within the study area were geo-coded. The UK Ordnance Survey MasterMap (OSM) data layers – the Topography Layer, Integrated Transport Network (ITN) Layer and Address Layer 2 – were employed to construct a set of built environment morphometrics, measured at the dwelling level as well as within multiple street network buffers around geo-coded individual dwelling units. GIS-based spatial analysis and network models were employed to construct more than 100 objectively measured built environmental morphometrics for each member of the study cohort. The land use morphometrics covered specific and general accessibility measures. Specific measures reflect the access of individuals to specific health-promoting and -detracting sources and included density, land use mix and network distance to health destinations. General accessibility measures captured systemic connectivity between an individual's home and every other destination. Two specific graph-theoretic metrics are used: closeness and betweenness. This analysis of street network accessibility was conducted using space syntax analysis and its successor technique spatial Design Network Analysis (sDNA), using ITN network data at multiple catchments around geo-coded individual dwelling units. Indices of the natural environment are also used, consisting of measures of slope variability and greenness in terms of satellite-derived NDVI. Other measures used include an index of area-level deprivation and dwelling-level morphometrics. The chapter thus aimed at capturing a highly detailed objective assessment of the built environment, with the objective of developing a multi-level data repository to be subsequently employed in the construction of well-formed spatially explicit epidemiological models of built environment–behaviour–health associations.

The relationship between the structure of configured urban space in a city and human behaviour and health has long been established. However, few studies have examined the impacts of the built environment configuration upon psychological disorders. Chapter 6 examines the impact of built environment configuration upon psychological distress and whether such association is moderated by the natural environment and area-level deprivation. Built environment morphological metrics derived from the sDNA-UH were related to change in psychological distress as measured by the General Health Questionnaire (GHQ-30). Participants consisted of 687 respondents in the Caerphilly Prospective Study, aged 65–83 years, participating in the study's fifth examination and for whom there were complete data. Environmental measures consisted of GIS-constructed land use and street network metrics, slope variability and a satellite-derived measure of greenness. The study employed a multi-level analytic framework, with individuals nested within lower super output areas (LSOAs). Given that the GHQ scale was semi-continuous, with a significant proportion of zeros, a two-part multi-level regression model was employed. In the first part, the prevalence of psychological distress was modelled as a two-level factor (case versus non-case) with the help of two-level logistic mixed effects models. In the second part, sensitivity analysis was performed upon the subset of the sample exhibiting a non-zero GHQ-30 score with the help of a two-level gamma mixed regression model. Subsequent to adjustments for confounding effects, higher degrees of land use mix (LUM) were associated with reduced odds of psychological distress. A higher density of bus stops and of business and offices was significantly related to increasing psychological distress. Higher local street network general accessibility ('betweenness') promoted better psychological health. Slope variability was directly associated with increased odds of psychological distress. Sensitivity analysis using the sub-population exhibiting symptoms of psychological distress (a non-zero GHQ score) indicated that none of the built environment variables was significant in explaining variation within the sub-population, while slope variability continued to be significantly associated with higher odds of psychological distress among this group. The findings support the hypothesis that built environment configuration is independently associated with psychological distress. The study thus underscores the need for effective intervention in the planning and design of residential built environments to achieve the goal of health-sustaining communities. The models point to the design factors to which attention should be paid.

There have been very few longitudinal studies assessing obesity trends of older adults in relation to the built environment. Chapter 7 employs cohort data of the third, fourth and fifth phases of the Caerphilly Prospective Study to present the first long-term longitudinal evidence relating the built environment to change in obesity in older people. Longitudinal trends in body mass index (BMI) were measured at three time points encompassing a 12-year period. The study consisted of 2052 observations at the three time points for 684 participants distributed over 35 LSOA census areas. Built environment attributes were assessed through five sets of 16 morphometrics derived from the sDNA-UH spatial model developed to implement an urban health niche model for the CaPS cohort. A three-level random effects modelling strategy was adopted wherein measurement occasions were nested within individuals and individuals were nested within LSOAs. BMI was observed to be significantly associated with a number of built environment factors. The study reported that seven of the 16 built environment morphometrics were significantly associated with BMI. Higher land use mix was associated with higher odds of obesity. The density of amenities, namely retail, churches, and recreation and leisure facilities, was observed to be inversely associated with BMI levels. Among the street network general accessibility variables, a higher city-scale street betweenness at 3000 metres was associated with improved BMI outcomes, while local-scale street choice at 1200 metres was associated with poorer weight outcomes. Higher slope variability, measured as standard deviation in slope within the defined buffer, was associated with improved BMI levels. Controlling for socio-demographic and lifestyle factors and for vascular diseases had negligible impact upon the influence of built environmental factors. A high degree of heterogeneity between individuals was reported subsequent to adjustments for other covariates. The study also found significant occasion-specific variance in the BMI over the 12-year duration. The increments in BMI over the three time points were consistently significant and positive. However, a negligible and non-significant heterogeneity in BMI between LSOAs was observed. The study demonstrates the importance of urban design and planning in devising community public health interventions towards a fit city, and the models point to specific urban configuration dimensions that are associated with obesity.

Chapter 8 tests the health effects of differential accessibility of an individual's dwelling with respect to multiple service and facility catchments at multiple spatial scales. The effects upon general health (expressed in terms of perceived health and disability) and hospital anxiety and depression in older adults of Caerphilly are examined. Built environment measures were derived from the spatial model sDNA-UH and consisted of both land use and spatial Design Network Analysis (sDNA) measured street network morphometrics, parameterized within 0.5 mile and 1 mile street network catchments. Dwelling-level density, dwelling type, density of community services, street network movement potential expressed in terms of a betweenness index, and neighbourhood-level deprivation were identified as the significant parameters. The study reported significant differences in point estimates and level of significance when comparing the two spatial scales of 0.5 and 1.0 mile network catchments. It thereby highlights the health impacts associated with differential physical accessibility as well as differential perceptions of accessibility to health-promoting capital.

The empirical studies of this book thus conclude that different attributes of objectively measured spatial morphometrics of land use and street network configuration appear to affect health outcomes in a population sample of older adults. This lends support to the book's principal hypothesis that the built environment influences individual health behaviour and eventually health. The key strengths of the three empirical studies reported include: the comprehensive nature of the data created, compiled and integrated on the basis of a holistic urban health niche model; the use of objectively assessed built environment morphometrics; the distinction between special and general accessibility effects; the distinction between these effects at different spatial scales; and the application of multi-level modelling to capture random effects across space and time. The application of UK Ordnance Survey data sets to extract land use and street network data layers as well as the subsequent GIS and space syntax and sDNA-based network modelling adds methodological novelty to this research. The studies also assessed the moderating effects of natural and social environments. With some of the associations we have been able to measure, causality may be reasonably inferred. Others remain statistical associations and open to alternative explanations such as migration effects (the association exists because certain types of people choose to self-select a specific type of neighbourhood). We have noted where this seems particularly likely.

9.2 AN URBAN HEALTH NICHE RESEARCH AGENDA

We foresee several potentially important directions of further research arising from this book, which extend the epidemiological evidence base of the association between attributes of the built environment and health, identifying causality as well as enabling the formulation of corresponding evidence-based policy and planning for effective interventions.

From a conceptual standpoint, there is an increasing need for closer collaboration between epidemiologists, public health planners and urban planners and policy makers for the design and delivery of effective public health interventions. For example, design and management of buildings, streets, neighbourhood services and domiciliary care for the elderly need to be conceptualized and implemented together and to be informed by evidence. Given the increasing focus on contextual variations in health outcomes, the exacerbating or mitigating role of a city's built environment must be incorporated in contemporary epidemiological and health economics frameworks. This is highlighted by our *urban health niche* framework. The framework has the potential to structure evidence-based knowledge gathered from epidemiological research into effective urban design and service management interventions.

From a methodological standpoint, firstly, future epidemiological studies of the contextual effects of attributes of the built environment on health should make more extensive application of emerging spatial analysis techniques to create detailed objective assessment of the built environment. As has been highlighted throughout this book, emerging spatial modelling and network analysis techniques have significant potential to contribute in the domain of spatial epidemiology by adding greater validity and reliability to such studies. More accurate measures will help resolve some of the ambiguities in knowledge arising from existing empirical studies. A more reliable model of socio-spatial distribution of health is a holistic one, which includes not only genetic, physiologic, lifestyle and social factors but also the built and natural environmental factors that shape behaviour and channel the interactions between exogenous and endogenous influences on health. Of special importance is the need to develop a perceptional behavioural theory – about how the built environment directly or indirectly modifies behaviour, lifestyle and social interactions and thereby health. The validity of the strength, direction and significance of associations in most studies may be further enhanced if corresponding retrospective data on health-influencing lifestyle and behaviour can also be collected and included in the models. In other words, in addition to the inclusion of measures of density of services and physical accessibility in epidemiological models, survey data on actual service utilization, objectively assessed physical activity (including within-household activity, transport and leisure activity measured through accelerometry) and eating behaviour (consumption of fresh versus fast food and calorific values) have the potential to enhance the methodological rigour of studies.

Secondly, studies are needed that employ a life-course approach to health for more reliable evidence (Ben-Shlomo and Kuh, 2002). In this direction, longitudinal study design would include not only prospective data on health and socio-demographic variables, but retrospective spatial data on the built and natural environment, compiled and integrated at individual and neighbourhood levels. Such studies have the potential to produce a more reliable assessment of the health impacts of sustained exposure to changes in the built environment. Furthermore, any environment–health model can benefit from significant increases in explanatory power to capture the unexplained variances in health by controlling for underlying genetic predispositions in addition to environmental and behavioural factors. In recent years, gene–environment (G–E) interaction models studying variances in disease after controlling for genetic variants and a set of environmental exposures have gained predominance (Hunter, 2005; Manolio et al., 2006). Genome-wide association studies (GWAS) have already provided considerable insights into the genetic and epigenetic complexities underlying chronic diseases by identifying the susceptibility loci for a diverse variety of traits (http://www.genome.gov/26525384). Introducing environmental risk factors within GWAS has the potential for robust causal inference, especially in terms of how the environment may play a role in modifying genetic risks. Thus, large-scale prospective G–E studies are presently required, as they have the potential to produce more reliable assessment of the health impacts of sustained environmental exposures, in terms both of significant increments in explanatory power and of causal inference (F.S. Collins, 2004; Manolio et al., 2006, 2012; Manolio and Collins, 2010). The UK Biobank is an example of a large-scale national resource which opens the door for such large-scale prospective G–E studies to unravel the interactions between genetic and environmental risks in disease aetiology (UK Biobank, 2007; R. Collins, 2012).

Thirdly, studies assessing the associations between neighbourhood built environment and health outcomes have generally depended upon regression-based approaches that essentially try to provide insights into complex interrelations between causal factors by identifying regularities (*lines/hyperplanes of best fit*) from a cloud of data points. Advanced statistical regression-based techniques such as multi-level modelling and discrete regression improve upon earlier regression approaches (linear, continuous, single level, etc.) and can, as we have shown, identify multi-level variances of contextual factors in both spatial and temporal domains. Nonetheless, causal inference in neighbourhood built environment–health studies still remains a considerable challenge. This is constrained primarily by the inherent systemic complexities operating in the public health domain. As highlighted in the urban health niche model, multiple multi-level factors, including physiological, genetic, social, behavioural, and built and natural environmental, may interact dynamically over time to produce health patterns in individuals and populations. Any single statistical approach will inevitably fail to take into account many aspects of such dynamic, often non-linear and reciprocal interactions (Galea et al., 2010). Other bottlenecks to unravelling causality include selective migration, cross-level interactions, and the confusion with mediating versus confounding effects of many of the individual and lifestyle variables in regression models (Diez Roux, 2002, 2004a). Such limitations in identifying disease aetiology can be gradually deconstructed by judicious use of the kinds of statistical techniques and dynamic research designs mentioned and also triangulation with qualitative data. Hybrid techniques can also bring quantitative and qualitative approaches together, for example agent-based complex adaptive systems models (N. Pearce and Merletti, 2006; Auchincloss and Diez Roux, 2008; Galea et al., 2010); and non-regression techniques such as dynamic equation models (Homer and Hirsch, 2006) and Bayesian network models can unravel associations and causality using analytical and probability techniques.

As a concluding thought experiment, a coupled four-tier suite of epidemiological models may be employed for a more accurate interpretation of causation, somewhat along the lines of the one proposed by Auchincloss and Diez Roux (2008). The first tier might consist of regression models on a large scale (large n) to identify the lines of fit and the determining variables. With large n models fitted to survey data we can recover the kind of weak but significant effects that we would predict of built environment factors. A second tier would comprise multi-level and structural equation models that aim to measure contextual and temporal variability and to add insights into causal pathways. Agent-based complex adaptive system models would constitute a third tier, deriving their inputs from the second tier of models. The main function of these individualistic models would be to conduct exploratory iterations and subsequent optimization of causal network pathways along which the multiple multi-level health-defining agents function. Such models would identify spatial urban health niches as a basis for making informed and targeted policy decisions. Software for agent-based modelling (Gilbert, 2007) such as Repast, Swarm and MASON may be customized for specific epidemiological applications. Drawing their inputs from the third tier, differential equation-based dynamic equation models in the uppermost tier would be used to simulate population-level processes, thereby providing deeper insights into the formation of *coalesced health niches*.

Another way to explore more effective causal modelling of urban health niches would be to devise case-controlled study designs with the objective of assessing the beneficial or detrimental effects of specific built environment attributes upon vulnerable versus normal individuals. Some authors advocate randomized controlled trials in order to study the health effects of differential built environments (Oakes, 2004). Although cost, logistics, politics and ethics make such designs problematic in practice, it may be that in certain circumstances they can be specifically employed at a smaller scale to study the effects of different micro-built environment configurations, for example in rehabilitation and recuperation of populations with varying degrees of disease prevalence. A comparatively more practical approach is to conduct prospective within-city, between-neighbourhood and between-cities, regional-level studies, including natural experiments testing before and after interventions.

A risk of writing a book such as this is that, by employing the medical language of public health scientists in some chapters, we lose or alienate urban planning readers, just as the methodological discussion about spatial analysis and urban form may disinterest public health and epidemiology readers. There is no other book, as far as we know, that gives an advanced, professional-level treatment of both fields, and we would like to think that our attempt to bring the two fields together may spark a deeper level of scholarly and practical engagement driven by a new cross-disciplinary appreciation.

What might urban planners make of a more rigorous evidence base for healthy city planning? We have commented on this at various stages in the book and earlier in this chapter. From an urban planner's perspective, the challenge is to devise effective interventions that may be expected, with some degree of probability, to improve the health of a city's residents. In this regard, the empirical chapters highlight the fact that there are *weak* but nonetheless *significant* associations between health and several policy-relevant attributes of built environmental configuration. Planners presenting high-density and mixed-use schemes to funders and city governments can and should argue their case with reference to health effects. There seems to be evidence, from multiple studies, for example, that mixed land uses tend to encourage walking and lower population obesity incidence, but that non-residential land uses if clustered into homogeneous blocks that are too large can act as barriers. This has important implications for the scale and spatial arrangement of land use mixing. We have found evidence in our own models that, for at least one population of elderly men, greater distance to green spaces tends to lower obesity – presumably because the walk to the facility is more important for physical health than the time spent in the facility (which may well involve sitting down). We have shown also that the topological structure of a neighbourhood's or whole city's road grid itself has an effect on physical and mental health. This is the most profound specific new insight developed and evidenced in this book, although it may not be the easiest to turn into practical advice for urban planners without more studies, particularly with larger numbers. The fundamental proposition, which we have tested as various-scale and health-outcome-specific hypotheses, is that being connected to other people and spaces and the opportunities for social and economic transactions that they provide *matters*. It matters for health as it matters for the economy, society and the polity. After all, as we emphasized in our first chapter, cities exist because of the advantages of human co-location. Apparently, the spatial patterns of that co-location have a bearing on individual and thence public health, just as they have a bearing on the economic efficiency or energy efficiency of a city. Urban configuration matters in optimizing urban health. The population and building density have long been known to affect public health, and so does the density of health care services or parks and gardens; but at the same time, independently of those effects, the density, shape and connectivity of the road and other communication channels through which human interactions are conveyed influence the health of a city's population.

Larger-scale studies are needed to extend these findings. The UK Biobank is a flagship epidemiology programme collecting data for half a million respondents. It is composed of more than 500000 individuals aged

40–69 years and living within 25 miles of any of the 21 study assessment centres spread all over the UK. The authors currently have a UK Biobank built environment project grant and an ESRC transformative research project grant to create a spatial database for the programme, adding a set of approximately 100 robust objectively measured morphometric variables for each of the 500 000 cohort members. These will include the same range of specific and general accessibility indicators used in the studies in this book, created following the sDNA-UH model and employing the sDNA tool. This will create a scientific basis for the largest study ever conducted of gene–(built) environment effects on individual health. From it, researchers will be able to test with consistent concepts, data, models and analysis all of the main hypotheses and findings emerging from the field surveyed in this book, and test them on a scale that will be able to identify the multiple weak but significant effects that will allow urban planners and public health planners to work together with a new understanding based on shared models and evidence.

Appendices

APPENDIX 1: ITEMS OF THE GENERAL HEALTH QUESTIONNAIRE (GHQ-30) SCALE

Serial no.	Items
1.	Could not concentrate
2.	Lost sleep
3.	Restless nights
4.	Not busy or occupied
5.	Not out of the house
6.	Not managing well
7.	Not doing things well
8.	Not satisfied with task
9.	No warmth and affection
10.	Could not get on with others
11.	Not chatting with others
12.	Not playing a useful part
13.	Could not make decisions
14.	Felt under strain
15.	Could not overcome difficulties
16.	Found life a struggle
17.	Not enjoying activities
18.	Taking things hard
19.	Scared or panicky
20.	Could not face problems
21.	Felt everything on top
22.	Unhappy or depressed
23.	Lost confidence
24.	Felt worthless
25.	Felt life hopeless
26.	Not hopeful about future
27.	Not feeling happy
28.	Nervous and strung up
29.	Felt life not worth living
30.	Nerves too bad

Note: Each of the items was assessed on a four-point scale, and the item scores were added together to produce the overall GHQ-30 score.

Source: Huppert et al. (1989, p. 179).

APPENDIX 2: ITEMS OF THE HOSPITAL ANXIETY AND DEPRESSION SCALE (HADS)

Anxiety items	Depression items
1. I feel tense or wound up.	2. I still enjoy the things I used to enjoy.
3. I get a sort of frightened feeling as if something awful is about to happen.	4. I can laugh and see the funny side of things.
5. Worrying thoughts go through my mind.	6. I feel cheerful.
7. I can sit at ease and feel relaxed.	8. I feel as if I am slowed down.
9. I get a sort of frightened feeling like 'butterflies' in the stomach.	10. I have lost interest in my appearance.
11. I feel restless as if I have to be on the move.	12. I look forward with enjoyment to things.
13. I get sudden feelings of panic.	14. I can enjoy a good book or TV programme.

Source: Moorey et al. (1991, p. 257).

References

Adam, E.K. and Chase-Lansdale, P.L. (2002), 'Home sweet home(s): parental separations, residential moves, and adjustment problems in low-income adolescent girls', *Developmental Psychology*, **38**, 792.

Addo, J., Smeeth, L. and Leon, D.A. (2007), 'Hypertension in sub-Saharan Africa: a systematic review', *Hypertension*, **50**, 1012–18.

Alker, H.S. (1969), 'A typology of ecological fallacies', in M. Dogan and S. Rokkan (eds), *Quantitative Ecological Analysis*, Cambridge, MA: MIT Press.

Allender, S. and Rayner, M. (2007), 'The burden of overweight and obesity-related ill health in the UK', *Obesity Reviews*, **8**, 467–73.

Allender, S., Foster, C., Scarborough, P. and Rayner, M. (2007), 'The burden of physical activity-related ill health in the UK', *Journal of Epidemiology and Community Health*, **61**, 344–8.

Allman-Farinelli, M.A., Chey, T., Merom, D., Bowles, H. and Bauman, A.E. (2009), 'The effects of age, birth cohort and survey period on leisure-time physical activity by Australian adults: 1990–2005', *British Journal of Nutrition*, **101**, 609–17.

Alonso, W. (1971), 'The economics of urban size', *Regional Science Association Papers*, **26**, 68–83.

Anderson, H.R. and Cook, D.G. (1997), 'Passive smoking and sudden infant death syndrome: review of the epidemiological evidence', *Thorax*, **52**, 1003–09.

Aneshensel, C.S., Wight, R.G., Miller-Martinez, D., Botticello, A.L., Karlamangla, A.S. and Seeman, T.E. (2007), 'Urban neighborhoods and depressive symptoms among older adults', *Journals of Gerontology, Series B: Psychological Sciences and Social Sciences*, **62**, S52–9.

Appleyard, D. and Lintell, M. (1972), 'The environmental quality of city streets', *Journal of the American Institute of Planners*, **38**, 84–101.

Araya, R., Montgomery, A., Rojas, G., Fritsch, R., Solis, J., Signorelli, A. and Lewis, G. (2007), 'Common mental disorders and the built environment in Santiago, Chile', *British Journal of Psychiatry*, **190**, 394–401.

Auchincloss, A.H. and Diez Roux, A.V. (2008), 'A new tool for epidemiology: the usefulness of dynamic-agent models in understanding place effects on health', *American Journal of Epidemiology*, **168**, 1–8.

Aylin, P., Morris, S., Wakefield, J., Grossinho, A., Jarup, L. and Elliott, P. (2001), 'Temperature, housing, deprivation and their relationship to excess winter mortality in Great Britain, 1986–1996', *International Journal of Epidemiology*, **30**, 1100–1108.

Babisch, W. (2000), 'Traffic noise and cardiovascular disease: epidemiological review and synthesis', *Noise and Health*, **2**, 9–32.

Babisch, W., Ising, H., Gallacher, J.E.J., Elwood, P.C., Sweetnam, P.M., Yarnell, J.W.G., Bainton, D. and Baker, I.A. (1990), 'Traffic noise, work noise and cardiovascular risk factors: the Caerphilly and Speedwell collaborative heart disease studies', *Environment International*, **16**, 425–35.

Babisch, W., Ising, H., Gallacher, J.E.J., Sweetnam, P.M. and Elwood, P.C. (1999), 'Traffic noise and cardiovascular risk: the Caerphilly and Speedwell studies, third phase – 10-year follow up', *Archives of Environmental Health*, **54**, 210–16.

Bafna, S. (2003), 'Space syntax: a brief introduction to its logic and analytical techniques', *Environment and Behavior*, **35**, 17–29.

Bairoch, P. (1988), *Cities and Economic Development: From the Dawn of History to the Present*, Chicago: University of Chicago Press.

Baker, M., McNicholas, A., Garrett, N., Jones, N., Stewart, J., Koberstein, V. and Lennon, D. (2000), 'Household crowding a major risk factor for epidemic meningococcal disease in Auckland children', *Pediatric Infectious Disease Journal*, **19**, 983–90.

Balfour, J.L. and Kaplan, G.J. (2002), 'Neighborhood environment and loss of physical function in older adults: evidence from the Alameda County Study', *American Journal of Epidemiology*, **155**, 507–15.

Ball, K., Lamb, K., Travaglini, N. and Ellaway, A. (2012), 'Street connectivity and obesity in Glasgow, Scotland: impact of age, sex and socioeconomic position', *Health and Place*, **18**, 1307–13.

Bandyopadhyay, A. and Merchant, A.N. (2006), 'Space syntax analysis of colonial houses in India', *Environment and Planning B: Planning and Design*, **33**, 923–42.

Baran, P.K., Rodríguez, D.A. and Khattak, A.J. (2008), 'Space syntax and walking in a New Urbanist and suburban neighbourhoods', *Journal of Urban Design*, **13**, 5–28.

Barker, D.J.P. (1994), *Mothers, Babies, and Disease in Later Life*, London: BMJ Publishing Group.

Bartlett, S. (1998), 'Does inadequate housing perpetuate children's poverty?', *Childhood*, **5**, 403–20.

Barton, H. (2009), 'Land use planning and health and well-being', *Land Use Policy*, **26**, S115–23.

Barton, H. and Tsourou, C. (2000), *Healthy Urban Planning: A WHO Guide to Planning for People*, London: Spon Press.

Barton, H., Grant, M., Mitcham, C. and Tsourou, C. (2009), 'Healthy urban planning in European cities', *Health Promotion International*, **24**, i91–9.

Barton, J. and Pretty, J. (2010), 'What is the best dose of nature and green exercise for improving mental health? A multi-study analysis', *Environmental Science and Technology*, **44**, 3947–55.

Bassett, D.R., Jr, Pucher, J., Buehler, R., Thompson, D.L. and Crouter, S.E. (2008), 'Walking, cycling, and obesity rates in Europe, North America and Australia', *Journal of Physical Activity and Health*, **5**, 795–814.

Bassuk, S.S., Glass, T.A. and Berkman, L.F. (1999), 'Social disengagement and incident cognitive decline in community-dwelling elderly persons', *Annals of Internal Medicine*, **131**, 165.

Basu, R. and Samet, J.M. (1999), 'A review of the epidemiological evidence on health effects of nitrogen dioxide exposure from gas stoves', *Journal of Environmental Medicine*, **1**, 173–87.

Bates, A. (2006), 'Methodology used for producing ONS's small area population estimates', *Population Trends*, **125**, 30–36.

Baum, A. and Davis, G.E. (1980), 'Reducing the stress of high-density living: an architectural intervention', *Journal of Personality and Social Psychology*, **38**, 471–81.

Baum, A. and Valins, S. (1979), 'Crowding and the regulation of social contact', in L. Berkowitz (ed.), *Advances in Experimental Social Psychology*, vol. 12, New York: Academic Press.

Baum, F. and Palmer, C. (2002), '"Opportunity structures": urban landscape, social capital and health promotion in Australia', *Health Promotion International*, **17**, 351–61.

Baum, F., Bush, R.A., Modra, C.C., Murray, C.J., Cox, E.M., Alexander, K.M. and Potter, R.C. (2000), 'Epidemiology of participation: an Australian community study', *Journal of Epidemiology and Community Health*, **54**, 414–23.

Bauman, A., Ford, I. and Armstrong, T. (2001), *Trends in Population Levels of Reported Physical Activity in Australia, 1997, 1999 and 2000*, Canberra: Australian Sports Commission.

Bean, J.F., Vora, A. and Frontera, W.R. (2004), 'Benefits of exercise for community-dwelling older adults', *Archives of Physical Medicine and Rehabilitation*, **85**, S31–42.

Beauchemin, K.M. and Hays, P. (1996), 'Sunny hospital rooms expedite recovery from severe and refractory depressions', *Journal of Affective Disorders*, **40**, 49–51.

Bell, A.C., Ge, K. and Popkin, B.M. (2002), 'The road to obesity or the path to prevention: motorized transportation and obesity in China', *Obesity Research*, **10**, 277–83.

Bell, M.L., Davis, D.L. and Fletcher, T. (2004), 'A retrospective assessment of mortality from the London smog episode of 1952: the role of influenza and pollution', *Environmental Health Perspectives*, **112**, 6–8.

Bellinger, D., Leviton, A., Waternaux, C., Needleman, H. and Rabinowitz, M. (1988), 'Low-level lead exposure, social class, and infant development', *Neurotoxicology and Teratology*, **10**, 497–503.

Ben-Shlomo, Y. and Kuh, D. (2002), 'A life course approach to chronic disease epidemiology: conceptual models, empirical challenges and interdisciplinary perspectives', *International Journal of Epidemiology*, **31**, 285–93.

Berke, E.M., Gottlieb, L.M., Moudon, A.V. and Larson, E.B. (2007), 'Protective association between neighborhood walkability and depression in older men', *Journal of the American Geriatrics Society*, **55**, 526–33.

Berke, E.M., Koepsell, T.D., Moudon, A.V., Hoskins, R.E. and Larson, E.B. (2007), 'Association of the built environment with physical activity and obesity in older persons', *American Journal of Public Health*, **97**, 486–92.

Berkman, L.F. and Kawachi, I. (2000), 'A historical framework for social epidemiology', in L.F. Berkman and I. Kawachi (eds), *Social Epidemiology*, New York: Oxford University Press.

Bernard, P., Charafeddine, R., Frohlich, K.L., Daniel, M., Kestens, Y. and Potvin, L. (2007), 'Health inequalities and place: a theoretical conception of neighbourhood', *Social Science and Medicine*, **65**, 1839–52.

Bernstein, K.T., Galea, S., Ahern, J., Tracy, M. and Vlahov, D. (2007), 'The built environment and alcohol consumption in urban neighborhoods', *Drug and Alcohol Dependence*, **91**, 244.

Besser, L.M. and Dannenberg, A.L. (2005), 'Walking to public transit: steps to help meet physical activity recommendations', *American Journal of Preventive Medicine*, **29**, 273–80.

Bierman, C.W. (1996), 'Environmental control of asthma', *Immunology and Allergy Clinics of North America*, **16**, 753–64.

Billings, C.G. and Howard, P. (1998), 'Damp housing and asthma', *Monaldi Archives of Chest Disease*, **53**, 43–9.

Bithell, J. (2006), 'An application of density estimation to geographical epidemiology', *Statistics in Medicine*, **9**, 691–701.

Björk, J., Albin, M., Grahn, P., Jacobsson, H., Ardö, J., Wadbro, J. and Ostergren, P.O. (2008), 'Recreational values of the natural environment in relation to neighbourhood satisfaction, physical activity, obesity and wellbeing', *Journal of Epidemiology and Community Health*, **62**.

Black, J.L., Macinko, J., Dixon, L.B. and Fryer, J.G.E. (2010), 'Neighborhoods and obesity in New York City', *Health and Place*, **16**, 489–99.

Blalock, H.M. and Wilken, P.H. (1979), *Intergroup Processes: A Micro–Macro Perspective*, New York: Free Press.

Blane, D., Mitchell, R. and Bartley, M. (2000), 'The "inverse housing law" and respiratory health', *Journal of Epidemiology and Community Health*, **54**, 745–9.

Blaxter, M. (1990), *Health and Lifestyles*, London: Tavistock/Routledge.

Bloom, D.E., Canning, D. and Fink, G. (2008), 'Urbanization and the wealth of nations', *Science*, **319**, 772–5.

BMA (2003), *Housing and Health: Building for the Future*, London: British Medical Association.

BMJ (1980), 'Blows from the winter wind', *British Medical Journal*, **280**, 137–8.

Boehmer, T.K., Hoehner, C.M., Deshpande, A.D., Brennan Ramirez, L.K. and Brownson, R.C. (2007), 'Perceived and observed neighborhood indicators of obesity among urban adults', *International Journal of Obesity*, **31**, 968–77.

Boer, R., Zheng, Y., Overton, A., Ridgeway, G.K. and Cohen, D.A. (2007), 'Neighborhood design and walking trips in ten U.S. metropolitan areas', *American Journal of Preventive Medicine*, **32**, 298–304.

Booth, C. (1889), *Life and Labour of the People*, first series (i): *East, Central and South London*, London: Macmillan (republished 1969).

Boyce, P.R. (1981), *Human Factors in Lighting*, London: Applied Science Publishers.

Branfman, E., Cohen, B. and Trubek, D. (1974), 'Measuring the invisible wall: land use controls and residential patterns of the poor', in D. Listokin (ed.), *Land Use Controls: Present Problems and Future Reform*, New Brunswick, NJ: Center for Urban Policy Research, Rutgers University.

Brauer, M., Hoek, G., Van Vliet, P., Meliefste, K., Fischer, P.H., Wijga, A., Koopman, L.P., Neijens, H.J., Gerritsen, J. and Kerkhof, M. (2002), 'Air pollution from traffic and the development of respiratory infections and asthmatic and allergic symptoms in children', *American Journal of Respiratory and Critical Care Medicine*, **166**, 1092–8.

Briggs, R. and Leonard, W.A., IV (1977), 'Mortality and ecological structure: a canonical approach', *Social Science and Medicine*, **11**, 757–62.

Britton, M., Fox, A.J., Goldblatt, P., Jones, G.R. and Rosato, M. (1990), *The Influence of Socio-economic and Environmental Factors on Geographic Variations in Mortality in OPCS*, London: HMSO.

Brown, B.B. and Werner, C.M. (2008), 'Before and after a new light rail stop: resident attitudes, travel behavior, and obesity', *Journal of the American Planning Association*, **75**, 5–12.

Brown, B.B., Yamada, I., Smith, K.R., Zick, C.D., Kowaleski-Jones,

L. and Fan, J.X. (2009), 'Mixed land use and walkability: variations in land use measures and relationships with BMI, overweight, and obesity', *Health and Place*, **15**, 1130–41.

Brown, S.C., Mason, C.A., Lombard, J.L., Martinez, F., Plater-Zyberk, E., Spokane, A.R., Newman, F.L., Pantin, H. and Szapocznik, J. (2009), 'The relationship of built environment to perceived social support and psychological distress in Hispanic elders: the role of "eyes on the street"', *Journals of Gerontology, Series B: Psychological Sciences and Social Sciences*, **64**, 234–46.

Brown, W.J. (2012), 'MCMC estimation in MLwiN v2.25', Centre for Multilevel Modelling, University of Bristol.

Brownson, R.C., Hoehner, C.M., Day, K., Forsyth, A. and Sallis, J.F. (2009), 'Measuring the built environment for physical activity: state of the science', *American Journal of Preventive Medicine*, **36**, S99–123.e12.

Buliung, R.N. and Kanaroglou, P.S. (2006), 'Urban form and household activity – travel behavior', *Growth and Change*, **37**, 172–99.

Burdette, H.L. and Whitaker, R.C. (2004), 'Neighborhood playgrounds, fast food restaurants, and crime: relationships to overweight in low-income preschool children', *Preventive Medicine*, **38**, 57–63.

Burgoine, T., Alvanides, S. and Lake, A.A. (2011), 'Assessing the obesogenic environment of North East England', *Health and Place*, **17**, 738–47.

Burr, M., St Leger, A. and Yarnell, J. (1981), 'Wheezing, dampness, and coal fires', *Journal of Public Health*, **3**, 205–09.

Buzzelli, M. and Su, J. (2006), 'Multi-level modelling in health research: a caution and rejoinder on temporally mismatched data', *Social Science and Medicine*, **62**, 1215–18.

Caballero, B. (2007), 'The global epidemic of obesity: an overview', *Epidemiologic Reviews*, **29**, 1–5.

CABE (2000), *By Design – Urban Design in the Planning System: Towards Better Practice*, London: Commission for Architecture and the Built Environment and Department of the Environment, Transport and the Regions.

CABE (2007), *Paved with Gold: The Real Value of Street Design*, London: Commission for Architecture and the Built Environment.

Cal/EPA (1997), *Health Effects of Exposure to Environmental Tobacco Smoke*, Smoking and Tobacco Control Monograph 10, Sacramento: Office of Environmental Health Hazard Assessment, California Environmental Protection Agency.

Canada Mortgage and Housing Corporation (1991), *Core Housing Need in Canada*, Ottawa: Canadian Government Printing.

Canadian Institute for Health Information (2006), *How Healthy Are Rural Canadians? An Assessment of Their Health Status and Health*

Determinants: Summary Report, Ottawa: Canadian Institute for Health Information.

Canguilhem, G. (1966), *Le normal et le pathologique*, Paris: Presses Universitaires de France.

Caspi, A., Taylor, A., Moffitt, T.E. and Plomin, R. (2000), 'Neighborhood deprivation affects children's mental health: environmental risks identified in a genetic design', *Psychological Science*, **11**, 338–42.

Cassel, J. (1976), 'The contribution of social epidemiology to host resistance', *American Journal of Epidemiology*, **104**, 107–23.

Cassel, J., Patrick, R. and Jenkins, D. (1960), 'Epidemiological analysis of health implications of cultural change: a conceptual model', *Annals of the New York Academy of Sciences*, **84**, 938–49.

Caughy, M.O., O'Campo, P.J. and Patterson, J. (2001), 'A brief observational measure for urban neighborhoods', *Health and Place*, **7**, 225–36.

Cerin, E., Leslie, E., Toit, L., Owen, N. and Frank, L.D. (2007), 'Destinations that matter: associations with walking for transport', *Health and Place*, **13**, 713–24.

Cerin, E., Macfarlane, D.J., Ko, H.H. and Chan, K.C.A. (2007), 'Measuring perceived neighbourhood walkability in Hong Kong', *Cities*, **24**, 209–17.

Cerin, E., Leslie, E., Owen, N. and Bauman, A. (2008), 'An Australian version of the neighborhood environment walkability scale: validity evidence', *Measurement in Physical Education and Exercise Science*, **12**, 31–51.

Cervero, R. (1988), 'Land-use mixing and suburban mobility', *Transportation Quarterly*, **42**, 429–46.

Cervero, R. (1989), *America's Suburban Centers: The Land Use–Transportation Link*, Boston, MA: Unwin-Hyman.

Cervero, R. (1996), 'Mixed land-uses and commuting: evidence from the American housing survey', *Transportation Research Part A: Policy and Practice*, **30**, 361–77.

Cervero, R. and Duncan, M. (2003), 'Walking, bicycling, and urban landscapes: evidence from the San Francisco Bay Area', *American Journal of Public Health*, **93**, 1478–83.

Cervero, R. and Kockelman, K. (1997), 'Travel demand and the 3Ds: density, diversity, and design', *Transportation Research Part D: Transport and Environment*, **2**, 199–219.

Chadwick, E. (1842), *Report on the Sanitary Condition of the Labouring Population of Great Britain*, Edinburgh: Edinburgh University Press (reprinted 1965).

Challen, A., King, D., Knapp, M. and McNally, S. (2008), *Foresight Mental Capital and Wellbeing Project: The Economic Consequences of*

Specific Learning Difficulties and the Cost-Effectiveness of Prevention Strategies, London: Government Office for Science.

Chandola, T. (2001), 'The fear of crime and area differences in health', *Health and Place*, **7**, 105–16.

Chiaradia, A., Hillier, B., Barnes, Y. and Schwander, C. (2009), 'Residential property value in London: space syntax spatial analysis', in *Proceedings of the 7th International Space Syntax Symposium*, Stockholm: Royal Institute of Technology (KTH).

Chiaradia, A., Hillier, B., Schwander, C. and Wedderburn, M. (2012), 'Compositional and urban form effects on centres in Greater London', *Proceedings of the ICE – Urban Design and Planning*, **165**, 21–42.

Chiaradia, A.J., Webster, C. and Crispin, C. (2012), 'sDNA: a software for spatial design network analysis, 1.7 specifications', available at: http://www.cardiff.ac.uk/sdna/.

Chiesura, A. (2004), 'The role of urban parks for the sustainable city', *Landscape and Urban Planning*, **68**, 129–38.

Clifton, K.J., Livi Smith, A.D. and Rodriguez, D. (2007), 'The development and testing of an audit for the pedestrian environment', *Landscape and Urban Planning*, **80**, 95–110.

Coetzee, N., Yach, D. and Joubert, G. (1988), 'Crowding and alcohol abuse as risk factors for tuberculosis in the Mamre population: results of a case-control study', *South African Medical Journal*, **74**, 352–4.

Cohen, D., Spear, M., Scribner, R., Kissenger, P., Mason, M. and Wildgen, J. (2000), '"Broken windows" and the risk of gonorrhea', *American Journal of Public Health*, **90**, 230–36.

Cohen, D.A., Mason, C., Bedimo, A., Scribner, R., Basolo, V. and Farley, T.A. (2003), 'Neighborhood physical conditions and health', *American Journal of Public Health*, **93**, 467–71.

Cohen, S. (2004), 'Social relationships and health', *American Psychologist*, **59**, 676–84.

Cohen, S., Evans, G.W., Stokols, D. and Krantz, D.S. (1986), *Behavior, Health, and Environmental Stress*, New York: Plenum Press.

Collins, F.S. (2004), 'The case for a US prospective cohort study of genes and environment', *Nature*, **429**, 475–7.

Collins, K.J. (1993), 'Cold and heat-related illnesses in the indoor environment', in R. Burridge and D. Ormandy (eds), *Unhealthy Housing: Research, Remedies and Reform*, New York: Spon Press.

Collins, R. (2012), 'What makes UK Biobank special?', *Lancet*, **379**, 1173–4.

Committee on Health Risks of Exposure to Radon (1999), *Health Effects of Exposure to Radon: BEIR VI*, Washington, DC: National Academies Press.

Comptroller and Auditor General (2010), *Management of NHS Hospital Productivity*, London: National Audit Office.

Cook, D.G. and Strachan, D.P. (1997), 'Health effects of passive smoking. 3. Parental smoking and prevalence of respiratory symptoms and asthma in school age children', *Thorax*, **52**, 1081–94.

Corburn, J. (2004), 'Confronting the challenges in reconnecting urban planning and public health', *American Journal of Public Health*, **94**, 541–6.

Corcoran, E., Nellemann, C., Baker, E., Bos, R., Osborn, D. and Savelli, H. (2010), *Sick Water? The Central Role of Wastewater Management in Sustainable Development*, Arendal, Norway: United Nations Environment Programme, UN-Habitat and GRID-Arendal.

Craig, C.L., Brownson, R.C., Cragg, S.E. and Dunn, A.L. (2002), 'Exploring the effect of the environment on physical activity: a study examining walking to work', *American Journal of Preventive Medicine*, **23**, 36–43.

Crucitti, P., Latora, V. and Porta, S. (2006a), 'Centrality in networks of urban streets', *Chaos*, **16**, 015113.

Crucitti, P., Latora, V. and Porta, S. (2006b), 'Centrality measures in spatial networks of urban streets', *Physical Review E*, **73**, 036125.

Cummins, S.K. and Jackson, R.J. (2001), 'The built environment and children's health', *Pediatric Clinics of North America*, **48**, 1241–52.

Cunningham, G.O., Michael, Y.L., Farquhar, S.A. and Lapidus, J. (2005), 'Developing a reliable senior walking environmental assessment tool', *American Journal of Preventive Medicine*, **29**, 215–17.

Curtis, C. and Scheurer, J. (2010), 'Planning for sustainable accessibility: developing tools to aid discussion and decision-making', *Progress in Planning*, **74**, 53–106.

Curwen, M. (1991), 'Excess winter mortality: a British phenomenon?', *Health Trends*, **22**, 169–75.

Cutumisu, N. and Spence, J.C. (2009), 'Exploring associations between urban environments and children's physical activity: making the case for space syntax', *Journal of Science and Medicine in Sport*, **12**, 537–8.

Dadvand, P., de Nazelle, A., Figueras, F., Basagaña, X., Su, J., Amoly, E., Jerrett, M., Vrijheid, M., Sunyer, J. and Nieuwenhuijsen, M.J. (2012), 'Green space, health inequality and pregnancy', *Environment International*, **40**, 110–15.

Dales, R., Liu, L., Wheeler, A.J. and Gilbert, N.L. (2008), 'Quality of indoor residential air and health', *Canadian Medical Association Journal*, **179**, 147–52.

Dannenberg, A.L., Jackson, R.J., Frumkin, H., Schieber, R.A., Pratt, M., Kochtitzky, C. and Tilson, H.H. (2003), 'The impact of community design and land-use choices on public health: a scientific research agenda', *American Journal of Public Health*, **93**, 1500–1508.

Darby, S.C. and Hill, D.C. (2003), 'Health effects of residential radon: a European perspective at the end of 2002', *Radiation Protection Dosimetry*, **104**, 321–9.

Darby, S., Hill, D. and Doll, R. (2001), 'Radon: a likely carcinogen at all exposures', *Annals of Oncology*, **12**, 1341–51.

Davey Smith, G., Shipley, M., Hole, D.J., Hart, C.L., Watt, G.C.M., Gillis, C.R., Marmot, M.G. and Hawthorne, V. (1995), 'Explaining male mortality differentials between the West of Scotland and the South of England', abstract, *Journal of Epidemiology and Community Health*, **49**, 541.

Davey Smith, G., Hart, C., Watt, G., Hole, D. and Hawthorne, V. (1998), 'Individual social class, area-based deprivation, cardiovascular disease risk factors, and mortality: the Renfrew and Paisley study', *Journal of Epidemiology and Community Health*, **52**, 399–405.

Dawber, T.R. (1980), *The Framingham Study: The Epidemiology of Coronary Heart Disease*, Cambridge, MA: Harvard University Press.

Day, K., Boarnet, M., Alfonzo, M. and Forsyth, A. (2006), The Irvine–Minnesota Inventory to measure built environments: development', *American Journal of Preventive Medicine*, **30**, 144–52.

Dedman, D., Gunnell, D., Smith, G.D. and Frankel, S. (2001), 'Childhood housing conditions and later mortality in the Boyd Orr cohort', *Journal of Epidemiology and Community Health*, **55**, 10–15.

Delgard, O.S. and Tambs, K. (1997), 'Urban environment and mental health: a longitudinal study', *British Journal of Psychiatry*, **171**, 530–36.

Dengel, D.R., Hearst, M.O., Harmon, J.H., Forsyth, A. and Lytle, L.A. (2009), 'Does the built environment relate to the metabolic syndrome in adolescents?', *Health and Place*, **15**, 946–51.

Department of the Environment (1977a), *Inner Area Studies: Liverpool, Birmingham and Lambeth: Summaries of Consultant's Final Report*, London: HMSO.

Department of the Environment (1977b), *Unequal City: Final Report of the Birmingham Inner Area Study*, London: HMSO.

Department of the Environment (1977c), *White Paper: Policy for the Inner Cities*, Cmnd 6845, London: HMSO.

Department of Health (2005), *Choosing Activity: A Physical Activity Action Plan*, Cm 6374, London: Department of Health.

Department of Health (2008), *Healthy Weight, Healthy Lives: A Cross-Government Strategy for England*, London: Department of Health.

Department of Health and Social Security (1980), *Inequalities in Health: Report of a Working Group Chaired by Sir Douglas Black*, London: DHSS.

Diehr, P., Koepsell, T., Cheadle, A., Psaty, B.M., Wagner, E. and Curry, S. (1993), 'Do communities differ in health behaviors?', *Journal of Clinical Epidemiology*, **46**, 1141–9.

Diez-Roux, A.V. (1998), 'Bringing context back into epidemiology: variables and fallacies in multilevel analysis', *American Journal of Public Health*, **88**, 216–22.

Diez Roux, A.V. (2001), 'Investigating neighborhood and area effects on health', *American Journal of Public Health*, **91**, 1783–9.

Diez Roux, A.V. (2002), 'Invited commentary: places, people, and health', *American Journal of Epidemiology*, **155**, 516–19.

Diez Roux, A.V. (2004a), 'Estimating neighborhood health effects: the challenges of causal inference in a complex world', *Social Science and Medicine*, **58**, 1953–60.

Diez Roux, A.V. (2004b), 'The study of group-level factors in epidemiology: rethinking variables, study designs, and analytical approaches', *Epidemiologic Reviews*, **26**, 104–11.

Diez Roux, A.V. (2007), 'Integrating social and biologic factors in health research: a systems view', *Annals of Epidemiology*, **17**, 569–74.

Diez-Roux, A.V., Nieto, F.J., Muntaner, C., Tyroler, H.A., Comstock, G.W., Shahar, E., Cooper, L.S., Watson, R.L. and Szklo, M. (1997), 'Neighborhood environments and coronary heart disease: a multilevel analysis', *American Journal of Epidemiology*, **146**, 48–63.

Diez Roux, A.V., Merkin, S.S., Arnett, D., Chambless, L., Massing, M., Nieto, F.J., Sorlie, P., Szklo, M., Tyroler, H.A. and Watson, R.L. (2001), 'Neighborhood of residence and incidence of coronary heart disease', *New England Journal of Medicine*, **345**, 99–106.

Diez Roux, A.V., Evenson, K.R., McGinn, A.P., Brown, D.G., Moore, L., Brines, S. and Jacobs, D.R., Jr (2007), 'Availability of recreational resources and physical activity in adults', *American Journal of Public Health*, **97**, 493–9.

Doll, R. and Hill, A.B. (1950), 'Smoking and carcinoma of the lung: preliminary report', *British Medical Journal*, **2**, 739–48.

Doll, R. and Hill, A.B. (1956), 'Lung cancer and other causes of death in relation to smoking', *British Medical Journal*, **2**, 1071–81.

Doll, R. and Peto, R. (1981), *The Causes of Cancer: Quantitative Estimates of Avoidable Risks of Cancer in the United States Today*, Oxford: Oxford University Press.

Doyle, J.T., Dawber, T.R., Kannel, W.B., Heslin, A.S. and Kahn, H.A. (1962), 'Cigarette smoking and coronary heart disease', *New England Journal of Medicine*, **266**, 796–801.

Doyle, S., Kelly-Schwartz, A., Schlossberg, M. and Stockard, J. (2006), 'Active community environments and health: the relationship of walkable and safe communities to individual health', *Journal of the American Planning Association*, **72**, 19–32.

Drechsel, P., Scott, C.A., Raschid-Sally, L., Redwood, M. and Bahri, A. (2010), *Wastewater Irrigation and Health: Assessing and Mitigating Risk in Low-Income Countries*, London: Earthscan.

Duckitt, J. (1983), 'Household crowding and psychological well-being in a South African coloured community', *Journal of Social Psychology*, **121**, 231–8.

Duffy, J. (1990), *The Sanitarians: A History of American Public Health*, Chicago: University of Illinois Press.

Duhl, L.J. and Sanchez, A.K. (1999), *Healthy Cities and the City Planning Process: A Background Document on the Links between Health and Urban Planning*, Copenhagen: World Health Organization.

Duncan, C., Jones, K. and Moon, G. (1993), 'Do places matter? A multilevel analysis of regional variations in health-related behaviour in Britain', *Social Science and Medicine*, **37**, 725–33.

Duncan, C., Jones, K. and Moon, G. (1995), 'Psychiatric morbidity: a multilevel approach to regional variations in the UK', *Journal of Epidemiology and Community Health*, **49**, 290–95.

Duncan, C., Jones, K. and Moon, G. (1998), 'Context, composition and heterogeneity: using multilevel models in health research', *Social Science and Medicine*, **46**, 97–117.

Duncan, M. and Mummery, K. (2005), 'Psychosocial and environmental factors associated with physical activity among city dwellers in regional Queensland', *Preventive Medicine*, **40**, 363–72.

Dunstan, F., Weaver, N., Araya, R., Bell, T., Lannon, S., Lewis, G., Patterson, J., Thomas, H., Jones, P. and Palmer, S. (2005), 'An observation tool to assist with the assessment of urban residential environments', *Journal of Environmental Psychology*, **25**, 293–305.

Eames, M., Ben-Shlomo, Y. and Marmot, M.G. (1993), 'Social deprivation and premature mortality: regional comparison across England', *British Medical Journal*, **307**, 1097–1102.

Eastwood, P. (2010), *Statistics on Obesity, Physical Activity and Diet: England, 2010*, Leeds: NHS Information Centre, Lifestyles Statistics.

Ebbeling, C.B., Pawlak, D.B. and Ludwig, D.S. (2002), 'Childhood obesity: public-health crisis, common sense cure', *Lancet*, **360**, 473–82.

Echeverria, S.E., Diez-Roux, A.V. and Link, B.G. (2004), 'Reliability of self-reported neighborhood characteristics', *Journal of Urban Health*, **81**, 682–701.

Editorial (2009), 'Editorial – what is health? The ability to adapt', *Lancet*, **373**, 781.

Edwards, J.N., Edwards, P.K. and Booth, A. (1982), 'Housing type, stress, and family relations', *Social Forces*, **61**, 241–57.
Edwards, R.D. (2008), 'Public transit, obesity, and medical costs: assessing the magnitudes', *Preventive Medicine*, **46**, 14–21.
Ellaway, A. and Macintyre, S. (1998), 'Does housing tenure predict health in the UK because it exposes people to different levels of housing related hazards in the home or its surroundings?', *Health and Place*, **4**, 141–50.
Ellaway, A., Macintyre, S. and Bonnefoy, X. (2005), 'Graffiti, greenery, and obesity in adults: secondary analysis of European cross sectional survey', *British Medical Journal*, **331**, 611–12.
Elliott, S.J., Cole, D.C., Krueger, P., Voorberg, N. and Wakefield, S. (1999), 'The power of perception: health risk attributed to air pollution in an urban industrial neighbourhood', *Risk Analysis*, **19**, 621–34.
Ellis, C.D., Lee, S.W. and Kweon, B.S. (2006), 'Retail land use, neighborhood satisfaction and the urban forest: an investigation into the moderating and mediating effects of trees and shrubs', *Landscape and Urban Planning*, **74**, 70–78.
Elton, C. (1927), *Animal Ecology*, London: Sidgwick & Jackson.
Elton, P. and Packer, J. (1986), 'A prospective randomised trial of the value of rehousing on the grounds of mental ill-health', *Journal of Chronic Diseases*, **39**, 221–7.
Elwood, P.C. (1984), 'Caerphilly and Speedwell collaborative heart disease studies', *Journal of Epidemiology and Community Health*, **38**, 259–62.
Emery, J., Crump, C. and Bors, P. (2003), 'Reliability and validity of two instruments designed to assess the walking and bicycling suitability of sidewalks and roads', *American Journal of Health Promotion*, **18**, 38–46.
Engels, F. ([1845] 1987), *The Condition of the Working Class in England*, Harmondsworth: Penguin Books.
Enström, R. and Netzell, O. (2008), 'Can space syntax help us in understanding the intraurban office rent pattern? Accessibility and rents in downtown Stockholm', *Journal of Real Estate Finance and Economics*, **36**, 289–305.
Eurostat (1996), *The European Community Household Panel (ECHP): Survey Methodology and Implementation*, Luxembourg: Office for Official Publications of the European Union.
Evans, A.S. (1976), 'Causation and disease: the Henle–Koch postulates revisited', *Yale Journal of Biology and Medicine*, **49**, 175–95.
Evans, B., Crookes, L. and Coaffee, J. (2012), 'Obesity/fatness and the city: critical urban geographies', *Geography Compass*, **6**, 100–110.
Evans, G.W. and Kantrowitz, E. (2002), 'Socioeconomic status and health: the potential role of environmental risk exposure', *Annual Review of Public Health*, **23**, 303–31.

Evans, G.W. and Lepore, S.J. (1993), 'Household crowding and social support: a quasiexperimental analysis', *Journal of Personality and Social Psychology*, **65**, 308–16.

Evans, G.W. and Maxwell, L. (1997), 'Chronic noise exposure and reading deficits: the mediating effects of language acquisition', *Environment and Behavior*, **29**, 638–56.

Evans, G.W., Palsane, M.N., Lepore, S.J. and Martin, J. (1989), 'Residential density and psychological health: the mediating effects of social support', *Journal of Personality and Social Psychology*, **57**, 994.

Evans, G.W., Hygge, S. and Bullinger, M. (1995), 'Chronic noise and psychological stress', *Psychological Science*, **6**, 333–9.

Evans, G.W., Lepore, S.J. and Schroeder, A. (1996), 'The role of interior design elements in human responses to crowding', *Journal of Personality and Social Psychology*, **70**, 41–6.

Evans, G.W., Wells, N.M., Chan, H.Y.E. and Saltzmand, H. (2000), 'Housing quality and mental health', *Journal of Consulting and Clinical Psychology*, **68**, 526–30.

Evans, G.W., Kantrowitz, E. and Eshelman, P. (2002), 'Housing quality and psychological well-being among the elderly population', *Journals of Gerontology, Series B: Psychological Sciences and Social Sciences*, **57**, P381–3.

Evans, G.W., Lercher, P. and Kofler, W.W. (2002), 'Crowding and children's mental health: the role of house type', *Journal of Environmental Psychology*, **22**, 221–31.

Evans, G.W., Wells, N.M. and Moch, A. (2003), 'Housing and mental health: a review of the evidence and a methodological and conceptual critique', *Journal of Social Issues*, **59**, 475–500.

Evans, J., Hyndman, S., Stewart-Brown, S., Smith, D. and Petersen, S. (2000), 'An epidemiological study of the relative importance of damp housing in relation to adult health', *Journal of Epidemiology and Community Health*, **54**, 677–86.

Ewing, R. and Cervero, R. (2001), 'Travel and the built environment: a synthesis', *Transportation Research Record: Journal of the Transportation Research Board*, **1780**, 87–114.

Ewing, R. and Handy, S. (2009), 'Measuring the unmeasurable: urban design qualities related to walkability', *Journal of Urban Design*, **14**, 65–84.

Ewing, R., Haliyur, P. and Page, G. (1994), 'Getting around a traditional city, a suburban PUD, and everything in-between', *Transportation Research Record*, **1466**, 53–62.

Ewing, R., Pendall, R. and Chen, D. (2003), 'Measuring sprawl and its transportation impacts', *Transportation Research Record: Journal of the Transportation Research Board*, **1831**, 175–83.

Ewing, R., Schmid, T., Killingsworth, R., Zlot, A. and Raudenbush, S. (2003), 'Relationship between urban sprawl and physical activity, obesity, and morbidity', *American Journal of Health Promotion*, **18**, 47–57.

Ewing, R., Schroeer, W. and Greene, W. (2004), 'School location and student travel: analysis of factors affecting mode choice', *Transportation Research Record: Journal of the Transportation Research Board*, **1895**, 55–63.

Ewing, R., Handy, S., Brownson, R.C., Clemente, O. and Winston, E. (2006), 'Identifying and measuring urban design qualities related to walkability', *Journal of Physical Activity and Health*, **3**, 223.

Ewing, R., Greenwald, M.J., Zhang, M., Walters, J., Feldman, M., Cervero, R. and Thomas, J. (2009), *Measuring the Impact of Urban Form and Transit Access on Mixed Use Site Trip Generation Rates: Portland Pilot Study*, Washington, DC: Environmental Protection Agency.

Ezzati, M. (2005), 'Indoor air pollution and health in developing countries', *Lancet*, **366**, 104–06.

Fanning, D. (1967), 'Families in flats', *British Medical Journal*, **4**, 382–6.

Faris, R.E.L. and Dunham, H.W. (1939), *Mental Disorders in Urban Areas: An Ecological Study of Schizophrenia and Other Psychoses*, New York: Hafner.

Farr, W. (1885), *Vital Statistics: A Memorial Volume of Selections from the Reports and Writings of William Farr*, ed. N.A. Humphreys, London: Royal Sanitary Institute of Great Britain, pp. 166–205 (reproduced in *Bulletin of World Health Organization*, 2000, **78** (1)).

Federal Highway Administration (1994), *The National Bicycling and Walking Study: Transportation Choices for a Changing America*, Publication No. FWHA-PD-94–023, Washington, DC: US Department of Transportation.

Feng, J., Glass, T.A., Curriero, F.C., Stewart, W.F. and Schwartz, B.S. (2010), 'The built environment and obesity: a systematic review of the epidemiologic evidence', *Health and Place*, **16**, 175–90.

Festinger, L. (1963), *Social Pressures in Informal Groups: A Study of Human Factors in Housing*, Stanford, CA: Stanford University Press.

Field, A., Witten, K., Robinson, E. and Pledger, M. (2004), 'Who gets to what? Access to community resources in two New Zealand cities', *Urban Policy and Research*, **22**, 189–205.

Fisk, W.J. (2001), 'Estimates of potential nationwide productivity and health benefits from better indoor environments: an update', in J.D. Spengler, J.M. Samet and J.F. McCarthy (eds), *Indoor Air Quality Handbook*, New York: McGraw-Hill.

Flegal, K.M., Graubard, B.I., Williamson, D.F. and Gail, M.H. (2007),

'Cause-specific excess deaths associated with underweight, overweight, and obesity', *Journal of the American Medical Association*, **298**, 2028–37.

Flowerdew, R., Manley, D.J. and Sabel, C.E. (2008), 'Neighbourhood effects on health: does it matter where you draw the boundaries?', *Social Science and Medicine*, **66**, 1241–55.

Fone, D.L. and Dunstan, F. (2006), 'Mental health, places and people: a multilevel analysis of economic inactivity and social deprivation', *Health and Place*, **12**, 332–44.

Fone, D., Dunstan, F., White, J., Webster, C., Rodgers, S., Lee, S., Shiode, N., Orford, S., Weightman, A. and Brennan, I. (2012), 'Change in alcohol outlet density and alcohol-related harm to population health (CHALICE)', *BMC Public Health*, **12**, 428.

Fonseca, W., Kirkwood, B.R., Victora, C.G., Fuchs, S., Flores, J. and Misago, C. (1996), 'Risk factors for childhood pneumonia among the urban poor in Fortaleza, Brazil: a case-control study', *Bulletin of the World Health Organization*, **74**, 199–208.

Forsdahl, A. (1977), 'Are poor living conditions in childhood and adolescence an important risk factor for arteriosclerotic heart disease?', *British Journal of Preventive and Social Medicine*, **31**, 91–5.

Forsyth, A., Hearst, M., Oakes, J.M. and Schmitz, K.H. (2008), 'Design and destinations: factors influencing walking and total physical activity', *Urban Studies*, **45**, 1973–96.

Foster, C. and Hillsdon, M. (2004), 'Changing the environment to promote health-enhancing physical activity', *Journal of Sports Sciences*, **22**, 755–69.

Fox, A.J. and Goldblatt, P.O. (1982), *Longitudinal Study: Socio-demographic Mortality Differentials: A First Report on Mortality in 1971–1975 (According to 1971 Census Characteristics, Based on Data Collected in the OPCS Longitudinal Study)*, London: HMSO.

Fox, A.J., Jones, D.R. and Goldblatt, P.O. (1984), 'Approaches to studying the effect of socio-economic circumstances on geographic differences in mortality in England and Wales', *British Medical Bulletin*, **40**, 309–14.

Frank, L. and Pivo, G. (1994), 'The impacts of mixed use and density on the utilization of three modes of travel: the single occupant vehicle, transit, and walking', *Transportation Research Record*, **1466**, 44–52.

Frank, L.D., Engelke, P.O. and Schmid, T.L. (2003), *Health and Community Design: The Impact of the Built Environment on Physical Activity*, Washington, DC: Island Press.

Frank, L.D., Andresen, M.A. and Schmid, T.L. (2004), 'Obesity relationships with community design, physical activity, and time spent in cars', *American Journal of Preventive Medicine*, **27**, 87–96.

Frank, L.D., Sallis, J.F., Conway, T.L., Chapman, J.E., Saelens, B.E. and

Bachman, W. (2006), 'Many pathways from land use to health: associations between neighborhood walkability and active transportation, body mass index, and air quality', *Journal of the American Planning Association*, **72**, 75–87.

Frank, L., Kerr, J., Rosenberg, D. and King, A. (2010), 'Healthy aging and where you live: community design relationships with physical activity and body weight in older Americans', *Journal of Physical Activity and Health*, **7**, S82–90.

Freeman, L.C. (1977), 'A set of measures of centrality based on betweenness', *Sociometry*, **40**, 35–41.

Frost, W.H. (1941), *Papers of Wade Hampton Frost, M.D.: A Contribution to Epidemiological Method*, ed. K.F. Maxcy, New York: Commonwealth Fund.

Frumkin, H. (2002), 'Urban sprawl and public health', *Public Health Reports*, **117**, 201.

Frumkin, H., Frank, L.D. and Jackson, R. (2004), *The Public Health Impacts of Sprawl*, Washington, DC: Island Press.

Fuller, T.D., Edwards, J.N., Vorakitphokatorn, S. and Sermsri, S. (1996), 'Chronic stress and psychological well-being: evidence from Thailand on household crowding', *Social Science and Medicine*, **42**, 265–80.

Fullilove, M.T. and Fullilove, R.E., III (2000), 'What's housing got to do with it?', *American Journal of Public Health*, **90**, 183–4.

Gabe, J. and Williams, P. (1987), 'Women, housing, and mental health', *International Journal of Health Services*, **17**, 667–79.

Gabe, J. and Williams, P. (1993), 'Women, crowding and mental health', in R.O.D. Burridge (ed.), *Unhealthy Housing*, London: Chapman & Hall.

Galdston, I. (ed.) (1949), *Social Medicine: Its Derivatives and Objectives*, New York Academy of Medicine, New York: Commonwealth Fund.

Gale, C.R., Sayer, A.A., Cooper, C., Dennison, E.M., Starr, J.M., Whalley, L.J., Gallacher, J.E., Ben-Shlomo, Y., Kuh, D. and Hardy, R. (2011), 'Factors associated with symptoms of anxiety and depression in five cohorts of community-based older people: the HALCyon (Healthy Ageing across the Life Course) Programme', *Psychological Medicine*, **41**, 2057–73.

Galea, S., Ahern, J., Rudenstine, S., Wallace, Z. and Vlahov, D. (2005), 'Urban built environment and depression: a multilevel analysis', *Journal of Epidemiology and Community Health*, **59**, 822–7.

Galea, S., Freudenberg, N. and Vlahov, D. (2005), 'Cities and population health', *Social Science and Medicine*, **60**, 1017–33.

Galea, S., Hall, C. and Kaplan, G.A. (2009), 'Social epidemiology and complex system dynamic modelling as applied to health behaviour and drug use research', *International Journal of Drug Policy*, **20**, 209–16.

Galea, S., Riddle, M. and Kaplan, G.A. (2010), 'Causal thinking and

complex system approaches in epidemiology', *International Journal of Epidemiology*, **39**, 97–106.
Garden, F.L. and Jalaludin, B.B. (2009), 'Impact of urban sprawl on overweight, obesity, and physical activity in Sydney, Australia', *Journal of Urban Health*, **86**, 19–30.
Gauvin, L., Richard, L., Craig, C.L., Spivock, M., Riva, M., Forster, M., Laforest, S., Laberge, S., Fournel, M.C. and Gagnon, H. (2005), 'From walkability to active living potential: an "ecometric" validation study', *American Journal of Preventive Medicine*, **28**, 126–33.
Gemmell, I. (2001), 'Indoor heating, house conditions, and health', *Journal of Epidemiology and Community Health*, **55**, 928–9.
Giddens, A. (1984), *The Constitution of Society*, Berkeley: University of California Press.
Gil, J., Stutz, C. and Chiaradia, A. (2007), 'Confeego: tool set for spatial configuration studies', presented at 6th International Space Syntax Symposium, Istanbul, in A. Turner (ed.), *New Developments in Space Syntax Software*, Istanbul: ITU Faculty of Architecture, pp. 15–22.
Gilbert, N. (2007), *Agent-Based Models*, Quantitative Applications in the Social Sciences, Thousand Oaks, CA: Sage.
Giles-Corti, B. and King, A.C. (2009), 'Creating active environments across the life course: "thinking outside the square"', *British Journal of Sports Medicine*, **43**, 109–13.
Giles-Corti, B., Macintyre, S., Clarkson, J.P., Pikora, T. and Donovan, R.J. (2003), 'Environmental and lifestyle factors associated with overweight and obesity in Perth, Australia', *American Journal of Health Promotion*, **18**, 93–102.
Giles-Corti, B., Timperio, A., Cutt, H., Pikora, T.J., Bull, F.C.L., Knuiman, M., Bulsara, M., Van Niel, K. and Shilton, T. (2006), 'Development of a reliable measure of walking within and outside the local neighborhood: RESIDE's Neighborhood Physical Activity Questionnaire', *Preventive Medicine*, **42**, 455–9.
Gillis, A.R. (1974), 'Population density and social pathology: the case of building type, social allowance and juvenile delinquency', *Social Forces*, **53**, 306–14.
Gillis, A. (1977), 'High-rise housing and psychological strain', *Journal of Health and Social Behavior*, **18**, 418–31.
Ginns, S.E. and Gatrell, A.C. (1996), 'Respiratory health effects of industrial air pollution: a study in east Lancashire, UK', *Journal of Epidemiology and Community Health*, **50**, 631–5.
Girman, J.R., Chang, Y.L., Hayward, S.B. and Liu, K.S. (1998), 'Causes of unintentional deaths from carbon monoxide poisonings in California', *Western Journal of Medicine*, **168**, 158–65.

Glass, T.A. and Balfour, J.L. (eds) (2003), *Neighborhoods, Ageing, and Functional Limitations*, New York: Oxford University Press.

Glass, T.A., De Leon, C.F.M., Bassuk, S.S. and Berkman, L.F. (2006), 'Social engagement and depressive symptoms in late life longitudinal findings', *Journal of Aging and Health*, **18**, 604–28.

Glass, T.A., Rasmussen, M.D. and Schwartz, B.S. (2006), 'Neighborhoods and obesity in older adults: the Baltimore Memory Study', *American Journal of Preventive Medicine*, **31**, 455–63.

GLLAMM (2010), 'Stata programs for estimating, predicting, simulating generalized linear latent and mixed models', available at: http://www.gllamm.org.

Godish, T. (2000), *Organic Contaminants: Indoor Environmental Quality*, Boca Raton, FL: CRC Press.

Goldberg, D. and Williams, P. (1988), *A User Guide to the General Health Questionnaire*, Windsor, UK: NEFR-Nelson.

Goldberger, J., Wheeler, G.A. and Sydenstricker, E. (1920), 'A study of the relation of diet to pellagra incidence in seven textile-mill communities of South Carolina in 1916', *Public Health Reports*, **35**, 648–713.

Gómez, L.F., Parra, D.C., Buchner, D., Brownson, R.C., Sarmiento, O.L., Pinzón, J.D., Ardila, M., Moreno, J., Serrato, M. and Lobelo, F. (2010), 'Built environment attributes and walking patterns among the elderly population in Bogotá', *American Journal of Preventive Medicine*, **38**, 592–9.

Gómez-Jacinto, L. and Hombrados-Mendieta, I. (2002), 'Multiple effects of community and household crowding', *Journal of Environmental Psychology*, **22**, 233–46.

Gordon, T. and Kannel, W. (1970), 'The Framingham, Massachusetts study – 20 years later', in I.I. Kessler and M.L. Levin (eds), *The Community as an Epidemiologic Laboratory: A Casebook of Community Studies*, Baltimore, MD: Johns Hopkins University Press.

Gordon-Larsen, P., Nelson, M.C., Page, P. and Popkin, B.M. (2006), 'Inequality in the built environment underlies key health disparities in physical activity and obesity', *Pediatrics*, **117**, 417–24.

Gove, W.R. and Hughes, M. (1979), 'Possible causes of the apparent sex differences in physical health: an empirical investigation', *American Sociological Review*, **44**, 126–46.

Gove, W.R. and Hughes, M. (1983), *Overcrowding in the Household*, New York: Academic Press.

Gove, W.R., Hughes, M. and Galle, O.R. (1979), 'Overcrowding in the home: an empirical investigation of its possible pathological consequences', *American Sociological Review*, **44**, 59–80.

Graham, N.M.H. (1990), 'The epidemiology of acute respiratory infections in children and adults: a global perspective', *Epidemiologic Reviews*, **12**, 149–78.

Grahn, P. and Stigsdotter, U.A. (2003), 'Landscape planning and stress', *Urban Forestry and Urban Greening*, **2**, 1–18.

Graunt, J. (1662), *Natural and Political Observations Made upon the Bills of Mortality, London, England*, printed by T. Roycraft, reprinted 1939, Baltimore, MD: Johns Hopkins University Press.

Greenberg, M., Popper, F., West, B. and Krueckeberg, D. (1994), 'Linking city planning and public health in the United States', *Journal of Planning Literature*, **8**, 235–9.

Greenwood, M. (1935), *Epidemics and Crowd-Diseases: An Introduction to the Study of Epidemiology*, London: Williams & Norgate.

Grinnell, J. (1917), 'Field tests of theories concerning distributional control', *American Naturalist*, **51**, 115–28.

Guite, H.F., Clark, C. and Ackrill, G. (2006), 'The impact of the physical and urban environment on mental well-being', *Public Health*, **120**, 1117–26.

Haan, M., Kaplan, G.A. and Camacho, T. (1987), 'Poverty and health: prospective evidence from the Alameda County study', *American Journal of Epidemiology*, **125**, 989–98.

Hackshaw, A.K., Law, M.R. and Wald, N.J. (1997), 'The accumulated evidence on lung cancer and environmental tobacco smoke', *British Medical Journal*, **315**, 980–88.

Haines, M.M., Stansfeld, S.A., Brentnall, S., Head, J., Berry, B., Jiggins, M. and Hygge, S. (2001a), 'The West London schools study: the effects of chronic aircraft noise exposure on child health', *Psychological Medicine*, **31**, 1385–96.

Haines, M.M., Stansfeld, S.A., Job, R.F.S., Berglund, B. and Head, J. (2001b), 'Chronic aircraft noise exposure, stress responses, mental health and cognitive performance in school children', *Psychological Medicine*, **31**, 265–77.

Hall, P. (1975), *Urban and Regional Planning*, Harmondsworth: Penguin Books.

Halpern, D. (1995), *Mental Health and the Built Environment: More than Bricks and Mortar?*, London: Taylor & Francis.

Hancock, T. and Duhl, L. (1988), *Promoting Health in the Urban Context*, WHO Healthy Cities Papers No. 1, Copenhagen: WHO Regional Office for Europe.

Handy, S.L. (1992), 'Regional versus local accessibility: neo-traditional development and its implications for non-work travel', *Built Environment*, **18**, 253–67.

Handy, S. (1996), 'Methodologies for exploring the link between urban form and travel behavior', *Transportation Research Part D: Transport and Environment*, **1**, 151–65.

Handy, S.L. and Niemeier, D.A. (1997), 'Measuring accessibility: an exploration of issues and alternatives', *Environment and Planning A*, **29**, 1175–94.

Handy, S., Cao, X. and Mokhtarian, P.L. (2006), 'Self-selection in the relationship between the built environment and walking: empirical evidence from Northern California', *Journal of the American Planning Association*, **72**, 55–74.

Hannay, D. (1981), 'Mental health and high flats', *Journal of Chronic Diseases*, **34**, 431–2.

Harpham, T. (2009), 'Urban health in developing countries: what do we know and where do we go?', *Health and Place*, **15**, 107–16.

Hartig, T., Evans, G., Jamner, L.D., Davis, D.S. and Garling, T. (2003), 'Tracking restoration in natural and urban field settings', *Journal of Environmental Psychology*, **23**, 109–23.

Haskell, W.L., Blair, S.N. and Hill, J.O. (2009), 'Physical activity: health outcomes and importance for public health policy', *Preventive Medicine*, **49**, 280–82.

Hassen, R. (1977), 'Social and psychological implications of high population density', *Civilisations*, **27**, 230–36.

He, J., Vupputuri, S., Allen, K., Prerost, M.R., Hughes, J. and Whelton, P.K. (1999), 'Passive smoking and the risk of coronary heart disease – a meta-analysis of epidemiologic studies', *New England Journal of Medicine*, **340**, 920–26.

Healthy Spaces and Places (2009), *Healthy Spaces and Places: A National Guide to Designing Places for Healthy Living*, Kingston, Canberra: Planning Institute of Australia.

Healy, J.D. (2003), 'Policy review', *Housing Studies*, **18**, 409–24.

Heimlich, R.E. and Anderson, W.D. (2001), *Development at the Urban Fringe and Beyond: Impacts on Agriculture and Rural Land*, Washington, DC: Economic Research Service, US Department of Agriculture.

Henderson, J.V. (1986), 'Efficiency of resource usage and city size', *Journal of Urban Economics*, **19**, 47–70.

Henderson, J.V. (1988), *Urban Development: Theory, Fact, and Illusion*, Oxford: Oxford University Press.

Henle, J. (1840), *Pathologische Untersuchingen*, Berlin: Hirschwald.

Henle, J. ([1840] 1938), *On Miasmata and Contagia*, trans. G. Rosen, Baltimore, MD: Johns Hopkins University Press.

Herrick, C. (2009), 'Designing the fit city: public health, active lives, and the (re)instrumentalization of urban space', *Environment and Planning A*, **41**, 2437–54.

Hicks, J. and Allen, G. (1999), *A Century of Change: Trends in UK Statistics since 1900*, Research Paper RP99/111, London: Social and General Statistics Section, House of Commons Library, available at: http://www.parliament.uk/briefing-papers/RP99–111.

Hillier, B. (1996), *Space Is the Machine: A Configurational Theory of Architecture*, Cambridge: Cambridge University Press.

Hillier, B. (1999), 'The hidden geometry of deformed grids: or, why space syntax works, when it looks as though it shouldn't', *Environment and Planning B: Planning and Design*, **26**, 169–91.

Hillier, B. (2004), 'Can streets be made safe?', *Urban Design International*, **9**, 31–45.

Hillier, B. (2012), 'Studying cities to learn about minds: some possible implications of space syntax for spatial cognition', *Environment and Planning B: Planning and Design*, **39**, 12–32.

Hillier, B. and Hanson, J. (1984), *The Social Logic of Space*, Cambridge: Cambridge University Press.

Hillier, B. and Iida, S. (2005), 'Network and psychological effects in urban movement', *Lecture Notes in Computer Science*, **3693**, 553–64.

Hillier, B., Hanson, J., Peponis, J., Hudson, J. and Burdet, R. (1983), 'Space syntax: a new urban perspective', *Architect's Journal*, **30**, 51–63.

Hillier, B., Hanson, J. and Graham, H. (1987), 'Ideas are in things: an application of the space syntax method to discovering house genotypes', *Environment and Planning B: Planning and Design*, **14**, 363–85.

Hillier, B., Penn, A., Hanson, J., Grajewski, T. and Xu, J. (1993), 'Natural movement: or, configuration and attraction in urban pedestrian movement', *Environment and Planning B: Planning and Design*, **20**, 29–66.

Hippocrates (1948), *Airs, Waters, Places*, trans. W.H.S. Jones, vol. I, Cambridge, MA: Harvard University Press, pp. 71–137.

Hodgson, M. (2002), 'Indoor environmental exposures and symptoms', *Environmental Health Perspectives*, **110**, Suppl. 4, 663–7.

Hoehner, C.M., Brennan, L.K., Brownson, R.C., Handy, S.L. and Killingsworth, R. (2003), 'Opportunities for integrating public health and urban planning approaches to promote active community environments', *American Journal of Health Promotion*, **18**, 14–20.

Hoehner, C.M., Brennan Ramirez, L.K., Elliott, M.B., Handy, S.L. and Brownson, R.C. (2005), 'Perceived and objective environmental measures and physical activity among urban adults', *American Journal of Preventive Medicine*, **28**, 105–16.

Hollander, A.E.M. de and Staatsen, B.A.M. (2003), 'Health, environment and quality of life: an epidemiological perspective on urban development', *Landscape and Urban Planning*, **65**, 53–62.

Homer, J.B. and Hirsch, G.B. (2006), 'System dynamics modeling for public health: background and opportunities', *American Journal of Public Health*, **96**, 452–8.

Hoppin, J.A., Ulmer, R. and London, S.J. (2004), 'Phthalate exposure and pulmonary function', *Environmental Health Perspectives*, **112**, 571–4.

Hopton, J.L. and Hunt, S.M. (1996), 'Housing conditions and mental health in a disadvantaged area in Scotland', *Journal of Epidemiology and Community Health*, **50**, 56–61.

Horton, F.E. and Reynolds, D.R. (1971), 'Effects of urban spatial structure on individual behavior', *Economic Geography*, **47**, 36–48.

Hosen, H. (1978), 'Moulds in allergy', *Journal of Asthma Research*, **15**, 151–6.

Howard, E. (1902), *Garden Cities of Tomorrow*, London: Swan Sonnenschein & Co.

Howard, M. (1993), 'The effects on human health of pest infestations in houses', in R. Burridge and D. Ormandy (eds), *Unhealthy Housing: Research, Remedies and Reforms*, London: Chapman & Hall.

Howden-Chapman, P. (2004), 'Housing standards: a glossary of housing and health', *Journal of Epidemiology and Community Health*, **58**, 162–8.

Howden-Chapman, P., Pierse, N., Nicholls, S., Gillespie-Bennett, J., Viggers, H., Cunningham, M., Phipps, R., Boulic, M., Fjällström, P., Free, S., Chapman, R., Lloyd, B., Wickens, K., Shields, D., Baker, M., Cunningham, C., Woodward, A., Bullen, C. and Crane, J. (2008), 'Effects of improved home heating on asthma in community dwelling children: randomised controlled trial', *British Medical Journal*, **337**, 852–5.

Hu, F.B. (2011), 'Globalization of diabetes: the role of diet, lifestyle, and genes', *Diabetes Care*, **34**, 1249–57.

Hu, G., Pekkarinen, H., Hänninen, O., Yu, Z., Guo, Z. and Tian, H. (2002), 'Commuting, leisure-time physical activity, and cardiovascular risk factors in China', *Medicine and Science in Sports and Exercise*, **34**, 234–8.

Huang, S.-J., Hung, W.-C., Sharpe, P.A. and Wai, J.P. (2010), 'Neighborhood environment and physical activity among urban and rural schoolchildren in Taiwan', *Health and Place*, **16**, 470–76.

Huber, M., Knottnerus, J.A., Green, L., Horst, H., Jadad, A.R., Kromhout, D., Leonard, B., Lorig, K., Loureiro, M.I. and Meer, J.W.M. (2011), 'How should we define health?', *British Medical Journal*, **343**, 235–7.

Hulka, B.S., Wilcosky, T.C. and Griffith, J.D. (1990), *Biological Markers in Epidemiology*, New York: Oxford University Press.

Humpel, N., Owen, N. and Leslie, E. (2002), 'Environmental factors associated with adults' participation in physical activity: a review', *American Journal of Preventive Medicine*, **22**, 188–99.

Humphreys, K. and Carr-Hill, R. (1991), 'Area variations in health outcomes: artefact or ecology', *International Journal of Epidemiology*, **20**, 251–8.

Hunter, D.J. (2005), 'Gene–environment interactions in human diseases', *Nature Reviews Genetics*, **6**, 287–98.

Huppert, F.A., Walters, D.E., Day, N.E. and Elliott, B.J. (1989), 'The factor structure of the General Health Questionnaire (GHQ-30): a reliability study on 6317 community residents', *British Journal of Psychiatry*, **155**, 178–85.

Husaini, B.A., Moore, S.T. and Castor, R.S. (1991), 'Social and psychological well-being of black elderly living in high-rises for the elderly', *Journal of Gerontological Social Work*, **16**, 57–78.

Hutchinson, G.E. (1957), 'Concluding remarks', *Cold Springs Harbor Symposia on Quantitative Biology*, **22**, 415–27.

Hygge, S., Evans, G.W. and Bullinger, M. (2002), 'A prospective study of some effects of aircraft noise on cognitive performance in schoolchildren', *Psychological Science*, **13**, 469–74.

Hyndman, S.J. (1990), 'Housing dampness and health amongst British Bengalis in East London', *Social Science and Medicine*, **30**, 131–41.

ICSU (2012), *Report of the ICSU Planning Group on Health and Wellbeing in the Changing Urban Environment: A Systems Analysis Approach*, Paris: International Council for Science.

Inagami, S., Cohen, D.A., Finch, B.K. and Asch, S.M. (2006), 'You are where you shop: grocery store locations, weight, and neighborhoods', *American Journal of Preventive Medicine*, **31**, 10–17.

Ineichen, B. and Hooper, D. (1974), 'Wives' mental health and children's behaviour problems in contrasting residential areas', *Social Science and Medicine*, **8**, 369–74.

Institute of Medicine (2000), *Clearing the Air: Asthma and Indoor Air Exposure*, Committee on the Assessment of Asthma and Indoor Air, Division of Health Promotion and Disease Prevention, Institute of Medicine, Washington, DC: National Academies Press.

Institute of Medicine (2001), *Rebuilding the Unity of Health and the Environment: A New Vision of Environmental Health for the 21st Century*, Washington, DC: National Academies Press.

Jaakkola, J.J.K., Øie, L., Nafstad, P., Botten, G., Samuelsen, S.O. and Magnus, P. (1999), 'Interior surface materials in the home and the development of bronchial obstruction in young children in Oslo, Norway', *American Journal of Public Health*, **89**, 188–92.

Jaakkola, J.J.K., Verkasalo, P.K. and Jaakkola, N. (2000), 'Plastic wall materials in the home and respiratory health in young children', *American Journal of Public Health*, **90**, 797–9.

Jackson, K.T. (1985), *Crabgrass Frontier: The Suburbanization of the United States*, New York: Oxford University Press.

Jadad, A.R. and O'Grady, L. (2008), 'How should health be defined?', *British Medical Journal*, **337**.

Jain, U. (1987), *The Psychological Consequences of Crowding*, New Delhi: Sage.

James, S.A. and Kleinbaum, D.G. (1976), 'Socioecologic stress and hypertension related mortality rates in North Carolina', *American Journal of Public Health*, **66**, 354–8.

James, W.P. (1998), 'What are the health risks? The medical consequences of obesity and its health risks', *Experimental and Clinical Endocrinology and Diabetes: Official Journal, German Society of Endocrinology [and] German Diabetes Association*, **106**, Suppl. 2, 1–6.

Jenkins, H.S., Devalia, J.L., Mister, R.L., Bevan, A.M., Rusznak, C. and Davies, R.J. (1999), 'The effect of exposure to ozone and nitrogen dioxide on the airway response of atopic asthmatics to inhaled allergen: dose- and time-dependent effects', *American Journal of Respiratory and Critical Care Medicine*, **160**, 33–9.

Jenkins, R., Meltzer, H., Jones, P.B., Brugha, T., Bebbington, P., Farrell, M., Crepaz-Keay, D. and Knapp, M. (2008), *Mental Health: Future Challenges*, Foresight Mental Capital and Wellbeing Project, London: Government Office for Science.

Jensen, J.R. (2005), *Introductory Digital Image Processing: A Remote Sensing Perspective*, New York: Prentice Hall.

Jerrett, M., McConnell, R., Chang, C.C.R., Wolch, J., Reynolds, K., Lurmann, F., Gilliland, F. and Berhane, K. (2010), 'Automobile traffic around the home and attained body mass index: a longitudinal cohort study of children aged 10–18 years', *Preventive Medicine*, **50**, S50–58.

Jha, P. (1999), *Curbing the Epidemic: Governments and the Economics of Tobacco Control*, Washington, DC: World Bank.

Jilcott, S.B., Evenson, K.R., Laraia, B.A. and Ammerman, A.S. (2007), 'Association between physical activity and proximity to physical activity resources among low-income, midlife women', *Preventing Chronic Disease*, **4**.

Johnson, M.P., Ladd, H.F. and Ludwig, J. (2002), 'The benefits and costs of residential mobility programs for the poor', *Housing Studies*, **17**, 125–38.

Jones, D.M., Song, X. and Rockwood, K. (2004), 'Operationalizing a frailty index from a standardized comprehensive geriatric assessment', *Journal of the American Geriatrics Society*, **52**, 1929–33.

Jones, K. and Duncan, C. (1995), 'Individuals and their ecologies: analysing the geography of chronic illness within a multilevel modelling framework', *Health and Place*, **1**, 27–40.

Kaczynski, A.T., Johnson, A.J. and Saelens, B.E. (2010), 'Neighborhood land use diversity and physical activity in adjacent parks', *Health and Place*, **16**, 413–15.

Kaplan, R. (2001), 'The nature of the view from home psychological benefits', *Environment and Behavior*, **33**, 507–42.

Karim, Y.G., Ijaz, M.K., Sattar, S.A. and Johnson-Lussenburg, C.M. (1985), 'Effect of relative humidity on the airborne survival of rhinovirus-14', *Canadian Journal of Microbiology*, **31**, 1058–61.

Karimi, K. (2012), 'A configurational approach to analytic urban design: "space syntax" methodology', *Urban Design International*, **17**, 297–318.

Karimi, K., Amir, A., Shaiei, K., Raford, N., Abdul, E., Zhang, J. and Mavridou, M. (2007), 'Evidence-based spatial intervention for regeneration of informal settlements: the case of Jeddah central unplanned areas', in *Proceedings of the 6th International Space Syntax Symposium*, Istanbul Technical University, Istanbul.

Kashef, M. (2011), 'Walkability and residential suburbs: a multidisciplinary perspective', *Journal of Urbanism*, **4**, 39–56.

Katzmarzyk, P.T. and Janssen, I. (2004), 'The economic costs associated with physical inactivity and obesity in Canada: an update', *Canadian Journal of Applied Physiology*, **29**, 90–115.

Kawachi, I. and Berkman, L.F. (2001), 'Social ties and mental health', *Journal of Urban Health*, **78**, 458–67.

Kearns, G. (1988), 'The urban penalty and the population history of England', in A. Brandstrom and L.G. Tederbrand (eds), *Society, Health and Population during the Demographic Transition*, Stockholm: Almquist and Wiskell International.

Kellett, J.M. (1993), 'Crowding and mortality in London boroughs', in R. Burridge and D. Ormandy (eds), *Unhealthy Housing: Research, Remedies and Reforms*, London: Chapman & Hall.

Khoury, M.J., Beaty, T.H. and Cohen, B.H. (1993), *Fundamentals of Genetic Epidemiology*, New York: Oxford University Press.

Kidd, S. (2007), 'Towards a framework of integration in spatial planning: an exploration from a health perspective', *Planning Theory and Practice*, **8**, 161–81.

Kimokoti, R.W. and Millen, B.E. (2011), 'Diet, the global obesity epidemic, and prevention', *Journal of the American Dietetic Association*, **111**, 1137–40.

King, A.C., Sallis, J.F., Frank, L.D., Saelens, B.E., Cain, K., Conway, T.L., Chapman, J.E., Ahn, D.K. and Kerr, J. (2011), 'Aging in neighborhoods differing in walkability and income: associations with physical activity and obesity in older adults', *Social Science and Medicine*, **73**, 1525–33.

King, W.C., Belle, S.H., Brach, J.S., Simkin-Silverman, L.R., Soska, T. and Kriska, A.M. (2005), 'Objective measures of neighborhood environment and physical activity in older women', *American Journal of Preventive Medicine*, **28**, 461.

Kligerman, M., Sallis, J.F., Ryan, S., Frank, L.D. and Nader, P.R. (2007), 'Association of neighborhood design and recreation environment variables with physical activity and body mass index in adolescents', *American Journal of Health Promotion*, **21**, 274–7.

Knave, B. (1994), 'Electric and magnetic fields and health outcomes – an overview', *Scandinavian Journal of Work, Environment and Health*, **20**, 78–89.

Knox, P. (1982), 'Residential structure, facility location and patterns of accessibility', in K. Cox and R. Johnston (eds), *Conflict, Politics and the Urban Scene*, London: Longman.

Kockelman, K.M. (1997), 'Travel behavior as a function of accessibility, land use mixing, and land use balance: evidence from the San Francisco Bay Area', *Transportation Research Record: Journal of the Transportation Research Board*, **1607**, 116–25.

Koenig, J.G. (1980), 'Indicators of urban accessibility: theory and application', *Transportation*, **9**, 145–72.

Koopman, J.S. and Lynch, J.W. (1999), 'Individual causal models and population system models in epidemiology', *American Journal of Public Health*, **89**, 1170–74.

Kopelman, P.G. (2000), 'Obesity as a medical problem', *Nature*, **404**, 635–43.

Koskenvuo, M., Kaprio, J., Kesäniemi, A. and Sarna, S. (1980), 'Differences in mortality from ischemic heart disease by marital status and social class', *Journal of Chronic Diseases*, **33**, 95–106.

Krieger, J. and Higgins, D.L. (2002), 'Housing and health: time again for public health action', *American Journal of Public Health*, **92**, 758–68.

Krieger, N. (1992), 'Overcoming the absence of socioeconomic data in medical records: validation and application of a census-based methodology', *American Journal of Public Health*, **82**, 703–10.

Krieger, N. (1994), 'Epidemiology and the web of causation: has anyone seen the spider?', *Social Science and Medicine*, **39**, 887–903.

Krieger, N. (2001), 'Theories for social epidemiology in the 21st century: an ecosocial perspective', *International Journal of Epidemiology*, **30**, 668–77.

Krieger, N., Rowley, D.L., Herman, A.A., Avery, B. and Phillips, M.T. (1993), 'Racism, sexism, and social class: implications for studies of health, disease, and well-being', *American Journal of Preventive Medicine*, **9**, 82–122.

Krzyzanowski, M., Quackenboss, J.J. and Lebowitz, M.D. (1990), 'Chronic respiratory effects of indoor formaldehyde exposure', *Environmental Research*, **52**, 117–25.

Kubzansky, L.D., Subramanian, S.V., Kawachi, I., Fay, M.E., Soobader, M.J. and Berkman, L.F. (2005), 'Neighborhood contextual influences on depressive symptoms in the elderly', *American Journal of Epidemiology*, **162**, 253–60.

Kuh, D. and Ben-Shlomo, Y. (2004), *A Life Course Approach to Chronic Disease Epidemiology*, New York: Oxford University Press.

Kulle, T.J. (1993), 'Acute odor and irritation response in healthy nonsmokers with formaldehyde exposure', *Inhalation Toxicology*, **5**, 323–32.

Kunzli, N., Kaiser, R., Medina, S., Studnicka, M., Chanel, O., Filliger, P., Herry, M., Horak, F., Jr, Puybonnieux-Texier, V. and Quenel, P. (2000), 'Public-health impact of outdoor and traffic-related air pollution: a European assessment', *Lancet*, **356**, 795–801.

Kutner, M.H., Nachtsheim, C.J. and Neter, J. (2004), *Applied Linear Regression Models*, Irwin, NY: McGraw-Hill.

Lachowycz, K. and Jones, A. (2011), 'Greenspace and obesity: a systematic review of the evidence', *Obesity Reviews*, **12**, e183–9.

Lakoff, G. and Johnson, M. (1980), *Metaphors We Live By*, Chicago: Chicago University Press.

Landsbergis, P.A., Schnall, P.L., Belkić, K.L., Baker, D., Schwartz, J.E. and Pickering, T.G. (2003), *The Workplace and Cardiovascular Disease: Relevance and Potential Role for Occupational Health Psychology*, Washington, DC: American Psychological Association.

Lang, T., Fouriaud, C. and Jacquinet-Salord, M.C. (1992), 'Length of occupational noise exposure and blood pressure', *International Archives of Occupational and Environmental Health*, **63**, 369–72.

Lauer, R.M., Lee, J. and Clarke, W.R. (1988), 'Factors affecting the relationship between childhood and adult cholesterol levels: the Muscatine Study', *Pediatrics*, **82**, 309–18.

Lawton, M.P. (1980), *Environment and Aging*, Monterey, CA: Brooks/Cole.

Lebowitz, B.D., Pearson, J.L., Schneider, L.S., Reynolds, C.F., III, Alexopoulos, G.S., Bruce, M.L., Conwell, Y., Katz, I.R., Meyers, B.S., Morrison, M.F., Mossey, J., Niederehe, G. and Parmelee, P. (1997), 'Diagnosis and treatment of depression in late life: consensus statement update', *Journal of the American Medical Association*, **278**, 1186–90.

Leckie, G. and Charlton, C. (2011), 'Runmlwin: Stata module for fitting multilevel models in the MLwiN software package', Centre for Multilevel Modelling, University of Bristol.

Lee, A.H. and Xiang, L. (2011), 'Mixture analysis of heterogeneous physical activity outcomes', *Annals of Epidemiology*, **21**, 780–86.
Lee, A.H., Zhao, Y., Yau, K.K.W. and Xiang, L. (2010), 'How to analyze longitudinal multilevel physical activity data with many zeros?', *Preventive Medicine*, **51**, 476–81.
Lee, C. and Moudon, A.V. (2006a), 'The 3Ds + R: quantifying land use and urban form correlates of walking', *Transportation Research Part D: Transport and Environment*, **11**, 204–15.
Lee, C. and Moudon, A.V. (2006b), 'Correlates of walking for transportation or recreation purposes', *Journal of Physical Activity and Health*, **3**, S77–98.
Lee, I.M., Ewing, R. and Sesso, H.D. (2009), 'The built environment and physical activity levels: the Harvard Alumni Health Study', *American Journal of Preventive Medicine*, **37**, 293–8.
Lee, S., Seo, J.G. and Webster, C. (2006), 'The decentralising metropolis: economic diversity and commuting in the US suburbs', *Urban Studies*, **43**, 2525–49.
Leech, J.A., Nelson, W.C., Burnett, R.T., Aaron, S. and Raizenne, M.E. (2002), 'It's about time: a comparison of Canadian and American time-activity patterns', *Journal of Exposure Analysis and Environmental Epidemiology*, **12**, 427–32.
Lehmann, I., Thoelke, A., Weiss, M., Schlink, U., Schulz, R., Diez, U., Sierig, G., Emmrich, F., Jacob, B., Belcredi, P., Bolte, G., Heinrich, J., Herbarth, O., Wichmann, H.E. and Borte, M. (2002), 'T cell reactivity in neonates from an East and a West German city – results of the LISA study', *Allergy: European Journal of Allergy and Clinical Immunology*, **57**, 129–36.
Lenthe, F.J. van, Brug, J. and Mackenbach, J.P. (2005), 'Neighbourhood inequalities in physical inactivity: the role of neighbourhood attractiveness, proximity to local facilities and safety in the Netherlands', *Social Science and Medicine*, **60**, 763–75.
Lepore, S.J., Evans, G.W. and Schneider, M.L. (1991), 'Dynamic role of social support in the link between chronic stress and psychological distress', *Journal of Personality and Social Psychology*, **61**, 899.
Lercher, P., Evans, G.W., Meis, M. and Kofler, W.W. (2002), 'Ambient neighbourhood noise and children's mental health', *Occupational and Environmental Medicine*, **59**, 380–86.
Leslie, E. and Cerin, E. (2008), 'Are perceptions of the local environment related to neighbourhood satisfaction and mental health in adults?', *Preventive Medicine*, **47**, 273–8.
Leslie, E., Coffee, N., Frank, L., Owen, N., Bauman, A. and Hugo, G. (2007), 'Walkability of local communities: using geographic information

systems to objectively assess relevant environmental attributes', *Health and Place*, **13**, 111–22.
Leyden, K.M. (2003) 'Social capital and the built environment: the importance of walkable neighborhoods', *American Journal of Public Health*, **93**, 1546–51.
Li, F., Fisher, K.J., Bauman, A., Ory, M.G., Chodzko-Zajko, W., Harmer, P., Bosworth, M. and Cleveland, M. (2005), 'Neighborhood influences on physical activity in middle-aged and older adults: a multilevel perspective', *Journal of Aging and Physical Activity*, **13**, 87–114.
Li, F., Fisher, K.J., Brownson, R.C. and Bosworth, M. (2005), 'Multilevel modelling of built environment characteristics related to neighbourhood walking activity in older adults', *Journal of Epidemiology and Community Health*, **59**, 558–64.
Li, F., Harmer, P.A., Cardinal, B.J., Bosworth, M., Acock, A., Johnson-Shelton, D. and Moore, J.M. (2008), 'Built environment, adiposity, and physical activity in adults aged 50–75', *American Journal of Preventive Medicine*, **35**, 38–46.
Li, F., Harmer, P., Cardinal, B.J., Bosworth, M., Johnson-Shelton, D., Moore, J.M., Acock, A. and Vongjaturapat, N. (2009), 'Built environment and 1-year change in weight and waist circumference in middle-aged and older adults: Portland neighborhood environment and health study', *American Journal of Epidemiology*, **169**, 401–08.
Li, F., Harmer, P., Cardinal, B.J. and Vongjaturapat, N. (2009), 'Built environment and changes in blood pressure in middle aged and older adults', *Preventive Medicine*, **48**, 237–41.
Li, R. and Klippel, A. (2010), 'Using space syntax to understand knowledge acquisition and wayfinding in indoor environments', in *Proceedings of the 9th IEEE International Conference on Cognitive Informatics*, Beijing, China.
Link, B.G. and Phelan, J. (1995), 'Social conditions as fundamental causes of disease', *Journal of Health and Social Behavior*, **35**, 80–94.
Litman, T. (2003), 'Measuring transportation: traffic, mobility and accessibility', *ITE Journal* (Institute of Transportation Engineers), **73**, 28–32.
Lobstein, T., Baur, L. and Uauy, R. (2004), 'Obesity in children and young people: a crisis in public health', *Obesity Reviews*, **5**, 4–85.
Logan, T.H. (1972), 'The invention of zoning in the emerging planning profession of late nineteenth century Germany', Ph.D. thesis, University of North Carolina at Chapel Hill.
Logue, E.E. and Jarjoura, D. (1990), 'Modeling heart disease mortality with census tract rates and social class mixtures', *Social Science and Medicine*, **31**, 545–50.
Loomis, D. and Wing, S. (1990), 'Is molecular epidemiology a germ

theory for the end of the twentieth century?', *International Journal of Epidemiology*, **19**, 1–3.

Lopez, A.D. (1993), 'Assessing the burden of mortality from cardiovascular diseases', *World Health Statistics Quarterly/Rapport trimestriel de statistiques sanitaires mondiales*, **46**, 91–6.

Lopez, R. (2004), 'Urban sprawl and risk for being overweight or obese', *American Journal of Public Health*, **94**, 1574–9.

Lopez Moreno, E. and Warah, R. (2006), 'The State of the World's Cities Report 2006/7 – urban and slum trends in the 21st century', *UN Chronicle*, **43**, 24.

Lovett, A., Haynes, R., Sünnenberg, G. and Gale, S. (2002), 'Car travel time and accessibility by bus to general practitioner services: a study using patient registers and GIS', *Social Science and Medicine*, **55**, 97–111.

Lowry, S. (1989), 'Health and housing: noise, space, and light', *British Medical Journal*, **299**, 1439.

Lund, H. (2002), 'Pedestrian environments and sense of community', *Journal of Planning Education and Research*, **21**, 301–12.

Luo, W. and Wang, F. (2003), 'Measures of spatial accessibility to health care in a GIS environment: synthesis and a case study in the Chicago region', *Environment and Planning B: Planning and Design*, **30**, 865–84.

Lynch, J.W., Davey Smith, G., Kaplan, G.A. and House, J.S. (2000), 'Income inequality and mortality: importance to health of individual income, psychosocial environment, or material conditions', *British Medical Journal*, **320**, 1200–1204.

Lynch, K. (1960), *The Image of the City*, Cambridge, MA: MIT Press.

Maantay, J. (2001), 'Zoning, equity, and public health', *American Journal of Public Health*, **91**, 1033.

Maas, C.J.M. and Hox, J.J. (2004), 'Robustness issues in multilevel regression analysis', *Statistica Neerlandica*, **58**, 127–37.

Maas, J., Verheij, R.A., Groenewegen, P.P., Vries S. de and Spreeuwenberg, P. (2006), 'Green space, urbanity, and health: how strong is the relation?', *Journal of Epidemiology and Community Health*, **60**, 587–92.

McCahill, C. and Garrick, N.W. (2008), 'The applicability of space syntax to bicycle facility planning', *Transportation Research Record*, **2074**, 46–51.

McCarthy, D. and Saegert, S. (1979), 'Residential density, social overload, and social withdrawal', in J. Aiello and A. Baum (eds), *Residential Crowding and Density*, New York: Plenum.

McCarthy, P., Byrne, D., Harrison, S. and Keithley, J. (1985), 'Housing type, housing location and mental health', *Social Psychiatry and Psychiatric Epidemiology*, **20**, 125–30.

MacCormac, E.R. (1985), *A Cognitive Theory of Metaphor*, Cambridge, MA: MIT Press.

McGeehin, M.A. and Mirabelli, M. (2001), 'The potential impacts of climate variability and change on temperature-related morbidity and mortality in the United States', *Environmental Health Perspectives*, **109**, 185.

McGoldrick, J.D., Graubard, S. and Horowitz, R. (1944), *Building Regulations in New York City*, New York: Commonwealth Fund.

Macintyre, S. (1997), 'The Black Report and beyond: what are the issues?', *Social Science and Medicine*, **44**, 723–45.

Macintyre, S., MacIver, S. and Sooman, A. (1993), 'Area, class and health: should we be focusing on places or people?', *Journal of Social Policy*, **22**, 213–34.

Macintyre, S., Ellaway, A., Der, G., Ford, G. and Hunt, K. (1998), 'Do housing tenure and car access predict health because they are simply markers of income or self esteem? A Scottish study', *Journal of Epidemiology and Community Health*, **52**, 657–64.

Macintyre, S., Hiscock, R., Kearns, A. and Ellaway, A. (2001), 'Housing tenure and car access: further exploration of the nature of their relations with health in a UK setting', *Journal of Epidemiology and Community Health*, **55**, 330–31.

Macintyre, S., Ellaway, A. and Cummins, S. (2002), 'Place effects on health: how can we conceptualise, operationalise and measure them?', *Social Science and Medicine*, **55**, 125–39.

McKeown, T. (1979), *The Role of Medicine: Dream, Mirage or Nemesis?*, Princeton, NJ: Princeton University Press.

McKinlay, A.F., Whillock, M. and Meulemans, C.C.E. (1989), *Ultraviolet Radiation and Blue Light Emissions from Spotlights Incorporating Tungsten Halogen Lamps*, Chilton, Oxfordshire: National Radiological Protection Board.

McKinlay, J.B. (1994), 'Towards appropriate levels of analysis, research methods and health public policy', International Symposium on Quality of Life and Health: Theoretical and Methodological Considerations, Berlin.

McMichael, A.J. (1994), 'Invited commentary – "molecular epidemiology": new pathway or new travelling companion?', *American Journal of Epidemiology*, **140**, 1–11.

McMichael, A.J. (1999), 'Prisoners of the proximate: loosening the constraints on epidemiology in an age of change', *American Journal of Epidemiology*, **149**, 887–97.

McMichael, A.J., Woodruff, R.E. and Hales, S. (2006), 'Climate change and human health: present and future risks', *Lancet*, **367**, 859–69.

McQueen, D.V. and Siegrist, J. (1982), 'Social factors in the etiology of chronic disease: an overview', *Social Science and Medicine*, **16**, 353–67.
Manolio, T.A. and Collins, R. (2010), 'Enhancing the feasibility of large cohort studies', *Journal of the American Medical Association*, **304**, 2290–91.
Manolio, T.A., Bailey-Wilson, J.E. and Collins, F.S. (2006), 'Genes, environment and the value of prospective cohort studies', *Nature Reviews Genetics*, **7**, 812–20.
Manolio, T.A., Weis, B.K., Cowie, C.C., Hoover, R.N., Hudson, K., Kramer, B.S., Berg, C., Collins, R., Ewart, W. and Gaziano, J.M. (2012), 'New models for large prospective studies: is there a better way?', *American Journal of Epidemiology*, **175**, 859–66.
Mantel, N. and Haenszel, W. (1959), 'Statistical aspects of the analysis of data from retrospective studies of disease', *Journal of the National Cancer Institute*, **22**, 719–48.
Markus, T.A. (1993), 'Cold, condensation and housing poverty', in R. Burridge and D. Ormandy (eds), *Unhealthy Housing: Research, Remedies and Reforms*, London: Chapman & Hall.
Marmot, M.G. and Syme, S.L. (1976), 'Acculturation and coronary heart disease in Japanese Americans', *American Journal of Epidemiology*, **104**, 225–47.
Marmot, M.G., Adelstein, A.M., Robinson, N. and Rose, G.A. (1978), 'Changing social-class distribution of heart disease', *British Medical Journal*, **2**, 1109–12.
Marmot, M.G., Shipley, M.J. and Rose, G. (1984), 'Inequalities in death: specific explanations of a general pattern?', *Lancet*, **1**, 1003–06.
Marmot, M.G., Smith, G.D., Stansfeld, S., Patel, C., North, F., Head, J., White, I., Brunner, E. and Feeney, A. (1991), 'Health inequalities among British civil servants: the Whitehall II Study', *Lancet*, **337**, 1387–93.
Marsella, A.J., Escudero, M. and Gordon, P. (1970), 'The effects of dwelling density on mental disorders in Filipino men', *Journal of Health and Social Behavior*, **11**, 288–94.
Marsh, A., Gordon, D., Pantazis, C. and Heslop, P. (1999), *Home Sweet Home? The Impact of Poor Housing on Health*, Bristol: Policy Press.
Martin, C.J., Platt, S.D. and Hunt, S.M. (1987), 'Housing conditions and ill health', *British Medical Journal* (Clinical Research edn), **294**, 1125–7.
Martin, D. (1997), 'From enumeration districts to output areas: experiments in the automated creation of a census output geography', *Population Trends*, **88**, 36–42.
Martin, D. (1998), 'Optimizing census geography: the separation of collection and output geographies', *International Journal of Geographical Information Science*, **12**, 673–85.

Materia, E. and Baglio, G. (2005), 'Health, science, and complexity', *Journal of Epidemiology and Community Health*, **59**, 534–5.

Matthews, J.W. and Turnbull, G.K. (2007), 'Neighborhood street layout and property value: the interaction of accessibility and land use mix', *Journal of Real Estate Finance and Economics*, **35**, 111–41.

Mehta, N.K. and Chang, V.W. (2008), 'Weight status and restaurant availability: a multilevel analysis', *American Journal of Preventive Medicine*, **34**, 127.

Meininghaus, R., Kirchner, S., Maupetit, F., Sallée, H. and Quenard, D. (2000), 'Gravimetric studies on VOC adsorption by indoor materials under near-ambient conditions', *Indoor and Built Environment*, **9**, 277–83.

Merlo, J. (2003), 'Multilevel analytical approaches in social epidemiology: measures of health variation compared with traditional measures of association', *Journal of Epidemiology and Community Health*, **57**, 550–52.

Michael, Y.L. and Yen, I.H. (2009), 'Invited commentary: built environment and obesity among older adults – can neighborhood-level policy interventions make a difference?', *American Journal of Epidemiology*, **169**, 409–12.

Miles, L. (2007), 'Physical activity and health', *Nutrition Bulletin*, **32**, 314–63.

Millington, C., Ward Thompson, C., Rowe, D., Aspinall, P., Fitzsimons, C., Nelson, N. and Mutrie, N. (2009), 'Development of the Scottish Walkability Assessment Tool (SWAT)', *Health and Place*, **15**, 474–81.

Milne, A., Allwood, G.K. and Moyes, C.D. (1987), 'A seroepidemiological study of the prevalence of hepatitis B infections in a hyperendemic New Zealand community', *International Journal of Epidemiology*, **16**, 84–90.

Mitchell, Richard, Blane, D. and Bartley, M. (2002), 'Elevated risk of high blood pressure: climate and the inverse housing law', *International Journal of Epidemiology*, **31**, 831–8.

Mitchell, Richard and Popham, F. (2008), 'Effect of exposure to natural environment on health inequalities: an observational population study', *Lancet*, **372** (9650), 1655–60.

Mitchell, Robert E. (1971), 'Some social implications of high density housing', *American Sociological Review*, **36**, 18–29.

Mobley, L.R., Root, E.D., Finkelstein, E.A., Khavjou, O., Farris, R.P. and Will, J.C. (2006), 'Environment, obesity, and cardiovascular disease risk in low-income women', *American Journal of Preventive Medicine*, **30**, 327–32.e1.

Montello, D.R. (1991), 'Spatial orientation and the angularity of urban routes: a field study', *Environment and Behavior*, **23**, 47–69.

Moomaw, R.L. (1981), 'Productivity and city size: a critique of the evidence', *Quarterly Journal of Economics*, **96**, 675–88.
Moorcroft, P. and Lewis, M.A. (2006), *Mechanistic Home Range Analysis*, Princeton, NJ: Princeton University Press.
Moorey, S., Greer, S., Watson, M., Gorman, C., Rowden, L., Tunmore, R., Robertson, B. and Bliss, J. (1991), 'The factor structure and factor stability of the Hospital Anxiety and Depression Scale in patients with cancer', *British Journal of Psychiatry*, **158**, 255–9.
Morland, K., Diez Roux, A.V. and Wing, S. (2006), 'Supermarkets, other food stores, and obesity: the Atherosclerosis Risk in Communities Study', *American Journal of Preventive Medicine*, **30**, 333–9.
Morris, J.N. (1955), 'Uses of epidemiology', *British Medical Journal*, **2**, 395–401.
Morris, J.N. (1957), *Uses of Epidemiology*, Edinburgh: Livingstone.
Morris, J.N., Blane, D.B. and White, I.R. (1996), 'Levels of mortality, education, and social conditions in the 107 local education authority areas of England', *Journal of Epidemiology and Community Health*, **50**, 15–17.
Motulsky, A.G. (1957), 'Drug reactions, enzymes, and biochemical reactions', *Journal of the American Medical Association*, **165**, 835–7.
Mueller, B.A., Rivara, F.P., Lii, S.M. and Weiss, N.S. (1990), 'Environmental factors and the risk for childhood pedestrian–motor vehicle collision occurrence', *American Journal of Epidemiology*, **132**, 550–60.
Mujahid, M.S., Diez Roux, A.V., Morenoff, J.D., Raghunathan, T.E., Cooper, R.S., Ni, H. and Shea, S. (2008), 'Neighborhood characteristics and hypertension', *Epidemiology*, **19**, 590–98.
Mujahid, M.S., Diez Roux, A.V., Shen, N., Gowda, D., Sanchez, B., Shea, S., Jacobs, D.R., Jr and Jackson, S.A. (2008), 'Relation between neighborhood environments and obesity in the multi-ethnic study of atherosclerosis', *American Journal of Epidemiology*, **167**, 1349–57.
Murray, C.J.L. and Lopez, A.D. (eds) (1996), *The Global Burden of Disease: A Comprehensive Assessment of Mortality and Disability from Diseases, Injuries and Risk Factors in 1990 and Projected to 2020*, Global Burden of Disease and Injury Series, vol. 1, Cambridge, MA: Harvard University Press.
Murtagh, P., Cerqueiro, C., Halac, A., Avila, M., Salomón, H. and Weissenbacher, M. (1993), 'Acute lower respiratory infection in Argentinian children: a 40 month clinical and epidemiological study', *Pediatric Pulmonology*, **16**, 1–8.
Muzet, A. (2007), 'Environmental noise, sleep and health', *Sleep Medicine Reviews*, **11**, 135–42.
Nagel, C.L., Carlson, N.E., Bosworth, M. and Michael, Y.L. (2008), 'The

relation between neighborhood built environment and walking activity among older adults', *American Journal of Epidemiology*, **168**, 461–8.

Nasar, J.L. and Julian, D.A. (1995), 'The psychological sense of community in the neighborhood', *Journal of the American Planning Association*, **61**, 178–84.

National Heart Forum (2007), *Building Health: Creating and Enhancing Places for Healthy, Active Lives: Blueprint for Action*, ed. N. Cavill, London: National Heart Forum.

National Heart Foundation of Australia (2004), *Healthy by Design: A Planners' Guide to Environments for Active Living*, Melbourne: Victorian Division, National Heart Foundation of Australia.

Neas, L.M., Dockery, D.W., Ware, J.H., Spengler, J.D., Speizer, F.E. and Ferris B.G., Jr (1991), 'Association of indoor nitrogen dioxide with respiratory symptoms and pulmonary function in children', *American Journal of Epidemiology*, **134**, 204–19.

Needleman, H.L., Schell, A., Bellinger, D., Leviton, A. and Allred, E.N. (1990), 'The long-term effects of exposure to low doses of lead in childhood: an 11-year follow-up report', *New England Journal of Medicine*, **322**, 83–8.

Nelson, M.C., Gordon-Larsen, P., Song, Y. and Popkin, B.M. (2006), 'Built and social environments: associations with adolescent overweight and activity', *American Journal of Preventive Medicine*, **31**, 109–17.

Neutens, T., Van de Weghe, N., Witlox, F. and De Maeyer, P. (2008), 'A three-dimensional network-based space–time prism', *Journal of Geographical Systems*, **10**, 89–107.

Newman, O. (1972), *Defensible Space*, New York: Macmillan.

New York City Board of Estimate and Apportionment (1916), *New York City Zoning Regulations*, New York: New York City Board of Estimate and Apportionment.

NICE (2008), *Promoting and Creating Built or Natural Environments That Encourage and Support Physical Activity*, NICE Public Health Guidance 8, London: National Institute for Health and Clinical Excellence.

NIEHS (1993), 'Genetic susceptibility', *Environmental Health Perspectives*, **101**, 364–5.

NIEHS (1994), 'Biomarkers: the clues to genetic susceptibility', *Environmental Health Perspectives*, **102**, 2–8.

Nielsen, T.S. and Hansen, K.B. (2007), 'Do green areas affect health? Results from a Danish survey on the use of green areas and health indicators', *Health and Place*, **13**, 839–50.

Norback, D., Bjornsson, E., Janson, C., Widstrom, J. and Boman, G. (1995), 'Asthmatic symptoms and volatile organic compounds, formaldehyde, and carbon dioxide in dwellings', *Occupational and Environmental Medicine*, **52**, 388–95.

Norberg-Schulz, C. (1971), *Existence, Space, and Architecture*, New York: Praeger.

Nordling, E., Berglind, N., Melén, E., Emenius, G., Hallberg, J., Nyberg, F., Pershagen, G., Svartengren, M., Wickman, M. and Bellander, T. (2008), 'Traffic-related air pollution and childhood respiratory symptoms, function and allergies', *Epidemiology*, **19**, 401–08.

Norman, G.J., Nutter, S.K., Ryan, S., Sallis, J.F., Calfas, K.J. and Patrick, K. (2006), 'Community design and access to recreational facilities as correlates of adolescent physical activity and body-mass index', *Journal of Physical Activity and Health*, **3**, S118–28.

Norris, T. and Pittman, M. (2000), 'The Healthy Communities movement and the coalition for healthier cities and communities', *Public Health Reports*, **115**, 118–24.

Northridge, M.E., Sclar, E.D. and Biswas, P. (2003), 'Sorting out the connections between the built environment and health: a conceptual framework for navigating pathways and planning healthy cities', *Journal of Urban Health*, **80**, 556–68.

Oakes, J.M. (2004), 'The (mis)estimation of neighborhood effects: causal inference for a practicable social epidemiology', *Social Science and Medicine*, **58**, 1929–52.

Obasanjo, O.O. (1999), 'The impact of the physical environment on adolescents in the inner city', doctoral dissertation, University of Michigan, Ann Arbor.

O'Campo, P. (2003), 'Invited commentary: advancing theory and methods for multilevel models of residential neighborhoods and health', *American Journal of Epidemiology*, **157**, 9–13.

Oda, M., Taniguchi, K., Wen, M. and Higurashi, M. (1989), 'Effects of high-rise living on physical and mental development of children', *Journal of Human Ergology*, **18**, 231–5.

Office of Population Censuses and Surveys (OPCS) (1980), *Classification of Occupations*, London: HMSO.

Oftedal, B., Nafstad, P., Magnus, P., Bjoørkly, S. and Skrondal, A. (2003), 'Traffic related air pollution and acute hospital admission for respiratory diseases in Drammen, Norway 1995–2000', *European Journal of Epidemiology*, **18**, 671–5.

Ogden, C.L., Yanovski, S.Z., Carroll, M.D. and Flegal, K.M. (2007), 'The epidemiology of obesity', *Gastroenterology*, **132**, 2087–2102.

Ohar, J., Sterling, D.A., Bleecker, E. and Donohue, J. (2004), 'Changing patterns in asbestos-induced lung disease', *Chest*, **125**, 744–53.

Oja, P., Vuori, I. and Paronen, O. (1998), 'Daily walking and cycling to work: their utility as health-enhancing physical activity', *Patient Education and Counseling*, **33**, S87–94.

Önder, D.E. and Gigi, Y. (2010), 'Reading urban spaces by the space-syntax method: a proposal for the South Haliç Region', *Cities*, **27**, 260–71.

Ordnance Survey UK (2011), 'OS MasterMap Address Layer 2: technical specification, v1.6 – 01/2011', available at: http://www.ordnancesurvey.co.uk/oswebsite/products/os-mastermap/address-layer-2/index.html (accessed 15 February 2011).

Orford, S., Dorling, D., Mitchell, R., Shaw, M. and Smith, G.D. (2002), 'Life and death of the people of London: a historical GIS of Charles Booth's inquiry', *Health and Place*, **8**, 25–35.

Ortega-Andeane, P., Jiménez-Rosas, E., Mercado-Doménech, S. and Estrada-Rodríguez, C. (2005), 'Space syntax as a determinant of spatial orientation perception', *International Journal of Psychology*, **40**, 11–18.

Osborn, F.J. and Whittick, A. (1977), *New Towns: Their Origins, Achievements and Progress*, London: International Textbook Company.

Ott, W.R. and Roberts, J.W. (1998), 'Everyday exposure to toxic pollutants', *Scientific American*, **278**, 86–91.

Owen, N., De Bourdeaudhuij, I., Sugiyama, T., Leslie, E., Cerin, E., Van Dyck, D. and Bauman, A. (2010), 'Bicycle use for transport in an Australian and a Belgian city: associations with built-environment attributes', *Journal of Urban Health*, **87**, 189–98.

Packer, C.N., Stewart-Brown, S. and Fowle, S.E. (1994), 'Damp housing and adult health: results from a lifestyle study in Worcester, England', *Journal of Epidemiology and Community Health*, **48**, 555–9.

Paine, T. (2005), 'The meaning of health', *British Journal of General Practice*, **55**, 554.

Pan, S.Y., Cameron, C., Desmeules, M., Morrison, H., Craig, C.L. and Jiang, X. (2009), 'Individual, social, environmental, and physical environmental correlates with physical activity among Canadians: a cross-sectional study', *BMC Public Health*, **9**.

Papas, M.A., Alberg, A.J., Ewing, R., Helzlsouer, K.J., Gary, T.L. and Klassen, A.C. (2007), 'The built environment and obesity', *Epidemiologic Reviews*, **29**, 129–43.

Paquet, C., Cargo, M., Kestens, Y. and Daniel, M. (2010), 'Reliability of an instrument for direct observation of urban neighbourhoods', *Landscape and Urban Planning*, **97**, 194–201.

Parra, D.C., Gomez, L.F., Sarmiento, O.L., Buchner, D., Brownson, R., Schimd, T., Gomez, V. and Lobelo, F. (2010), 'Perceived and objective neighbourhood environment attributes and health related quality of life among the elderly in Bogotá, Colombia', *Social Science and Medicine*, **70**, 1070–76.

Partonen, T. and Lönnqvist, J. (1998), 'Seasonal affective disorder', *Lancet*, **352**, 1369–74.

Passchier-Vermeer, W. and Passchier, W.F. (2000), 'Noise exposure and public health', *Environmental Health Perspectives*, **108**, 123–31.

Patterson, P.K. and Chapman, N.J. (2004), 'Urban form and older residents' service use, walking, driving, quality of life, and neighborhood satisfaction', *American Journal of Health Promotion*, **19**, 45–52.

Patz, J.A., Campbell-Lendrum, D., Holloway, T. and Foley, J.A. (2005), 'Impact of regional climate change on human health', *Nature*, **438**, 310–17.

Pearce, J., Witten, K. and Bartie, P. (2006), 'Neighbourhoods and health: a GIS approach to measuring community resource accessibility', *Journal of Epidemiology and Community Health*, **60**, 389–95.

Pearce, N. (1996), 'Traditional epidemiology, modern epidemiology, and public health', *American Journal of Public Health*, **86**, 678–83.

Pearce, N. (2000), 'The ecological fallacy strikes back', *Journal of Epidemiology and Community Health*, **54**, 326–7.

Pearce, N. and Merletti, F. (2006), 'Complexity, simplicity, and epidemiology', *International Journal of Epidemiology*, **35**, 515–19.

Peponis, J., Ross, C. and Rashid, M. (1997), 'The structure of urban space, movement and co-presence: the case of Atlanta', *Geoforum*, **28**, 341–58.

Perera, F.P. and Weinstein, I.B. (1982), 'Molecular epidemiology and carcinogen-DNA adduct detection: new approaches to studies of human cancer causation', *Journal of Chronic Diseases*, **35**, 581–600.

Perera, F.P. and Weinstein, I.B. (2000), 'Molecular epidemiology: recent advances and future directions', *Carcinogenesis*, **21**, 517–24.

Perkins, D., Meeks, J. and Taylor, R. (1992), 'The physical environment of street blocks and resident perceptions of crime and disorder: implications for theory and measurement', *Journal of Environmental Psychology*, **12**, 21–34.

Perkins, D., Wandersman, A.H., Rich, R.C. and Taylor, R.B. (1993), 'The physical environment of street crime: defensible space, territoriality and incivilities', *Journal of Environmental Psychology*, **13**, 29–49.

Perry, C.A. (1929a), 'City planning for neighborhood life', *Social Forces*, **8**, 98.

Perry, C.A. (1929b), *The Neighborhood Unit: A Scheme of Arrangement for the Family-Life Community*, Regional Study of New York and Its Environs, vol. VII, pp. 2–140, New York: Regional Plan of New York and Its Environs.

Peterson, J. (2003), *The Birth of City Planning in the United States, 1840–1917*, Baltimore, MD: Johns Hopkins University Press.

Petty, W. and Hull, C.H. (eds) (1899), *The Economic Writings of Sir William*

Petty, together with the Observations upon the Bills of Mortality More Probably by Captain John Graunt, Cambridge: Cambridge University Press.

Phipatanakul, W., Eggleston, P.A., Wright, E.C. and Wood, R.A. (2000), 'Mouse allergen. II. The relationship of mouse allergen exposure to mouse sensitization and asthma morbidity in inner-city children with asthma', *Journal of Allergy and Clinical Immunology*, **106**, 1075–80.

Pickett, K.E. and Pearl, M. (2001), 'Multilevel analyses of neighbourhood socioeconomic context and health outcomes: a critical review', *Journal of Epidemiology and Community Health*, **55**, 111–22.

Pikora, T.J., Bull, F.C., Jamrozik, K., Knuiman, M., Giles-Corti, B. and Donovan, R.J. (2002), 'Developing a reliable audit instrument to measure the physical environment for physical activity', *American Journal of Preventive Medicine*, **23**, 187.

Pi-Sunyer, F. Xavier (2002), 'The medical risks of obesity', *Obesity Surgery*, **12**, 6S–11S.

Platt, S.D., Martin, C.J., Hunt, S.M. and Lewis, C.W. (1989), 'Damp housing, mould growth, and symptomatic health state', *British Medical Journal*, **298**, 1673–8.

Platt, S.D., Martin, C.J. and Hunt, S.M. (1990), 'The mental health of women with children living in deprived areas of Great Britain: the role of living conditions, poverty and unemployment', in D. Goldberg and D. Tantam (eds), *The Public Health Impact of Mental Disorder*, Gottingen: Hogrefe & Huber.

Pollack, C.E. and Knesebeck, O. von dem (2004), 'Social capital and health among the aged: comparisons between the United States and Germany', *Health and Place*, **10**, 383–91.

Pollard, W.L. (1931), 'Outline of the law of zoning in the United States', *Annals of the American Academy of Political and Social Science*, **155**, 15–33.

Porta, S., Crucitti, P. and Latora, V. (2006), 'The network analysis of urban streets: a dual approach', *Physica A: Statistical Mechanics and Its Applications*, **369**, 853–66.

Pouliou, T. and Elliott, S.J. (2010), 'Individual and socio-environmental determinants of overweight and obesity in urban Canada', *Health and Place*, **16**, 389–98.

Pretty, J., Peacock, J., Sellens, M. and Griffin, M. (2005), 'The mental and physical health outcomes of green exercise', *International Journal of Environmental Health Research*, **15**, 319–37.

Prince, M., Patel, V., Saxena, S., Maj, M., Maselko, J., Phillips, M.R. and Rahman, A. (2007), 'No health without mental health', *Lancet*, **370**, 859–77.

Propper, C., Jones, K., Bolster, A., Burgess, S., Johnston, R. and Sarker, R. (2005), 'Local neighbourhood and mental health: evidence from the UK', *Social Science and Medicine*, **61**, 2065–83.

Public Health Advisory Committee (2008), *Re-thinking Urban Environments and Health*, Wellington, New Zealand: Public Health Advisory Committee.

Pucher, J., Buehler, R., Bassett, D.R. and Dannenberg, A.L. (2010), 'Walking and cycling to health: a comparative analysis of city, state, and international data', *American Journal of Public Health*, **100**, 1986–92.

Pujades-Rodríguez, M., McKeever, T., Lewis, S., Whyatt, D., Britton, J. and Venn, A. (2009), 'Effect of traffic pollution on respiratory and allergic disease in adults: cross-sectional and longitudinal analyses', *BMC Pulmonary Medicine*, **9**, 42.

Radford, N., Chiaradia, A. and Jorge, G. (2007), 'Space syntax: the role of urban form in cyclist route choice in Central London', Paper UCB-TSC-TR-2007–5, Safe Transportation Research and Education Center, Institute of Transportation Studies, University of California, Berkeley, available at: http://escholarship.org/uc/item/8qz8m4fz.

Raffestin, C. and Lawrence, R. (1990), 'Ecological perspective on housing, health and well-being', *Journal of Sociology and Social Welfare*, **17**, 143–60.

Raford, N. and Ragland, D. (2004), 'Space syntax: innovative pedestrian volume modeling tool for pedestrian safety', *Transportation Research Record*, **1878**, 66–74.

Raleigh, V.S. and Kiri, V.A. (1997), 'Life expectancy in England: variations and trends by gender, health authority, and level of deprivation', *Journal of Epidemiology and Community Health*, **51**, 649–58.

Ramirez, L.K.B., Hoehner, C.M., Brownson, R.C., Cook, R., Orleans, C.T., Hollander, M., Barker, D.C., Bors, P., Ewing, R. and Killingsworth, R. (2006), 'Indicators of activity-friendly communities', *American Journal of Preventive Medicine*, **31**, 515–24.

Rand, G. (1984), 'Crime and environment: a review of the literature and its implications for urban architecture and planning', *Journal of Architectural and Planning Research*, **1**, 3–19.

Raschke, F. (2004), 'Arousals and aircraft noise – environmental disorders of sleep and health in terms of sleep medicine', *Noise and Health*, **6**, 15–26.

Ratti, C. (2004), 'Urban texture and space syntax – some inconsistencies', *Environment and Planning B: Planning and Design*, **31**, 487–99.

Raw, G.J., Aizlewood, C.E. and Hamilton, R.M. (eds) (2001), *Building Regulation, Health and Safety: A Report Concerning the Influence on the Health and Safety of Building Users of Fabric and Services Controlled or Controllable by Regulation of Buildings*, report for Building Research Establishment, London: Construction Research Communications.

Reeder, L. (1972), 'Social epidemiology: an appraisal', in E.G. Jaco (ed.), *Patients, Physicians and Illness: A Sourcebook in Behavioral Science and Health*, 2nd edn, New York: Free Press.

Richard, L., Gauvin, L., Gosselin, C. and Laforest, S. (2009), 'Staying connected: neighbourhood correlates of social participation among older adults living in an urban environment in Montreal, Quebec', *Health Promotion International*, **24**, 46–57.

Richardson, H.W. (1978), *Regional and Urban Economics*, London: Penguin Books.

Richman, N. (1977), 'Behaviour problems in pre-school children: family and social factors', *British Journal of Psychiatry*, **131**, 523–7.

Riley, M.W. (1963), *Sociological Research*, New York: Harcourt, Brace & World.

Roberts, J.W. and Dickey, P. (1995), 'Exposure of children to pollutants in house dust and indoor air', *Reviews of Environmental Contamination and Toxicology*, **143**, 59–78.

Robinson, W.S. (2011), 'Ecological correlations and the behavior of individuals', *International Journal of Epidemiology*, **40**, 1134, reprinted from *American Sociological Review*, **15**, 351–7.

Rockwood, K., Song, X., MacKnight, C., Bergman, H., Hogan, D.B., McDowell, I. and Mitnitski, A. (2005), 'A global clinical measure of fitness and frailty in elderly people', *Canadian Medical Association Journal*, **173**, 489–95.

Rodin, J. (1977), 'Crowding, perceived choice, and response to controllable and uncontrollable outcomes', *Journal of Experimental Social Psychology*, **12**, 564–78.

Röösli, M. (2008), 'Radiofrequency electromagnetic field exposure and non-specific symptoms of ill health: a systematic review', *Environmental Research*, **107**, 277–87.

Rose, G. (1985), 'Sick individuals and sick populations', *International Journal of Epidemiology*, **14**, 32–8.

Rose, G. (1992), *The Strategy of Preventive Medicine*, Oxford: Oxford University Press.

Rose, G. (2001), 'Sick individuals and sick populations', *International Journal of Epidemiology*, **30**, 427–32.

Rosen, G. (1947), 'What is social medicine? A genetic analysis of the concept', *Bulletin of the History of Medicine*, **21**, 674–733.

Rosen, G. (1958), *A History of Public Health*, New York: MD Publications.

Rosen, G. (1973), 'Health, history and the social sciences', *Social Science and Medicine*, **7**, 233–48.

Rosenstreich, D.L., Eggleston, P., Kattan, M., Baker, D., Slavin, R.G., Gergen, P., Mitchell, H., McNiff-Mortimer, K., Lynn, H., Ownby, D. and Malveaux, F. (1997), 'The role of cockroach allergy and exposure to cockroach allergen in causing morbidity among inner-city children with asthma', *New England Journal of Medicine*, **336**, 1356–63.

Rosenthal, N.E., Sack, D.A. and Carpenter, C.J. (1985), 'Antidepressant effects of light in seasonal affective disorder', *American Journal of Psychiatry*, **142**, 163–70.

Ross, C.L. and Dunning, A.E. (1997), *Land Use Transportation Interaction: An Examination of the 1995 NPTS Data*, Atlanta, GA: US Department of Transportation, Federal Highway Administration.

Rossum, E. van, Frederiks, C., Philipsen, H., Portengen, K., Wiskerke, J. and Knipschild, P. (1993), 'Effects of preventive home visits to elderly people', *British Medical Journal*, **307**, 27–32.

Rothman, R.A. (1992), *Inequality and Stratification: Class, Color, and Gender*, Englewood Cliffs, NJ: Prentice Hall.

Roubenoff, R. (2004), 'Sarcopenic obesity: the confluence of two epidemics', *Obesity Research*, **12**, 887–8.

RTPI (2009), *Delivering Healthy Communities*, RTPI Good Practice Note 5, London: Royal Town Planning Institute, available at: www.rtpi.org.uk/item/325/23/5/3.

Rudge, J. and Nicol, F. (2000), *Cutting the Cost of Cold: Affordable Warmth for Healthier Homes*, Abingdon: Routledge.

Rumchev, K.B., Spickett, J.T., Bulsara, M.K., Phillips, M.R. and Stick, S.M. (2002), 'Domestic exposure to formaldehyde significantly increases the risk of asthma in young children', *European Respiratory Journal*, **20**, 403–08.

Rundle, A., Diez Roux, A.V., Freeman, L.M., Miller, D., Neckerman, K.M. and Weiss, C.C. (2007), 'The urban built environment and obesity in New York City: a multilevel analysis', *American Journal of Health Promotion*, **21**, 326–34.

Rutt, C.D. and Coleman, K.J. (2005), 'Examining the relationships among built environment, physical activity, and body mass index in El Paso, TX', *Preventive Medicine*, **40**, 831–41.

Ryan, D., Levy, B., Pollack, S. and Walker, B., Jr (1999), 'Protecting children from lead poisoning and building healthy communities', *American Journal of Public Health*, **89**, 822–4.

Rydin, Y., Bleahu, A., Davies, M., Dávila, J.D., Friel, S., De Grandis, G., Groce, N., Hallal, P.C., Hamilton, I. and Howden-Chapman, P. (2012), 'Shaping cities for health: complexity and the planning of urban environments in the 21st century', *Lancet*, **379**, 2079–2108.

Ryle, J.A. (1948), *Changing Disciplines: Lectures on the History, Method, and Motives of Social Pathology*, London: Oxford University Press.

Saarloos, D., Alfonso, H., Giles-Corti, B., Middleton, N. and Almeida, O.P. (2011), 'The built environment and depression in later life: the Health in Men Study', *American Journal of Geriatric Psychiatry*, **19**, 461–70.

Saegert, S. (1982a), 'Environment and children's mental health: residential density and low income children', *Handbook of Psychology and Health*, **2**, 247–71.

Saegert, S. (1982b), 'Environments and children's mental health: residential density and low income children', in A. Baum and J.E. Singer (eds), *Handbook of Psychology and Health*, Hillsdale, NJ: Erlbaum.

Saelens, B.E. and Handy, S.L. (2008), 'Built environment correlates of walking: a review', *Medicine and Science in Sports and Exercise*, **40**, S550–66.

Saelens, B.E., Sallis, J.F., Black, J.B. and Chen, D. (2003), 'Neighborhood-based differences in physical activity: an environment scale evaluation', *American Journal of Public Health*, **93**, 1552–8.

Saelens, B.E., Sallis, J.F. and Frank, L.D. (2003), 'Environmental correlates of walking and cycling: findings from the transportation, urban design, and planning literatures', *Annals of Behavioral Medicine*, **25**, 80–91.

Sallis, J.F., Hovell, M.F., Hofstetter, C.R., Elder, J.P., Hackley, M., Caspersen, C.J. and Powell, K.E. (1990), 'Distance between homes and exercise facilities related to frequency of exercise among San Diego residents', *Public Health Reports*, **105**, 179–85.

Sallis, J.F., Frank, L.D., Saelens, B.E. and Kraft, M.K. (2004), 'Active transportation and physical activity: opportunities for collaboration on transportation and public health research', *Transportation Research Part A: Policy and Practice*, **38**, 249–68.

Sallis, J.F., Bowles, H.R., Bauman, A., Ainsworth, B.E., Bull, F.C., Craig, C.L., Sjöström, M., De Bourdeaudhuij, I., Lefevre, J., Matsudo, V., Matsudo, S., Macfarlane, D.J., Gomez, L.F., Inoue, S., Murase, N., Volbekiene, V., McLean, G., Carr, H., Heggebo, L.K., Tomten, H. and Bergman, P. (2009), 'Neighborhood environments and physical activity among adults in 11 countries', *American Journal of Preventive Medicine*, **36**, 484–90.

Sallis, J.F., Saelens, B.E., Frank, L.D., Conway, T.L., Slymen, D.J., Cain, K.L., Chapman, J.E. and Kerr, J. (2009), 'Neighborhood built environment and income: examining multiple health outcomes', *Social Science and Medicine*, **68**, 1285–93.

Sallis, J.F., Floyd, M.F., Rodríguez, D.A. and Saelens, B.E. (2012), 'Role of built environments in physical activity, obesity, and cardiovascular disease', *Circulation*, **125**, 729–37.

Salome, C.M., Marks, G.B., Savides, P., Xuan, W. and Woolcock, A.J.

(2000), 'The effect of insecticide aerosols on lung function, airway responsiveness and symptoms in asthmatic subjects', *European Respiratory Journal*, **16**, 38–43.

Samimi, A. and Mohammadian, A.K. (2009), 'Health impacts of urban development and transportation systems', *Journal of Urban Planning and Development*, **136**, 208–13.

Sampson, R.J., Raudenbush, S.W. and Earls, F. (1997), 'Neighborhoods and violent crime: a multilevel study of collective efficacy', *Science*, **277**, 918–24.

Santana, P., Santos, R. and Nogueira, H. (2009), 'The link between local environment and obesity: a multilevel analysis in the Lisbon Metropolitan Area, Portugal', *Social Science and Medicine*, **68**, 601–09.

Sargent, J.D., Brown, M.J., Freeman, J.L., Bailey, A., Goodman, D. and Freeman D.H., Jr (1995), 'Childhood lead poisoning in Massachusetts communities: its association with sociodemographic and housing characteristics', *American Journal of Public Health*, **85**, 528–34.

Sarkar, C. (2013), 'The science of healthy cities: deciphering the associations between urban morphometrics and health outcomes', Ph.D. thesis, Cardiff University.

Sarkar, C., Gallacher, J. and Webster, C. (2013a), 'Built environment configuration and change in body mass index: the Caerphilly Prospective Study (CaPS)', *Health and Place*, **19**, 33–44.

Sarkar, C., Gallacher, J. and Webster, C. (2013b), 'Urban built environment configuration and psychological distress in older men: results from the Caerphilly study', *BMC Public Health*, **13**, 695.

Savitz, D.A. (1994), 'In defense of black box epidemiology', *Epidemiology*, **5**, 550–52.

Schelling, T.C. (1971), 'Dynamic models of segregation', *Journal of Mathematical Sociology*, **1**, 143–86.

Schelling, T.C. (2006), *Micromotives and Macrobehavior*, New York: W.W. Norton & Co.

Schlesselman, J.J. (1982), *Case-Control Studies: Design, Conduct, Analysis*, New York: Oxford University Press.

Schwartz, J. (1988), 'The relationship between blood lead and blood pressure in the NHANES II survey', *Environmental Health Perspectives*, **78**, 15–22.

Schwartz, S., Susser, E. and Susser, M. (1999), 'A future for epidemiology?', *Annual Review of Public Health*, **20**, 15–33.

Scotch, N.A. and Gierger, H.J. (1963), 'The epidemiology of essential hypertension II: psychologic and sociocultural factors in etiology', *Journal of Chronic Diseases*, **16**, 1183–1212.

Segal, D. (1976), 'Are there returns to scale in city size?', *Review of Economics and Statistics*, **58**, 339–50.

Self, P. (1972), 'Introduction', in H. Evans (ed.), *New Towns: The British Experience*, London: Charles Knight & Co., for the Town and Country Planning Association.

Seligman, M.E.P. (1975), *Helplessness*, San Francisco: Freeman.

Selvin, H.C. (1958), 'Durkheim's suicide and problems of empirical research', *American Journal of Sociology*, **63**, 607–19.

Sen, A. (2009), *The Idea of Justice*, London: Penguin Books.

Shannon, C.E. and Weaver, W. (1949), *The Mathematical Theory of Communication*, Urbana: University of Illinois Press.

Sharfstein, J., Sandel, M., Kahn, R. and Bauchner, H. (2001), 'Is child health at risk while families wait for housing vouchers?', *American Journal of Public Health*, **91**, 1191–2.

Shields, P.G. and Harris, C.C. (1991), 'Molecular epidemiology and the genetics of environmental cancer', *Journal of the American Medical Association*, **266**, 681–7.

Shouls, S., Congdon, P. and Curtis, S. (1996), 'Modelling inequality in reported long term illness in the UK: combining individual and area characteristics', *Journal of Epidemiology and Community Health*, **50**, 366–76.

Shriver, K., Planner, T. and Council, B. (2003), 'A walkable places survey: approach and results', in *Transportation Research Board Annual Meeting, Washington DC*, 03–4081.

Siegrist, J., Siegrist, K. and Weber, I. (1986), 'Sociological concepts in the etiology of chronic disease: the case of ischemic heart disease', *Social Science and Medicine*, **22**, 247–53.

Sloggett, A. and Joshi, H. (1994), 'Higher mortality in deprived areas: community or personal disadvantage?', *British Medical Journal*, **309**, 1470–74.

Sloggett, A. and Joshi, H. (1998), 'Deprivation indicators as predictors of life events 1981–1992 based on the UK ONS longitudinal study', *Journal of Epidemiology and Community Health*, **52**, 228–33.

Smith, K.R. (2002), 'Indoor air pollution in developing countries: recommendations for research', *Indoor Air*, **12**, 198–207.

Smith, K.R. and Mehta, S. (2003), 'The burden of disease from indoor air pollution in developing countries: comparison of estimates', *International Journal of Hygiene and Environmental Health*, **206**, 279–89.

Smith, K.R., Brown, B.B., Yamada, I., Kowaleski-Jones, L., Zick, C.D. and Fan, J.X. (2008), 'Walkability and body mass index: density, design, and new diversity measures', *American Journal of Preventive Medicine*, **35**, 237–44.

Snow, J. (1853), *On Continuous Molecular Changes, More Particular in Their Relation to Epidemic Diseases: Being the Oration Delivered at the 80th Anniversary of the Medical Society of London*, London: John Churchill, reprinted in *Reviews of Infectious Diseases*, 1985, **7** (3), 441–7.

Snow, J. (1936), 'On the mode of communication of cholera', 2nd edn, in *Snow on Cholera*, reprint, New York: Commonwealth Fund.

Song, Y., Gee, G.C., Fan, Y. and Takeuchi, D.T. (2007), 'Do physical neighborhood characteristics matter in predicting traffic stress and health outcomes?', *Transportation Research Part F: Traffic Psychology and Behaviour*, **10**, 164–76.

Sport England (2007), *Active Design: Promoting Opportunities for Sport and Physical Activity through Good Design*, study supported by CABE, Department of Health and Department for Culture, Media and Sport, London: Sport England.

Srinath Reddy, K., Shah, B., Varghese, C. and Ramadoss, A. (2005), 'Responding to the threat of chronic diseases in India', *Lancet*, **366**, 1744–9.

SS&CM (School of Social and Community Medicine, University of Bristol) (2007), 'Caerphilly Prospective Study', available at: http://www.bris.ac.uk/social-community-medicine/projects/caerphilly/about/ (accessed 10 June 2010).

Stafford, M. and Marmot, M. (2003), 'Neighbourhood deprivation and health: does it affect us all equally?', *International Journal of Epidemiology*, **32**, 357–66.

Stafford, M., Chandola, T. and Marmot, M. (2007), 'Association between fear of crime and mental health and physical functioning', *American Journal of Public Health*, **97**, 2076–81.

Stafford, M., Cummins, S., Ellaway, A., Sacker, A., Wiggins, R.D. and Macintyre, S. (2007), 'Pathways to obesity: identifying local, modifiable determinants of physical activity and diet', *Social Science and Medicine*, **65**, 1882–97.

Stamler, J. (1967), *Lectures in Preventive Cardiology*, New York: Grune & Stratton.

Stansfeld, S.A. and Matheson, M.P. (2003), 'Noise pollution: non-auditory effects on health', *British Medical Bulletin*, **68**, 243–57.

Stansfeld, S.A., Gallacher, J.E.J., Sharp, D.S. and Yarnell, J.W.G. (1991), 'Social factors and minor psychiatric disorder in middle-aged men: a validation study and a population survey', *Psychological Medicine*, **21**, 157–67.

Stansfeld, S., Gallacher, J., Babisch, W. and Shipley, M. (1996), 'Road traffic noise and psychiatric disorder: prospective findings from the Caerphilly study', *British Medical Journal*, **313**, 266–7.

Stansfeld, S., Haines, M. and Brown, B. (2000), 'Noise and health in the urban environment', *Reviews on Environmental Health*, **15**, 43–82.

Stansfeld, S.A., Berglund, B., Clark, C., Lopez-Barrio, I., Fischer, P., Öhrström, E., Haines, M.M., Head, J., Hygge, S., Kamp, I. van and Berry, B.F. (2005), 'Aircraft and road traffic noise and children's cognition and health: a cross-national study', *Lancet*, **365**, 1942–9.

Stein, L. (1950), 'A study of respiratory tuberculosis in relation to housing conditions in Edinburgh. I. The pre-war period', *British Journal of Social Medicine*, **4**, 143–69.

Stevens, J., Cai, J., Pamuk, E.R., Williamson, D.F., Thun, M.J. and Wood, J.L. (1998), 'The effect of age on the association between body-mass index and mortality', *New England Journal of Medicine*, **338**, 1–7.

Stewart, G.T. (1968), 'Limitations of the germ theory', *Lancet*, **1**, 1077–81.

Stewart, W.F.R. (1970), *Children in Flats: A Family Study*, London: National Society for the Prevention of Cruelty to Children.

Stokols, D. (1976), 'The experience of crowding in primary and secondary environments', *Environment and Behavior*, **8**, 49–86.

Stokols, D. (1978), 'A typology of crowding experiences', in A. Baum and Y. Epstein (eds), *Human Response to Crowding*, New York: John Wiley & Sons.

Strachan, D.P. and Cook, D.G. (1997), 'Health effects of passive smoking. 1. Parental smoking and lower respiratory illness in infancy and early childhood', *Thorax*, **52**, 905–14.

Strachan, D.P. and Cook, D.G. (1998), 'Parental smoking and childhood asthma: longitudinal and case-control studies', *Thorax*, **53**, 204–12.

Strawbridge, W.J., Deleger, S., Roberts, R.E. and Kaplan, G.A. (2002), 'Physical activity reduces the risk of subsequent depression for older adults', *American Journal of Epidemiology*, **156**, 328–34.

Subramanian, S.V., Kubzansky, L., Berkman, L., Fay, M. and Kawachi, I. (2006), 'Neighborhood effects on the self-rated health of elders: uncovering the relative importance of structural and service-related neighborhood environments', *Journals of Gerontology, Series B: Psychological Sciences and Social Sciences*, **61**, S153–60.

Sugiyama, T., Leslie, E., Giles-Corti, B. and Owen, N. (2008), 'Associations of neighbourhood greenness with physical and mental health: do walking, social coherence and local social interaction explain the relationships?', *Journal of Epidemiology and Community Health*, **62**.

Summerbell, C.D., Douthwaite, W., Whittaker, V., Ells, L.J., Hillier, F., Smith, S., Kelly, S., Edmunds, L.D. and Macdonald, I. (2009), 'The association between diet and physical activity and subsequent excess weight gain and obesity assessed at 5 years of age or older: a systematic review of the epidemiological evidence', *International Journal of Obesity*, **33**, Suppl. 3, S1–92.

Sundquist, K., Winkleby, M., Ahlén, H. and Johansson, S.E. (2004), 'Neighborhood socioeconomic environment and incidence of coronary heart disease: a follow-up study of 25,319 women and men in Sweden', *American Journal of Epidemiology*, **159**, 655–62.

Susser, M. (1991), 'What is a cause and how do we know one? A grammar for pragmatic epidemiology', *American Journal of Epidemiology*, **133**, 635–48.

Susser, M. (1993), 'Health as a human right: an epidemiologist's perspective on the public health', *American Journal of Public Health*, **83**, 418–26.

Susser, M. (1994a), 'The logic in ecological. I. The logic of analysis', *American Journal of Public Health*, **84**, 825–9.

Susser, M. (1994b), 'The logic in ecological. II. The logic of design', *American Journal of Public Health*, **84**, 830–35.

Susser, M. (1998), 'Does risk factor epidemiology put epidemiology at risk? Peering into the future', *Journal of Epidemiology and Community Health*, **52**, 608–11.

Susser, M. and Susser, E. (1996a), 'Choosing a future for epidemiology. I. Eras and paradigms', *American Journal of Public Health*, **86**, 668–73.

Susser, M. and Susser, E. (1996b), 'Choosing a future for epidemiology. II. From black box to Chinese boxes and eco-epidemiology', *American Journal of Public Health*, **86**, 674–7.

Szreter, S. and Mooney, G. (1998), 'Urbanization, mortality, and the standard of living debate: new estimates of the expectation of life at birth in nineteenth-century British cities', *Economic History Review*, **51**, 84–112.

Takano, T., Nakamura, K. and Watanabe, M. (2002), 'Urban residential environments and senior citizens' longevity in megacity areas: the importance of walkable green spaces', *Journal of Epidemiology and Community Health*, **56**, 913–18.

Talbot, J. (1998), 'Health and environment', Town and Country Planning Summer School, University of York, York.

Talen, E. (1999), 'Sense of community and neighbourhood form: an assessment of the social doctrine of new urbanism', *Urban Studies*, **36**, 1361–79.

Tan, J., Zheng, Y., Tang, X., Guo, C., Li, L., Song, G., Zhen, X., Yuan, D., Kalkstein, A.J. and Li, F. (2010), 'The urban heat island and its impact on heat waves and human health in Shanghai', *International Journal of Biometeorology*, **54**, 75–84.

Taubes, G. (1995), 'Epidemiology faces its limits', *Science*, **269**, 164–7.

Taylor, R.B. (1988), *Human Territorial Functioning*, New York: Cambridge University Press.

Taylor, R.B. and Harrell, A.V. (1996), *Physical Environment and Crime*, Rockville, MD: National Institute of Justice, US Department of Justice, available at: https://www.ncjrs.gov/App/Publications/abstract.aspx?ID=157311.

Taylor, S.M. (1984), 'A path model of aircraft noise annoyance', *Journal of Sound and Vibration*, **96**, 243–60.

Terris, M.E. (1964), *Goldberger on Pellagra*, Baton Rouge: Louisiana State University Press.

Thoerell, T. (1981), 'Life events, job stress and coronary heart disease', in J. Siegrist and M.J. Hulhuber (eds), *Myocardial Infarction and Psychosocial Risks*, Berlin: Springer.

Thomas, C.M. and Morris, S. (2003), 'Cost of depression among adults in England in 2000', *British Journal of Psychiatry*, **183**, 514–19.

Thomas, H., Weaver, N., Patterson, J., Jones, P., Bell, T., Playle, R., Dunstan, F., Palmer, S., Lewis, G. and Araya, R. (2007), 'Mental health and quality of residential environment', *British Journal of Psychiatry*, **191**, 500–505.

Thorndike, E.L. (1939), 'On the fallacy of imputing the correlations found for groups to the individuals or smaller groups composing them', *American Journal of Psychology*, **52**, 122–4.

Thun, M., Henley, J. and Apicella, L. (1999), 'Epidemiologic studies of fatal and nonfatal cardiovascular disease and ETS exposure from spousal smoking', *Environmental Health Perspectives*, **107**, 841–6.

Tilt, J.H., Unfried, T.M. and Roca, B. (2007), 'Using objective and subjective measures of neighborhood greenness and accessible destinations for understanding walking trips and BMI in Seattle, Washington', *American Journal of Health Promotion*, **21**, 371–9.

Timperio, A., Salmon, J., Telford, A. and Crawford, D. (2005), 'Perceptions of local neighbourhood environments and their relationship to childhood overweight and obesity', *International Journal of Obesity*, **29**, 170–75.

Tinetti, M.E. and Fried, T. (2004), 'The end of the disease era', *American Journal of Medicine*, **116**, 179–85.

Townsend, P., Davidson, N. and Whitehead, M. (1992), *Inequalities in Health and the Health Divide*, Harmondsworth: Penguin Books.

Townshend, T. and Lake, A.A. (2009), 'Obesogenic urban form: theory, policy and practice', *Health and Place*, **15**, 909–16.

Tripp, H.A. (1942), *Town Planning and Road Traffic*, London: Edward Arnold.

Troped, P.J., Wilson, J.S., Matthews, C.E., Cromley, E.K. and Melly, S.J. (2010), 'The built environment and location-based physical activity', *American Journal of Preventive Medicine*, **38**, 429–38.

Tsourou, C. (1998), 'Urban planning and health: implications of the WHO strategy for all for urban planning in Europe', Ph.D. thesis, Venice Institute of Architecture, University of Venice.

Turner, A. (2000), 'Angular analysis', in *Proceedings of the 3rd International Space Syntax Symposium*, Georgia Institute of Technology, Atlanta.

Turner, A. (2005), 'Could a road-centre line be an axial line in disguise?', in *Proceedings of the 5th International Space Syntax Symposium*, Delft University of Technology, Delft.

Turner, A. (2007), From axial to road-centre lines: a new representation for space syntax and a new model of route choice for transport network analysis', *Environment and Planning B: Planning and Design*, **34**, 539–55.

Tyroler, H.A. and Cassel, J. (1964), 'Health consequences of culture change. II. The effect of urbanization on coronary heart mortality in rural residents', *Journal of Chronic Diseases*, **17**, 167–77.

UK Biobank (2007), 'UK Biobank: protocol for a large-scale prospective epidemiological resource', available at: http://www.ukbiobank.ac.uk/wp-content/uploads/2011/11/UK-Biobank-Protocol.pdf.

Ulrich, R.S. (1984), 'View through a window may influence recovery from surgery', *Science*, **224**, 420–21.

UNFPA (2007), *State of the World Population 2007: Unleashing the Potential of Urban Growth*, New York: United Nations Population Fund.

Unilever (1976), *Port Sunlight Village*, Wirral, Merseyside: Unilever Services Company.

United Nations (2010), *World Urbanization Prospects: The 2009 Revision*, New York: Population Division, Department of Economic and Social Affairs, United Nations.

United Nations (2012), *World Urbanization Prospects: The 2011 Revision*, New York: Population Division, Department of Economic and Social Affairs, United Nations.

United Nations Commission on Human Settlements (1996), *An Urbanizing World: Global Report on Human Settlements*, New York: Oxford University Press.

United Nations Scientific Committee on the Effects of Atomic Radiation (2000), *Sources and Effects of Ionizing Radiation: UNSCEAR 2000 Report to the General Assembly, with Scientific Annexes*, vol. I, New York: United Nations.

USDHHS (US Department of Health and Human Services) (1996), *A Report from the Surgeon General (Physical Activity and Health)*, Atlanta, GA: Centers for Disease Control and Prevention, National Center for Chronic Disease Prevention and Health Promotion, President's Council on Physical Fitness and Sports.

USDHHS (US Department of Health and Human Services) (2006), *The Health Consequences of Involuntary Exposure to Tobacco Smoke: A Report of the Surgeon General*, Atlanta, GA: US Department of Health and Human Services, Centers for Disease Control and Prevention, Coordinating Center for Health Promotion, National Center for Chronic Disease Prevention and Health Promotion, Office on Smoking and Health.

USEPA (1992), *Respiratory Health Effects of Passive Smoking: Lung Cancer and Other Disorders*, EPA/600/6–90/006F, Washington, DC: US Environmental Protection Agency.

Üstün, T.B., Ayuso-Mateos, J.L., Chatterji, S., Mathers, C. and Murray, C.J.L. (2004), 'Global burden of depressive disorders in the year 2000', *British Journal of Psychiatry*, **184**, 386–92.

Vallarino, J.F. (2001), 'Fibers', in J.D. Spengler, J.M. Samet and J.F. McCarthy (eds), *Indoor Air Quality Handbook*, New York: McGraw-Hill.

Vallery-Radot, R. and Devonshire, R.L. (1901), *The Life of Pasteur*, London: Constable.

Vandenbroucke, J.P. (1988), 'Is "the causes of cancer" a miasma theory for the end of the twentieth century?', *International Journal of Epidemiology*, **17**, 708–09.

Van de Poel, E., O'Donnell, O. and Van Doorslaer, E. (2012), 'Is there a health penalty of China's rapid urbanization?', *Health Economics*, **21**, 367–85.

Van Dyck, D., Cardon, G., Deforche, B., Sallis, J.F., Owen, N. and De Bourdeaudhuij, I. (2010), 'Neighborhood SES and walkability are related to physical activity behavior in Belgian adults', *Preventive Medicine*, **50**, S74–9.

Vaughan, J.W. and Platts-Mills, T.A.E. (2000), 'New approaches to environmental control', *Clinical Reviews in Allergy and Immunology*, **18**, 325–39.

Vaughan, L. (2007), 'The spatial syntax of urban segregation', *Progress in Planning*, **67**, 205–94.

Vlahov, D. and Galea, S. (2003), 'Urban health: a new discipline', *Lancet*, **362**, 1091–2.

Vögele, J. (2000), 'Urbanization and the urban mortality change in Imperial Germany', *Health and Place*, **6**, 41–55.

Volchenkov, D. and Blanchard, P. (2008), 'Scaling and universality in city space syntax: between Zipf and Matthew', *Physica A: Statistical Mechanics and Its Applications*, **387**, 2353–64.

Von Korff, M., Koepsell, T., Curry, S. and Diehr, P. (1992), 'Multi-level analysis in epidemiologic research on health behaviors and outcomes', *American Journal of Epidemiology*, **135**, 1077–82.

Vries, S. de, Verheij, R.A., Groenewegen, P.P. and Spreeuwenberg, P. (2003), 'Natural environments – healthy environments? An exploratory analysis of the relationship between greenspace and health', *Environment and Planning A*, **35**, 1717–31.

Vuori, P.I. and Oja, P. (1999), *The Health Potential of Physical Activity through Transport by Walking and Cycling: A Scientific Review Prepared for the Charter on Transport, Environment and Health*, Copenhagen: World Health Organization.

Wachs, T.D. and Gruen, G. (1982), *Early Experience and Human Development*, New York: Plenum.

Waitzman, N.J. and Smith, K.R. (1998), 'Phantom of the area: poverty-area residence and mortality in the United States', *American Journal of Public Health*, **88**, 973–6.

Walker, E. and Hay, A. (1999), 'Carbon monoxide poisoning', *British Medical Journal*, **319**, 1082–3.

Wandersman, A. and Nation, M. (1998), 'Urban neighborhoods and mental health', *American Psychology*, **53**, 647–56.

Wang, Y. Claire, McPherson, K., Marsh, T., Gortmaker, S.L. and Brown, M. (2011), 'Health and economic burden of the projected obesity trends in the USA and the UK', *Lancet*, **378**, 815–25.

Wang, Youfa and Lobstein, T. (20060, 'Worldwide trends in childhood overweight and obesity', *International Journal of Pediatric Obesity*, **1**, 11–25.

Warburton, D.E.R., Nicol, C.W. and Bredin, S.S.D. (2006), 'Health benefits of physical activity: the evidence', *Canadian Medical Association Journal*, **174**, 801–09.

Webster, C. (2003), 'The Donald Robertson Memorial Prizewinner 2003: the nature of the neighbourhood', *Urban Studies*, **40**, 2591–612.

Webster, C. (2010), 'Pricing accessibility: urban morphology, design and missing markets', *Progress in Planning*, **73**, 77–111.

Webster, C. and Lai, L.W.C. (2003), *Property Rights, Planning and Markets: Managing Spontaneous Cities*, Cheltenham, UK and Northampton, MA, USA: Edward Elgar Publishing.

Webster, P. and Lipp, A. (2009), 'The evolution of the WHO city health profiles: a content review', *Health Promotion International*, **24**, i56–63.

Weich, S. and Lewis, G. (1998), 'Material standard of living, social class, and the prevalence of the common mental disorders in Great Britain', *Journal of Epidemiology and Community Health*, **52**, 8–14.

Weich, S., Burton, E., Blanchard, M., Prince, M., Sproston, K. and Erens, B. (2001), 'Measuring the built environment: validity of a site survey instrument for use in urban settings', *Health and Place*, **7**, 283–92.

Weich, S., Blanchard, M., Prince, M., Burton, E., Erens, B. and Sproston,

K. (2002), 'Mental health and the built environment: cross-sectional survey of individual and contextual risk factors for depression', *British Journal of Psychiatry*, **180**, 428–33.

Weinblatt, E., Ruberman, W., Goldberg, J.D., Frank, C.W., Shapiro, S. and Chaudhary, B.S. (1978), 'Relation of education to sudden death after myocardial infarction', *New England Journal of Medicine*, **299**, 60–65.

Wells, N.M. and Yang, Y. (2008), 'Neighborhood design and walking: a quasi-experimental longitudinal study', *American Journal of Preventive Medicine*, **34**, 313–19.

Welsh Local Government (2005), 'Welsh Index of Multiple Deprivation 2005: summary report', available at: http://wales.gov.uk/topics/statistics/publications/publication-archive/wimd2005/?lang=en.

Wener, R.E. and Evans, G.W. (2007), 'A morning stroll: levels of physical activity in car and mass transit commuting', *Environment and Behavior*, **39**, 62–74.

Weschler, C.J. (2004), 'Chemical reactions among indoor pollutants: what we've learned in the new millennium', *Indoor Air*, **14**, 184–94.

Weschler, C.J. and Shields, H.C. (1996), 'Production of the hydroxyl radical in indoor air', *Environmental Science and Technology*, **30**, 3250–58.

Weuve, J., Kang, J.H., Manson, J.E., Breteler, M.M.B., Ware, J.H. and Grodstein, F. (2004), 'Physical activity, including walking, and cognitive function in older women', *Journal of the American Medical Association*, **292**, 1454–61.

Whillock, M., Clark, I.E., McKinlay, A.F., Todd, C.D. and Mundy, E.J. (1988), *Ultraviolet Radiation Levels Associated with the Use of Fluorescent General Lighting, UV-A and UV-B Lamps in the Workplace and Home*, Chilton, Oxfordshire: National Radiological Protection Board.

Whitehead, M. and Dahlgren, G. (1991), 'What can be done about inequalities in health?', *Lancet*, **338**, 1059–63.

WHO (1987), *Health Impact of Low Indoor Temperatures*, Copenhagen: World Health Organization.

WHO (1990), *Indoor Environment: Health Aspects of Air Quality, Thermal Environment, Light and Noise*, Geneva: World Health Organization.

WHO (2005a), *Constitution of the World Health Organization*, New York: World Health Organization, available at: http://apps.who.int/gb/bd/PDF/bd47/EN/constitution-en.pdf.

WHO (2005b), *Preventing Chronic Diseases: A Vital Investment*, WHO Global Report, Geneva: World Health Organization.

WHO (2007), *Global Age-Friendly Cities: A Guide*, Geneva: World Health Organization.

WHO (2009), *Global Health Risks: Mortality and Burden of Disease*

Attributable to Selected Major Risks, Geneva: World Health Organization, available at: http://www.who.int/healthinfo/global_burden_disease/global_health_risks/en/.
WHO Europe (2009), *Zagreb Declaration for Healthy Cities*, Copenhagen: WHO Regional Office for Europe.
WHO Europe (2010), *Urban Planning, Environment and Health: From Evidence to Policy Action*, meeting report, Copenhagen: World Health Organization.
Wieslander, G., Norbäck, D., Björnsson, E., Janson, C. and Boman, G. (1997), 'Asthma and the indoor environment: the significance of emission of formaldehyde and volatile organic compounds from newly painted indoor surfaces', *International Archives of Occupational and Environmental Health*, **69**, 115–24.
Wight, R.G., Cummings, J.R., Karlamangla, A.S. and Aneshensel, C.S. (2009), 'Urban neighborhood context and change in depressive symptoms in late life', *Journals of Gerontology, Series B: Psychological Sciences and Social Sciences*, **64**, 247–51.
Wiles, N.J., Haase, A.M., Gallacher, J., Lawlor, D.A. and Lewis, G. (2007), 'Physical activity and common mental disorder: results from the Caerphilly study', *American Journal of Epidemiology*, **165**, 946–54.
Wilkinson, D. and Britain, G. (1998), *Poor Housing and Ill Health: A Summary of Research Evidence*, Edinburgh: Scottish Office Central Research Unit.
Williams, R.L. (2000), 'A note on robust variance estimation for cluster-correlated data', *Biometrics*, **56**, 645–6.
Wilson, P.W.F., D'Agostino, R.B., Levy, D., Belanger, A.M., Silbershatz, H. and Kannel, W.B. (1998), 'Prediction of coronary heart disease using risk factor categories', *Circulation*, **97**, 1837–47.
Wilson, W.J. (1991), 'Studying inner-city social dislocations: the challenge of public agenda research', *American Sociological Review*, **56**, 1–14.
Windham, G.C., Eaton, A. and Hopkins, B. (1999), 'Evidence for an association between environmental tobacco smoke exposure and birthweight: a meta-analysis and new data', *Paediatric and Perinatal Epidemiology*, **13**, 35–57.
Wing, S., Casper, M., Hayes, C.G., Dargent-Molina, P., Riggan, W. and Tyroler, H.A. (1987), 'Changing association between community occupational structure and ischaemic heart disease mortality in the United States', *Lancet*, **2**, 1067–70.
Wing, S., Barnett, E., Casper, M. and Tyroler, H.A. (1992), 'Geographic and socioeconomic variation in the onset of decline of coronary heart disease mortality in white women', *American Journal of Public Health*, **82**, 204–09.

Winkelstein, W., Jr (1995), 'A new perspective on John Snow's communicable disease theory', *American Journal of Epidemiology*, **142**, S3–9.

Wolch, J., Jerrett, M., Reynolds, K., McConnell, R., Chang, R., Dahmann, N., Brady, K., Gilliland, F., Su, J.G. and Berhane, K. (2011), 'Childhood obesity and proximity to urban parks and recreational resources: a longitudinal cohort study', *Health and Place*, **17**, 207–14.

Wolkoff, P. (2000), 'Formation of strong airway irritants in terpene/ozone mixtures', *Indoor Air*, **10**, 82–91.

Wood, L., Shannon, T., Bulsara, M., Pikora, T., McCormack, G. and Giles-Corti, B. (2008), 'The anatomy of the safe and social suburb: an exploratory study of the built environment, social capital and residents' perceptions of safety', *Health and Place*, **14**, 15–31.

Wood, L., Frank, L.D. and Giles-Corti, B. (2010), 'Sense of community and its relationship with walking and neighborhood design', *Social Science and Medicine*, **70**, 1381–90.

Woods, R. (2003), 'Urban–rural mortality differentials: an unresolved debate', *Population and Development Review*, **29**, 29–46.

Woods, W.I. and Woodward, J. (eds) (1984), *Urban Disease and Mortality in Nineteenth Century England*, London: Batsford.

Wright, F.L. (1935), 'Broadacre City: a new community plan', *Architectural Record*, **77**, 243–54.

Wrigley, E.A. (1969), *Société et population*, Paris, Collection l'Univers des Connaissances.

Wrigley, E.A., Davies, R.S., Oeppen, J.E. and Schofield, R.S. (1997), *English Population History from Family Reconstitution, 1580–1837*, Cambridge: Cambridge University Press.

Wu, F., He, S. and Webster, C. (2010), 'Path dependency and the neighbourhood effect: urban poverty in impoverished neighbourhoods in Chinese cities', *Environment and Planning A*, **42**, 134.

Yan, A.F., Voorhees, C.C., Clifton, K. and Burnier, C. (2010), '"Do you see what I see?" Correlates of multidimensional measures of neighborhood types and perceived physical activity-related neighborhood barriers and facilitators for urban youth', *Preventive Medicine*, **50**, S18–23.

Yankauer, A. (1950), 'The relationship of fetal and infant mortality to residential segregation: an inquiry into social epidemiology', *American Sociological Review*, **15**, 644–8.

Zahner, G., Kasl, S.V., White, M. and Will, J. (1985), 'Psychological consequences of infestation of the dwelling unit', *American Journal of Public Health*, **75**, 1303–07.

Zamboni, M., Mazzali, G., Fantin, F., Rossi, A. and Di Francesco, V. (2008), 'Sarcopenic obesity: a new category of obesity in the elderly', *Nutrition, Metabolism and Cardiovascular Diseases*, **18**, 388–95.

Zhang, J. and Smith, K.R. (1996), 'Hydrocarbon emissions and health risks from cookstoves in developing countries', *Journal of Exposure Analysis and Environmental Epidemiology*, **6**, 147–61.

Zhang, J. and Smith, K.R. (2003), 'Indoor air pollution: a global health concern', *British Medical Bulletin*, **68**, 209–25.

Zhang, J. and Smith, K.R. (2007), 'Household air pollution from coal and biomass fuels in China: measurements, health impacts, and interventions', *Environmental Health Perspectives*, **115**, 848–55.

Zhang, J., Smith, K.R., Ma, Y., Ye, S., Jiang, F., Qi, W., Liu, P., Khalil, M.A.K., Rasmussen, R.A. and Thorneloe, S.A. (2000), 'Greenhouse gases and other airborne pollutants from household stoves in China: a database for emission factors', *Atmospheric Environment*, **34**, 4537–49.

Zhao, H., Li, L. and Zhu, H. (2007), 'Application of extended space syntax in urban land grading', *Journal of Geomatics*, **32**, 9–11.

Zhao, Y., Zhang, S., Selvin, S. and Spear, R.C. (1991), 'A dose response relation for noise induced hypertension', *British Journal of Industrial Medicine*, **48**, 179–84.

Zigmond, A.S. and Snaith, R.P. (1983), 'The Hospital Anxiety and Depression Scale', *Acta Psychiatrica Scandinavica*, **67**, 361–70.

Zimring, C. (1983), 'The built environment as a source of psychological stress: impacts of buildings and cities on satisfaction and behavior', in G.W. Evans (ed.), *Environmental Stress*, Cambridge: Cambridge University Press.

Ziraba, A.K., Fotso, J.C. and Ochako, R. (2009), 'Overweight and obesity in urban Africa: a problem of the rich or the poor?', *BMC Public Health*, **9**, 465.

Zlunick, S. and Altman, I. (1972), 'Crowding and human behaviour', in J.F. Wohlwill and D.H. Carson (eds), *Environment and the Social Sciences: Perspectives and Applications*, Washington, DC: American Psychological Association.

Zock, J.P., Plana, E., Jarvis, D., Antó, J.M., Kromhout, H., Kennedy, S.M., Künzli, N., Villani, S., Olivieri, M., Torén, K., Radon, K., Sunyer, J., Dahlman-Hoglund, A., Norbäck, D. and Kogevinas, M. (2007), 'The use of household cleaning sprays and adult asthma: an international longitudinal study', *American Journal of Respiratory and Critical Care Medicine*, **176**, 735–41.

Index